Medicinal Plants and Foods

Medicinal Plants and Foods

Editor

Gema Nieto

MDPI • Basel • Beijing • Wuhan • Barcelona • Belgrade • Manchester • Tokyo • Cluj • Tianjin

Editor
Gema Nieto
Department of Food Technology,
Nutrition and Food Science,
Veterinary Faculty,
University of Murcia,
Regional Campus of International Excellence "Campus Mare Nostrum",
30100 Espinardo, Murcia,
Spain;
gnieto@um.es

Editorial Office
MDPI
St. Alban-Anlage 66
4052 Basel, Switzerland

This is a reprint of articles from the Special Issue published online in the open access journal *Medicines* (ISSN 2305-6320) (available at: https://www.mdpi.com/journal/medicines/special_issues/medicinal_plants).

For citation purposes, cite each article independently as indicated on the article page online and as indicated below:

LastName, A.A.; LastName, B.B.; LastName, C.C. Article Title. *Journal Name* **Year**, *Article Number*, Page Range.

ISBN 978-3-03943-398-8 (Hbk)
ISBN 978-3-03943-399-5 (PDF)

Contents

About the Editor vii

Gema Nieto
How Are Medicinal Plants Useful When Added to Foods?
Reprinted from: *Medicines* **2020**, *7*, 58, doi:10.3390/medicines7090058 1

Gabriela M. Chiocchetti, Elisabete A. De Nadai Fernandes, Anna A. Wawer, Susan Fairweather-Tait and Tatiana Christides
In Vitro Iron Bioavailability of Brazilian Food-Based by-Products
Reprinted from: *Medicines* **2018**, *5*, 45, doi:10.3390/medicines5020045 7

Agena Ghout, Amar Zellagui, Noureddine Gherraf, Ibrahim Demirtas, Yaglioglu Ayse Sahin, Meriem Boukhenaf, Mesbah Lahouel, Gema Nieto and Salah Akkal
Antiproliferative and Antioxidant Activities of Two Extracts of the Plant Species *Euphorbia dendroides* L.
Reprinted from: *Medicines* **2018**, *5*, 36, doi:10.3390/medicines5020036 19

Rubén Agregán, Paulo E. S. Munekata, Daniel Franco, Javier Carballo, Francisco J. Barba and José M. Lorenzo
Antioxidant Potential of Extracts Obtained from Macro- (*Ascophyllum nodosum, Fucus vesiculosus* and *Bifurcaria bifurcata*) and Micro-Algae (*Chlorella vulgaris* and *Spirulina platensis*) Assisted by Ultrasound
Reprinted from: *Medicines* **2018**, *5*, 33, doi:10.3390/medicines5020033 33

Mostefa Lefahal, Nabila Zaabat, Radia Ayad, El hani Makhloufi, Lakhdar Djarri, Merzoug Benahmed, Hocine Laouer, Gema Nieto and Salah Akkal
In Vitro Assessment of Total Phenolic and Flavonoid Contents, Antioxidant and Photoprotective Activities of Crude Methanolic Extract of Aerial Parts of *Capnophyllum peregrinum* (L.) Lange (Apiaceae) Growing in Algeria
Reprinted from: *Medicines* **2018**, *5*, 26, doi:10.3390/medicines5020026 43

Spyros Grigorakis and Dimitris P. Makris
Characterisation of Polyphenol-Containing Extracts from *Stachys mucronata* and Evaluation of Their Antiradical Activity
Reprinted from: *Medicines* **2018**, *5*, 14, doi:10.3390/medicines5010014 53

Sisse Jongberg, Mari Ann Tørngren and Leif H. Skibsted
Dose-Dependent Effects of Green Tea or Maté Extracts on Lipid and Protein Oxidation in Brine-Injected Retail-Packed Pork Chops
Reprinted from: *Medicines* **2018**, *5*, 11, doi:10.3390/medicines5010011 61

Sisse Jongberg, Mari Ann Tørngren and Leif H. Skibsted
Protein Oxidation and Sensory Quality of Brine-Injected Pork Loins Added Ascorbate or Extracts of Green Tea or Maté during Chill-Storage in High-Oxygen Modified Atmosphere
Reprinted from: *Medicines* **2018**, *5*, 7, doi:10.3390/medicines5010007 73

Fatemeh Shafiee, Elnaz Khoshvishkaie, Ali Davoodi, Ayat Dashti Kalantar, Hossein Bakhshi Jouybari and Ramin Ataee
The Determination of Blood Glucose Lowering and Metabolic Effects of *Mespilus germanica* L. Hydroacetonic Extract on Streptozocin-Induced Diabetic Balb/c Mice
Reprinted from: *Medicines* **2018**, *5*, 1, doi:10.3390/medicines5010001 87

Godwin Eneji Egbung, Item Justin Atangwho, Ochuole Diana Odey and Victor Ndubuisi Ndiodimma
The Lipid Lowering and Cardioprotective Effects of *Vernonia calvoana* Ethanol Extract in Acetaminophen-Treated Rats
Reprinted from: *Medicines* **2017**, *4*, 90, doi:10.3390/medicines4040090 . . . . **95**

Nidal Jaradat, Abdel Naser Zaid, Fatima Hussein, Maram Zaqzouq, Hadeel Aljammal and Ola Ayesh
Anti-Lipase Potential of the Organic and Aqueous Extracts of Ten Traditional Edible and Medicinal Plants in Palestine; a Comparison Study with Orlistat
Reprinted from: *Medicines* **2017**, *4*, 89, doi:10.3390/medicines4040089 . . . . **105**

Gema Nieto, Gaspar Ros and Julián Castillo
Antioxidant and Antimicrobial Properties of Rosemary (*Rosmarinus officinalis,* L.): A Review
Reprinted from: *Medicines* **2018**, *5*, 98, doi:10.3390/medicines5030098 . . . . **119**

Antonio Serrano, Gaspar Ros and Gema Nieto
Bioactive Compounds and Extracts from Traditional Herbs and Their Potential Anti-Inflammatory Health Effects
Reprinted from: *Medicines* **2018**, *5*, 76, doi:10.3390/medicines5030076 . . . . **133**

Lorena Martínez, Gaspar Ros and Gema Nieto
Hydroxytyrosol: Health Benefits and Use as Functional Ingredient in Meat
Reprinted from: *Medicines* **2018**, *5*, 13, doi:10.3390/medicines5010013 . . . . **143**

About the Editor

Gema Nieto completed his Ph.D. in 2009 at the University of Murcia and Postdoctoral studies in several centers, such as the University of Life Science (Denmark) and the University of Kentucky (USA). She is a young Researcher who has published numerous high-quality papers in different scientific journals in the field of food technology and human nutrition and has been invited as speaker in at several national and international conferences. At the moment, she is an Associate Professor at the University of Murcia and a member of the research group in Human Nutrition.

medicines

Editorial

How Are Medicinal Plants Useful When Added to Foods?

Gema Nieto

Department of Food Technology, Food Science and Nutrition, Faculty of Veterinary Sciences, Regional Campus of International Excellence "Campus Mare Nostrum", Espinardo, 30071 Murcia, Spain; gnieto@um.es

Received: 4 September 2020; Accepted: 7 September 2020; Published: 14 September 2020

Consumers are concerned about the use of synthetic additives in foods and this has forced food processors to find ways to produce food products without the use of these additives. Therefore there is a need in the food industry to find "clean label" products. In this context, the inclusion of medicinal plants into food products is an excellent strategy to produce functional foods, because plant-based extracts are rich in phytochemicals, with particular importance due to the health-beneficial effects.

Therefore, it is reasonable to imagine that, over the next few decades, the uses of natural extracts from medicinal plants will rapidly increase. In this sense, the search for new, effective and cheap sources of bioactive compounds is attracting food industry interest. However, it is important to study the implication on sensory characteristics of natural extracts of medicinal plants on foods to select specific raw materials; some of them of residual origin are especially promising due to their lower costs. Natural extracts from medicinal plants can be used as effective strategies for the production of functional foods, therefore achieving a significant increase in social and environmental sustainability. However, extensive research on sensory characteristics, antioxidant and antimicrobial sources, optimization of concentration of the extracts and a better knowledge of the mechanisms of the implication on shelf life of food, is still required.

This Special Issue of Medicines presents the current state of the art in medicinal plants and foods, collecting original manuscripts focused on topic-related research. The main objective is to publish original research work related to the chemistry of medicinal plants, and their application in food systems. Research work related mainly to the antimicrobial, antioxidant, and anti-inflammatory activities of medicinal plants and their applications in food systems is also included. The papers contribute significantly to furthering scientific knowledge in the above-mentioned scientific fields.

This Special Issue gives an overview of the current knowledge and recent trends in the use of medicinal plants as antimicrobials and antioxidants in foods, their potentials and challenges. It is critical to understand the effect of natural extracts and optimize their combinations for use in food preservation in order to better exploit their synergistic effects against both lipid oxidation and spoilage of pathogenic organisms. These considerations warrant the introduction of new species with high phenolic compound contents for beneficial applications by the food industry.

Medicinal plants or medicinal herbs have been identified and used since ancient times to improve the sensory characteristics of food. The main compounds found in plants correspond to four major biochemical classes: Polyphenols, terpenes, glycosides and alkaloids. Plants synthesize these compounds for a variety of purposes, including protection of the plant against fungi and bacteria, defense against insects and attraction of pollinators and dispersal agents to favor the dispersion of seeds and pollens.

Nowadays, there is also a growing interest in medicinal plants as natural alternatives to synthetic additives in foods because herbs and spices are generally recognized as safe (GRAS) and are excellent substitutes for chemical additives. The major activities of extracts and herbs from medicinal plants are antimicrobial, anti-inflammatory, bactericidal, antiviral, antifungal and preservative for foods. The use of natural preservatives to increase the shelf life of food systems is a promising technology since many vegetal substances show antioxidant and antimicrobial properties.

Taking into account all these considerations, recent changes in legislation controlling the use of animal feed additives and increased demand by consumers for healthier food products, if possible free of chemical additives, have stimulated interest in bioactive secondary metabolites from medicinal plants as alternative performance enhancers.

Since ancient times, medicinal plants have been added to improve the sensory characteristics of food. These plants have been gaining importance in recent years as potential sources of natural food preservatives due to the growing interest in the development of safe and effective natural food preservation. The use of vegetal substances with antimicrobial and antioxidant properties to increase the shelf life in foods is a promising technology.

The objective of including functional ingredients into foods is not only concerned with providing it with certain desirable properties, but also an attempt to change its image in these health-conscious days. In the market of functional food, rapid progress has been made in the development of this kind of food, based on the results of studies on food components providing positive health benefits over and above normal nutritional benefits.

The reduction or elimination of synthetic antioxidants in the elaboration of food could shorten the shelf-life, and this is the main concern for its marketing. As an alternative to synthetic antioxidants, natural extracts can be used, from plants such as grape, olive, sesame seed, tea, soybean, rosemary, thyme, etc., with antioxidant properties. Antioxidant compounds are usually added at a moderate dosage level since high levels of inclusion may mechanistically cause adverse effects through pro-oxidative action.

Between the strategies used to include natural additives, food can be modified by external addition in the elaboration of these products or by the addition into the animal diet of these extracts, where these ingredients are able to eliminate or reduce components that are considered harmful.

Work from our laboratory provides enough evidence for the use of natural extracts from medicinal plants in food preservation. Different studies found several interesting compounds in the plants and demonstrated the antioxidant and antimicrobial activity of natural extracts.

Nieto et al. [1]. reviewed the antioxidant and antimicrobial properties of rosemary. This review gives an overview on the on the use of natural extract from rosemary as a preservative in foods. Their use is limited due to their negative organoleptic properties, such as odour and taste. However, different new extraction methods have been developed in order to get colourless and odourless rosemary extracts. Several studies have reported that bioactive compounds, present in rosemary extracts and essential oils, delay lipid oxidation and microbiological spoilage, extending the shelf life of food. Taking into account all these aspects, rosemary extracts could be used in functional foods, pharmaceutical products, plant products and food preservation. The application of this natural extract can be complimented in different food systems such as meat, oils and dressing.

In the current publication, Serrano et al. [2] reviewed the potential anti-inflammatory health effects of traditional herbs. This review includes a summary of the dose–response anti-inflammatory activity of little-studied traditional botanical species, such as citrus fruit extracts rich in hesperidin, camu-camu (*Myrciaria dubia*), blackcurrant (*Ribes nigrum*), devil's claw (*Harpagophytum procumbens*) and cat's claw (*Uncaria tomentosa*). All these extracts reported greater or similiar effects than tea and cocoa. In addition, the known pathways of action and the potential synergistic effects of the constituent compounds of the extracts were also discussed.

Chiocchetti et al. [3] studied five agro-industrial food by-products, such as rice bran, pumpkin, peels from cucumber, cupuaçu seed peel and jackfruit, in order to establish alternative sources of nutrients. They determined the macronutrients, total and dialyzable Fe, the concentrations of iron-uptake inhibitors (phytic acid, tannins, fiber) and their correlation with iron bioavailability, several compounds that are interesting antifungal agents. These authors concluded that some by-products, in particular cucumber and pumpkin peels, could be valuable alternative sources of bioavailable Fe to reduce iron deficiency in at-risk populations and may contribute significantly to iron intake. This study showed the search for new by-products that can be used as alternative and inexpensive iron sources, and research into the development of new products based on cucumber and pumpkin peel.

Ghout et al. [4] describe their work to find biologically-active compounds from two extracts of the plant species *Euphorbia dendroides* L. They describe several compounds that are interesting antiproliferative and antioxidant antifungal agents, such as chlorogenic and gallic acids as major compounds. The two extracts exhibited antioxidant and anticancer activity. Based on the total phenolics and flavonoids contents, they concluded that the two extracts of *Euphorbia dendroides* L. display important reducing capacity, lipid peroxidation and antiradical activities.

Agregan et al. [5] provide a study of the the antioxidant potential of extracts obtained from three brown macroalgae, such as *Fucus vesiculosus, Ascophyllum nodosum* and *Bifurcaria bifurcata*, and two microalgae, such as *Spirulina platensis* and *Chlorella vulgaris* using a green and innovative extraction (ultrasound-assisted extraction using water/ethanol). Among the obtained macroalgae extracts, Bifurcaria bifurcata and the other macroalgaes were particularly suitable to be used as sources of phenolic antioxidants and to be included in products for human consumption.

Lefahal et al. [6]. describe their work to find biologically-active compounds from crude methanolic extract of aerial parts of *Capnophyllum peregrinum* (L.) Lange (Apiaceae) growing in Algeria. They describe several compounds that are interesting antifungal agents. The methanolic extract was found to have high flavonoid and phenolic contents as well as photoprotective and antioxidant activities. They could be used a sunscreen in pharmaceutical or cosmetic preparations and as a natural source of antioxidants.

Grigorakis et al. [7] describe their work to find biologically-active compounds, such as polyphenol, from *Stachys mucronata* and study of its antiradical activity. These authors reported as major constituents: apigenin analogues, derivatives of the flavone luteolin, chlorogenate conjugates and flavonol glycosides, being the most potent radical-scavenging compounds detected in the n-butanol fraction of the extracts, suggesting that they are the most active antioxidants in *Stachys mucronata.* This study showed valuable data for future studies that will aim at investigating the possible biological effects of *Stachys mucronata*, which remain unexamined to date.

Martínez et al. [8] describe in their work the search for biologically-active compounds from hydroxytyrosol (HXT) and their possible uses as functional ingredients in meat. They expose the health benefits provided by HXT consumption and the latest research about its use on meat. Due to its molecular structure, its regular consumption has several beneficial effects such as antioxidant, anti-inflammatory, anticancer, and as a protector of skin and eyes, etc. For these reasons, the use of HXT extract is a good strategy for use in meat products to replace synthetic additives. However, this extract has a strong odour and flavour, so it is necessary to previously treat this compound in order to not alter the organoleptic quality of the meat product when is added as an ingredient. For that reason, researchers have currently been focused on the encapsulation of this extract and the production of emulsion gels to prevent the sensorial alteration of meat products. In addition, the inclusion on meat endogenously, through the animal diet, or through its application in new packaging systems are the best strategies in order to introduce it into meat products.

Jongberg et al. [9] study in their work the effects of phenolic extracts from green tea (*Camellia sinensis*) and maté (*Ilex paraguariensis*) on the oxidative stability of modified atmosphere pork chops. They showed that phenolic plant extracts could be added as antioxidants in meat to prevent lipid oxidation, but depending on the concentration applied, may affect proteins either through covalent interactions or by serving as a prooxidant. They studied the oxidative stability in chops cut from injection-enhanced loins containing three different levels of green tea or maté extract. They concluded that Maté is a good source of antioxidants for the protection of both lipids and proteins in brine-injected pork, though the dose must be carefully selected.

Jongberg et al. [10] study in their work the protein oxidation and sensory quality of brine-injected pork loins added ascorbate or extracts of green tea or maté during chill-storage in a high-oxygen modified atmosphere. They showed that green tea and maté were found to equally protect against lipid oxidation-derived off-flavors, and maté showed less prooxidative activity towards proteins as compared to ascorbate, resulting in more tender meat. Based on present results, maté extract could be a potential substitution for ascorbate in the production of brine-injected pork, more so than green tea extract, as maté extract did not affect protein cross-linking, tenderness, or juiciness negatively throughout storage. Compared to green tea, maté extract generated no off-flavor, and, hence, based on the findings, is a valuable alternative as an antioxidant in brine-injected meat.They reported that maté is a valuable substitute for ascorbate in brine-injected pork chops.

Shafiee et al. [11] study the determination of blood glucose lowering and metabolic effects of *Mespilus germanica* L. hydroacetonic extract on streptozocin-induced diabetic BALB/c mice. The serum glucose lowering, normalization animal body weight, and antioxidative stress effects of *Mespilus germanica* L. leaf extract were investigated in normal and streptozotocin-induced BALB/c mice. The present study indicated that the *Mespilus germanica* leaf extract significantly decreased serum glucose and maintained normal body weight in BALB/c diabetic mice as compared with control groups. In addition, this extract decreased oxidative stress and lipid peroxidation. In conclusion, this species and other citable plants are very valuable and should be evaluated in experimental and clinical trials for their pharmacological efficacy and the discovery of new approved drugs for diabetes mellitus.

Egbung et al. [12] investigated the cardioprotective and hypolipidemic activity of *Vernonia calvoana* extract in paracetamol-treated rats. They suggested that the ethanol leaf extract of *Vernonia calvoana* reported cardioprotective and lipid-lowering effects and is a strategy to manage the toxicities induced by paracetamol.

Jaradat et al. [13] investigated new antilipase agents from ten traditional Palestinian edible and medicinal plants through inhibition of the absorption of dietary lipids. This effect was compared to Orlistat. Among all the extracts studied, Vitis vinifera and Rhus coriaria had the highest antilipase effects and could be considered a natural inhibitors of the pancreatic lipase enzyme and to be an excellent treatment of obesity players in obesity. These plants can be consumed in the diet or be prepared as natural supplements to treat or prevent obesity and control weight gain, and can be used for the treatment of hyperlipidemia.

The purpose of the current writing is to publish original research work related to the chemistry of medicinal plants, and their application in food systems. The research works published are related mainly to the antimicrobial, antioxidant, and anti-inflammatory activities of medicinal plants and their applications in food systems. The author of the current editorial encourages the modern use of extract from medicinal plants after performing trials of stability and sensory appreciation into foods.

Funding: This research received no external funding.

Conflicts of Interest: The author declares no conflict of interest.

References

1. Nieto, G.; Ros, G.; Sánchez, J.C. Antioxidant and Antimicrobial Properties of Rosemary (*Rosmarinus officinalis* L.): A Review. *Medicines* **2018**, *5*, 98. [CrossRef] [PubMed]
2. Serrano, A.; Ros, G.; Nieto, G. Bioactive Compounds and Extracts from Traditional Herbs and Their Potential Anti-Inflammatory Health Effects. *Medicines* **2018**, *5*, 76. [CrossRef] [PubMed]
3. Chiocchetti, G.M.; Fernandes, E.A.D.N.; Wawer, A.A.; Fairweather-Tait, S.J.; Christides, T. In Vitro Iron Bioavailability of Brazilian Food-Based by-Products. *Medicines* **2018**, *5*, 45. [CrossRef] [PubMed]
4. Ghout, A.; Zellagui, A.; Gherraf, N.; Demirtaş, I.; Yaglioglu, A.S.; Boukhenaf, M.; Lahouel, M.; Nieto, G.; Akkal, S. Antiproliferative and Antioxidant Activities of Two Extracts of the Plant Species *Euphorbia dendroides* L. *Medicines* **2018**, *5*, 36. [CrossRef] [PubMed]
5. Agregán, R.; Munekata, P.E.S.; Franco, D.; Carballo, J.; Barba, F.J.; Lorenzo, J.M. Antioxidant Potential of Extracts Obtained from Macro- (Ascophyllum nodosum, Fucus vesiculosus and Bifurcaria bifurcata) and Micro-Algae (Chlorella vulgaris and Spirulina platensis) Assisted by Ultrasound. *Medicines* **2018**, *5*, 33. [CrossRef] [PubMed]

6. Lefahal, M.; Zaabat, N.; Ayad, R.; Makhloufi, E.H.; Djarri, L.; Benahmed, M.; Laouer, H.; Nieto, G.; Akkal, S. In Vitro Assessment of Total Phenolic and Flavonoid Contents, Antioxidant and Photoprotective Activities of Crude Methanolic Extract of Aerial Parts of *Capnophyllum peregrinum* (L.) Lange (Apiaceae) Growing in Algeria. *Medicines* **2018**, *5*, 26. [CrossRef] [PubMed]
7. Grigorakis, S.; Makris, D.P. Characterisation of Polyphenol-Containing Extracts from Stachys mucronata and Evaluation of Their Antiradical Activity. *Medicines* **2018**, *5*, 14. [CrossRef] [PubMed]
8. Nieto, G.; Ros, G.; Nieto, G. Hydroxytyrosol: Health Benefits and Use as Functional Ingredient in Meat. *Medicines* **2018**, *5*, 13. [CrossRef]
9. Jongberg, S.; Tørngren, M.A.; Skibsted, L.H. Dose-Dependent Effects of Green Tea or Maté Extracts on Lipid and Protein Oxidation in Brine-Injected Retail-Packed Pork Chops. *Medicines* **2018**, *5*, 11. [CrossRef] [PubMed]
10. Jongberg, S.; Tørngren, M.A.; Skibsted, L.H. Protein Oxidation and Sensory Quality of Brine-Injected Pork Loins Added Ascorbate or Extracts of Green Tea or Maté during Chill-Storage in High-Oxygen Modified Atmosphere. *Medicines* **2018**, *5*, 7. [CrossRef] [PubMed]
11. Shafiee, F.; Khoshvishkaie, E.; Davoodi, A.; Kalantar, A.D.; Jouybari, H.B.; Ataee, R. The Determination of Blood Glucose Lowering and Metabolic Effects of *Mespilus germanica* L. Hydroacetonic Extract on Streptozocin-Induced Diabetic Balb/c Mice. *Medicines* **2018**, *5*, 1. [CrossRef] [PubMed]
12. Egbung, G.E.; Atangwho, I.J.; Odey, O.D.; Ndiodimma, V.N. The Lipid Lowering and Cardioprotective Effects of Vernonia calvoana Ethanol Extract in Acetaminophen-Treated Rats. *Medicines* **2017**, *4*, 90. [CrossRef] [PubMed]
13. Jaradat, N.; Zaid, A.N.; Hussein, F.; Zaqzouq, M.; Aljammal, H.; Ayesh, O. Anti-Lipase Potential of the Organic and Aqueous Extracts of Ten Traditional Edible and Medicinal Plants in Palestine; A Comparison Study with Orlistat. *Medicines* **2017**, *4*, 89. [CrossRef] [PubMed]

medicines

MDPI

Article

In Vitro Iron Bioavailability of Brazilian Food-Based by-Products

Gabriela M. Chiocchetti [1,†], Elisabete A. De Nadai Fernandes [1], Anna A. Wawer [2,‡], Susan Fairweather-Tait [2] and Tatiana Christides [3,*]

1 Centro de Energia Nuclear na Agricultura (CENA), Universidade de São Paulo (USP), Av. Centenário, 303, 13416-000 Piracicaba, SP, Brazil; gmchiocchetti@gmail.com (G.M.C.); lis@cena.usp.br (E.A.D.N.F.)
2 Norwich Medical School, University of East Anglia, Norwich NR4 7TJ, UK; aa.wawer@gmail.com (A.A.W.); s.fairweather-tait@uea.ac.uk (S.F.-T.)
3 Department of Life and Sports Sciences, Faculty of Engineering & Science, University of Greenwich, Medway Campus, Chatham Maritime, Kent ME4 4TB, UK
* Correspondence: t.christides@greenwich.ac.uk or ct33@gre.ac.uk; Tel.: +44-(0)20-8331-8427
† Current association: Instituto de Agroquímica y Tecnología de Alimentos (IATA-CSIC), Avenida Agustín Escardino 7, 46980 Paterna (Valencia), Spain.
‡ Current association: Discipline of Medicine, University of Adelaide, The Queen Elizabeth Hospital and the Basil Hetzel Institute for Translational Health Research, Woodville, SA 5011, Australia.

Received: 31 March 2018; Accepted: 7 May 2018; Published: 16 May 2018

Abstract: Background: Iron deficiency is a public health problem in many low- and middle-income countries. Introduction of agro-industrial food by-products, as additional source of nutrients, could help alleviate this micronutrient deficiency, provide alternative sources of nutrients and calories in developed countries, and be a partial solution for disposal of agro-industry by-products. **Methods**: The aim of this study was to determine iron bioavailability of 5 by-products from Brazilian agro-industry (peels from cucumber, pumpkin, and jackfruit, cupuaçu seed peel, and rice bran), using the in vitro digestion/Caco-2 cell model; with Caco-2 cell ferritin formation as a surrogate marker of iron bioavailability. Total and dialyzable Fe, macronutrients, the concentrations of iron-uptake inhibitors (phytic acid, tannins, fiber) and their correlation with iron bioavailability were also evaluated. **Results**: The iron content of all by-products was high, but the concentration of iron and predicted bioavailability were not related. Rice bran and cupuaçu seed peel had the highest amount of phytic acid and tannins, and lowest iron bioavailability. Cucumber peels alone, and with added extrinsic Fe, and pumpkin peels with extrinsic added iron, had the highest iron bioavailability. **Conclusion**: The results suggest that cucumber and pumpkin peel could be valuable alternative sources of bioavailable Fe to reduce iron deficiency in at-risk populations.

Keywords: Caco-2 cells; iron; bioavailability; phytic acid; agro by-products; food waste; waste utilization

---

1. Introduction

Iron deficiency (ID) is the most prevalent micronutrient deficiency in the world, affecting approximately 30% of the world's population [1,2]. Although ID is a public health issue in the developed world, especially in high-risk groups such as young children and pregnant women [3], its prevalence is particularly high in developing countries. Iron deficiency anemia (IDA) affects approximately one billion people [4] and is associated with diminished work productivity and an increase in maternal and neonatal mortality [1].

In Brazil, hunger and poverty remain serious population problems, and ID and IDA are significant public health concerns. It is estimated that about 7.2 million Brazilians suffer from hunger, and

4.8 million young Brazilian children suffer from IDA [5]. The underlying cause of this problem relates more to access to food within the context of distribution and waste rather than food production [6]. Waste in the food chain is approximately 61% of total food planted, occurring in all processing phases—planting, harvesting, transportation, storage, distribution—and consumer use [7]. Fruit and vegetable peels, seeds and leaves, which are classed as by-products of food processing, and deemed inedible, are not included in the waste data. However, these by-products may be a potential source of minerals and vitamins including iron, and thus might be useful in addressing ID/IDA in Brazil. Furthermore, recent rapid growth of the world's population has increased global demand for food sources [8]. Therefore, the transformation of food by-products to alternative food sources may be crucial not just in low and middle income countries, but worldwide.

Recently, uses for Brazilian agro-industrial food by-products have been investigated by several research centers as alternative sources of calories and micronutrients. These investigations resulted in the development of products such as biscuits, hamburgers and vegetable powders [9–12]; however, there is no data about the nutritional quality or bioavailability of the iron in these by-products. Some of them may potentially be nutritious and may contain high amounts of bioavailable iron [13,14] and thus could be considered possible sources for development of iron supplemental or fortificant products.

Iron absorption from foods is determined by a number of variables: the form of iron (i.e., heme versus non-heme iron); the modulating effect of dietary inhibitors and enhancers; and body iron status of the individual [15]. Non-heme iron is usually much less well absorbed than heme iron because its bioavailability is strongly influenced by the balance between iron inhibitors and enhancers [16]. Inhibitors include tannins, calcium, zinc, polyphenols, phytic acid and possibly fiber [15,16].

The primary aim of this study was to evaluate the non-heme iron (herein referred to as iron) bioavailability of 5 food processing by-products derived from fruits, vegetables and rice, from Brazilian agro-industrial sources, and thus their potential use as sources of supplemental iron. To achieve this, we employed the Caco-2 cell/in vitro digestion model to assess iron bioavailability, using absolute levels of cell ferritin as a surrogate marker for iron absorption, in the method developed by Glahn et al. [17]. This methodology has been validated and used in numerous studies in the last 20 years to evaluate iron bioavailability from foods and supplements [18–20].

The macronutrients composition, the concentration of iron absorption inhibitors (phytic acid, tannins and total dietary fiber) in the agro-industrial food-based by-products and their relation with iron bioavailability were also measured.

2. Materials and Methods

2.1. Samples

Samples of food processing by-products from fruits, vegetables and rice [cucumber peel, pumpkin peel, jackfruit peel (*Artocarpus heterophyllus*), cupuaçu seed peel (*Theobroma grandiflorum*), and rice bran] were collected directly from Brazilian agro-industries located in São Paulo and Amazonas states. The sample preparation was comprised of freeze-drying in a Thermo Savant ModulyoD lyophilizer (Thermo electron Corp., Waltham, MA, USA) and particle size reduction in a Retsch Grindomix GM200 knife mill (Retsch GmbH & Co, Haan, Germany), using polypropylene containers and a titanium knife to avoid contamination with iron.

2.2. Total Iron Content

The total amount of iron was determined by neutron activation analysis (NAA), recognized as a primary method of iron measurement in solid samples [21]. Analytical portions of 250 mg of food by-products were transferred to high-purity polyethylene capsules, specific for irradiation with neutrons. Ni–Cr alloy flux monitors with known composition and homogeneity [22] were intercalated with samples for monitoring neutron flux during the irradiation. Samples were irradiated for 8 h at a thermal neutron flux of 5.9×10^{12} cm^{-2} s^{-1}, in the nuclear research reactor IEA-R1 of the

Instituto de Pesquisas Energéticas e Nucleares, Comissão Nacional de Energia Nuclear (IPEN/CNEN), São Paulo. The induced radioactivity was measured after decay periods of 4, 7, 15 and 40 days, using an HPGe detector (GEM 45190, ORTEC, Aix en Provence, France) with 45% relative efficiency for the 1332 keV line of ^{60}Co. Chemical elements were calculated by the k_0-method using an in-house software package [23].

Use of certified reference materials (IAEA V-10 Hay Powder and INCT MPH-2 Mixed Polish Herbs) demonstrated a mean recovery of 101% for iron, which in within acceptable experimental standards.

2.3. Determination of Dialyzable Iron

The simulated digestion was according to the protocol described by Whittaker, Fox and Forbes [24]. All solutions were prepared fresh for each experiment, and all glassware used in experiments was soaked and cleaned in 10% nitric acid, followed by rinsing with 18 mΩ purity water.

The first step was gastric digestion simulation. Twenty g of each sample were homogenized in 100 mL of distilled H_2O, the pH was adjusted to 2.0 with HCl, followed by the addition of pepsin (2 mg/g, Sigma, Saint Louis, MO, USA); these prepared samples are herein referred to as digestas. The digestas were shaken at 37 °C, 200 RPM, for 2 h. In the following step, pH was adjusted to 7.0 with KOH and twenty g of this digesta was put inside a bag made of a dialysis membrane (15,000 Dalton molecular weight, Fisher Scientific, Waltham, MA, USA). This bag was submersed in 25 mL of a solution of 0.5 M $NaHCO_3$ for 30 min (shaken at 37 °C, 200 RPM). Past this time, a solution with bile (3 mg/g, Sigma, Saint Louis, MO, USA) and pancreatic digestive enzymes (0.5 mg/g, Sigma, Saint Louis, MO, USA) was added to the $NaHCO_3$ solution, and the digestas were shaken at 37 °C, 200 RPM, 2 h. The amount of iron in the $NaHCO_3$ solution was measured by inductively coupled plasma-optical emission spectrometry (ICP-OES).

2.4. Cell Culture

The TC7 Caco-2 cell clone was used for experiments between passages 39–51. This cell line has been validated for use in studies on iron metabolism and iron bioavailability [19].

Cells were grown in T75 tissue culture flasks in a humidified atmosphere with 5% of CO_2 at 37 °C and sub-cultured every 7 days. The culture medium used was Dulbecco's Modified Eagle Medium (DMEM) supplemented with 10% *v*/*v* fetal bovine serum, 1% penicillin–streptomycin, 4 mmol/L L-glutamine, 1% non-essential amino acids and Plasmocin 5 mg/mL and it was changed every 48 h. For experiments, cells were grown in six-well plates seeded at a density of $1 \times 10^4/cm^2$ and used 12–14 days after seeding as per the Glahn protocol [25].

Twenty-four hours prior to the initiation of in vitro digestion experiments, cell culture medium was changed to MEM without fetal bovine serum supplemented with 10 mmol/L PIPES [piperazine-*N*,*N*-bis-(2-ethanesulfonic acid)], 1% antibiotic/antimycotic solution, 11 µmol/L hydrocortisone, 0.87 µmol/L insulin, 0.02 µmol/L sodium selenite (Na_2SeO_3), 0.05 µmol/L triiodothyronine and 20 mg/L epidermal growth factor, in order to ensure adequate cell growth but low basal media iron levels.

2.5. In Vitro Digestion/Caco-2 Model to Measure Iron Bioavailability

Two experiments were carried out. In Experiment I, iron bioavailability from all the agro-industrial by-products samples was evaluated. Positive controls of Fe (25 µg) and Fe plus ascorbic acid (1:10 molar ratio) were carried out with each experiment, in addition to a "blank" control containing no food and no iron.

In Experiment II, the possible enhancing or inhibiting effects of the agro-industrial food by-products on extrinsically added iron bioavailability were investigated. For this purpose, all the agro- industrial by-products samples were analyzed with the addition of 25 µg of extrinsically added non-heme Fe (Fe solubilized in 1% HCL, High-Purity Standards, 100026-2). Controls were as in Experiment I.

The in vitro digestion followed a modified version of the protocol developed by Boato et al. [26]. All digestion solutions were prepared fresh for each experiment, and all glassware used in experiments was soaked and cleaned in 10% nitric acid, followed by rinsing with 18 mΩ purity water.

One g of each sample was added to 10 mL of pH 2 140 mmol/L NaCl and 5 mmol/L KCl followed by the addition of 0.5 mL pepsin solution (Chelex purified, concentration as previously noted), to simulate the peptic phase. The pH was readjusted to pH 2.0 with 1 mol/L HCl and the samples were shaken in a New Brunswick Orbital shaker at 37 °C, 200 RPM, for 1 h.

The intestinal digestion phase was initiated with the addition of 2.5 mL Chelex-purified bile/pancreatin solution (concentrations as previously noted) with subsequent adjustment of the pH to pH 6.9–7.0 with 1 mol/L $NaHCO_3$. Following this, 1.5 mL of the above digestas were placed in a chamber suspended over a layer of Caco-2 cells grown on the bottom of the tissue culture wells of a six-well plate. The upper chamber was created using a 15,000 Dalton molecular weight cut-off dialysis membrane (Tubing Spectra/Por 7 dialysis membrane, Fisher Scientific, Waltham, MA, USA) fitted over a modified Transwell insert (Fisher Scientific, Waltham, MA, USA; the necks of the rings were shortened by 0.1 mm to remove the original filter and prevent excessive pressure on the cell monolayer) and held in place with a silicon ring (Parker 2-023S0613, Web Seal). Plates were placed on a platform-fitted multi-function 3D rotator (Fisher Scientific PSM3D, Waltham, MA, USA) set at six oscillations per minute in a 37 °C incubator with a 5% CO_2 atmosphere at constant humidity for 60 min. Inserts were then removed, and an additional 1 mL of supplemented MEM was added to the cells, which were returned to the incubator for a further 22 h. Each food sample was tested in three separate experiments, $n = 6$ for each experiment.

At the end of each experiment, medium was removed from the wells and cells were rinsed twice with ice cold Phosphate Buffered Saline (PBS). 200 ml ice cold CelLytic (Sigma, Saint Louis, MO, USA) with 1% protease inhibitor was added to each well, and cell monolayers were removed with a cell scraper and placed in 1.8 mL Eppendorf tubes. Tubes were shaken for 15 min on a Stuart microtitre plate shaker at 1250 RPM and then spun at 6000 g for 6 min in a 5804R Eppendorf centrifuge. The supernatant was aspirated and stored at −80 °C until analysis.

The ferritin analysis was carried out using the SpectroFerritin MT Enzyme Linked Immunoassay (ELISA; RAMCO, Houston, TX, USA) on cell extraction supernatants. Absorption readings were performed at 492 nm with subtraction for background at 620 nm in a Thermo Multiscan Ascent Spectrophotometer. Protein concentration in each sample, to correct for differing cell counts per well, was measured using the Pierce Protein BCA Assay (Fisher Scientific, 23227, Waltham, MA, USA).

2.6. Macronutrients Composition and Analysis of Iron Absorption Inhibitors (Phytic Acid and Tannin)

Levels of macronutrients, phytic acid, tannin and total fiber were measured as follows. Phytic acid was determined according to the method described by Grynspan and Cheryan [27]. The samples were digested in 0.65 M HCl and the supernatant was eluted in an anionic resin and collected in a NaCl 0.7 M solution. Phytic acid levels were measured using the Wade's reagent ($FeCl_3 \cdot 6H_2O$ and sulfoalicylic acid), and quantified by absorption readings performed at 500 nm in a spectrophotometer Femto 700 plus.

The amount of tannin was determined by the methodology described by Price, Hagerman and Butler [28], through metal extraction and colorimetric reaction with vanillin solution at 1% methanol, 8% HCl in methanol (1:1 methanol), left at 30 °C for 20 min. Absorption readings were performed at 500 nm in a spectrophotometer Femto 700 plus. The concentration of tannins was obtained from a standard catechin curve, and the results were expressed as mg/100 g catechin.

The macronutrients composition were determined by the AOAC methods.

2.7. Statistical Analysis

The data generated was analyzed statistically by means of one-factor analysis of variance (ANOVA), followed by Tukey's post-hoc test to correct for multiple comparisons. Differences were considered significant at $p < 0.05$. Data analysis was performed using SigmaPlot (version 12.0, Systat Software, Inc., San Jose, CA, USA), except for data from ferritin formation, where the software Iron Data Manager (Excel version), provided by the University of Greenwich, was used.

Analysis of the relationship between ferritin formation, and inhibitors, and total iron levels, was carried out by non-linear regression and statistical significance was determined using the Delta method with $p < 0.05$ [29].

Because of ferritin level variation amongst the controls between experiments all data was normalized to the Fe Alone positive control according to the following equation:

$$y = f_e \times x$$

where y is the normalized value of x; and x is any given data point from experiment e; f_e is the mean value of the positive control (Fe Alone) across all experiments divided by the mean value of the positive control (Fe Alone) for experiment e only. This method has been used in previously published studies [19,30].

3. Results

3.1. Total Amount of Fe and Dialyzable Fe

Table 1 shows the data for total iron and dialyzable iron in samples of food processing by-products.

Table 1. Total iron (μg/g) and dialyzable iron (μg/g and percentage in respect to total Fe) in samples of food processing by-products.

Samples	Total Fe (μg/g)	Dialyzable Fe	
		μg/g	% in Respect Total Fe
Cupuaçu seed peel	829.7 ± 55.4 ^{a}	63.4 ± 5.12 ^{a}	7.64 ± 0.36 ^{b}
Jackfruit peel	379.1 ± 35.3 ^{b}	2.23 ± 0.46 ^{c}	0.59 ± 0.09 ^{d}
Pumpkin peel	117.8 ± 5.0 ^{c}	21.4 ± 0.76 ^{b}	18.1 ± 0.45 ^{a}
Cucumber peel	107.8 ± 2.9 ^{c}	2.47 ± 0.05 ^{c}	2.29 ± 0.03 ^{c}
Rice bran	96.7 ± 3.8 ^{c}	0.45 ± 0.02 ^{d}	0.63 ± 0.15 ^{d}

Values presented in dry weight (mean ± standard deviation, $n = 3$). Values within a column with unlike superscript letters are significantly different ($p < 0.05$). Total Fe jackfruit peel values have previously been published [14]; © Akadémiai Kiadó, Budapest, Hungary 2013 (with permission).

The levels of total iron varied for the tested samples. Cupuaçu seed peel had the highest level of total iron, followed by jackfruit peel, presenting 830 and 379 μg/g of iron, respectively. Pumpkin peel, cucumber peel and rice bran contained similar amounts of iron (around 95–120 μg/g), approximately 12 and 26% of the Fe present in cupuaçu seed peel and jackfruit peel samples, respectively.

Cupuaçu seed peel also contained the highest amount of dialyzable iron (63.4 μg/g), which represented 7.64% of the total amount of iron measured. Pumpkin peel had the highest percentage of dialyzable iron: 21.4 μg/g of the iron was in the dialyzable form, representing approximately 20% of the total iron. Cucumber peel contained approximately 2.5 μg/g of dialyzable iron. Jackfruit peel and rice bran had less than 1% of total iron presented in the dialyzable form.

3.2. Iron Bioavailability of Agro Industrial by-Products

Data on iron bioavailability from the in vitro digestion/Caco-2 cell model on a weight per weight basis (one gram of each sample was used per digesta) comparative basis are presented in Figure 1.

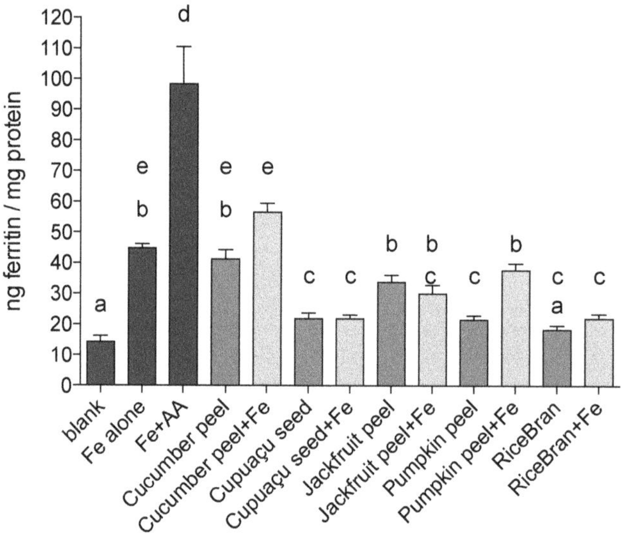

Figure 1. Ferritin formation (ng/mg protein) of Brazilian agro industrial by-products on a weight per weight comparative basis (one gram sample/digesta). Blank refers to digestas with no added sample, Fe alone is a positive control with the addition of inorganic Fe alone, and Fe + AA refers to iron plus ascorbic acid at a 1:10 molar ratio. All other samples are as referred to in the manuscript. Caco-2 cell ferritin formation was highest after exposure to cucumber peel + Fe. Cucumber peel, jackfruit peel, jackfruit peel + Fe and pumpkin peel + Fe treatments resulted in similar ferritin formation. In Pumpkin peel, cupuaçu seed peel, cupuaçu seed peel + Fe and rice Bran + Fe treatments, ferritin levels were similar and approximately 50% less than the response noted in the Fe alone positive control. Rice bran treated cells formed the lowest amount of ferritin: 75% less than the levels formed with Fe alone. Values are presented as means ± standard error of the mean (n = 18). Different letters show statistically significant differences ($p < 0.05$) between samples.

Cucumber peel and jackfruit peel treatments resulted in the greatest uptake of iron as measured by the ferritin assay (41.3 and 33.9 ng ferritin/mg protein, respectively). Ferritin formation by Caco-2 cells treated with pumpkin peel, cupuaçu seed peel and rice bran was approximately 50% less than Fe only positive control induced ferritin formation ($p < 0.0001$ in all instances).

When Fe was added to the by-product samples, Caco-2 ferritin formation in cells treated with cucumber peel + Fe was higher when compared to the treatment with cucumber peel only, although not statistically significant ($p = 0.0587$). A stronger effect was observed in pumpkin peel samples: addition of Fe increased ferritin formation by 68% ($p < 0.0001$). The addition of Fe to Cupuaçu seed peel, jackfruit peel or rice bran samples did not affect ferritin formation significantly when compared to treatments containing by-products only; cupuaçu seed peel, jackfruit peel and rice bran, respectively.

3.3. *Concentrations of Macronutrients and Iron Absorption Inhibitors in Agro-Industrial by-Products*

Table 2 shows the data for macronutrient and energy composition, and iron absorption inhibitors, namely phytic acid, tannin and total fiber in agro-industrial food-based by-products.

The level of phytic acid varied widely between samples; rice bran had the highest amount of phytic acid (1994 mg/100 g), followed by cupuaçu seed peel (1519 mg/100 g), and the second lowest ferritin levels. Cucumber peel and pumpkin peel presented similar amounts of phytic acid (approximately 200 mg/100 g). Jackfruit peel levels of phytic acid were below the limit of detection (BLD) (<139 mg/100 g).

Table 2. Food processing by-product sample macronutrient and energy composition and inhibitor amounts (phytic acid and tannin); values presented in dry weight.

Sample	Protein	Lipids	Carbohydrates	Total Fiber	Calories	Phytic Acid	Tannin
Cucumber peel	20.4 ± 0.1 [a]	2.34 ± 029 [c]	8.91 ± 1.66 [c]	46.5 ± 0.89 [a]	138 ± 5 [d]	233.5 ± 34.1 [c]	189.4 ± 15.7 [c]
Pumpkin peel	14.4 ± 0.3 [c]	4.10 ± 0.42 [b]	43.9 ± 1.4 [a]	24.1 ± 0.5 [c]	270 ± 2 [b]	201.1 ± 22.4 [c]	BDL *
Jackfruit peel	6.88 ± 0.04 [d]	4.12 ± 0.42 [b]	25.2 ± 1.2 [b]	50.4 ± 0.9 [a]	165 ± 9 [c]	BDL *	BDL *
Cupuaçu seed peel	17.0 ± 0.2 [b]	20.4 ± 1.1 [a]	25.1 ± 4.4 [b]	30.7 ± 1.9 [b]	352 ± 6 [a]	1519 ± 67 [b]	462 ± 4.7 [a]
Rice bran	13.0 ± 0.1 [c]	17.6 ± 0.6 [a]	27.5 ± 3.5 [b]	29.4 ± 1.5 [b]	320 ± 8 [a]	1994 ± 24 [a]	300 ± 27 [b]

Values are presented as g/100 g for protein, lipids, carbohydrates and total fiber, kcal/100 g for energy, and mg/100 g for phytic acid and tannin. Values are the mean ± standard deviation, n = 3. Different letters show statistically significant differences ($p < 0.05$) between samples * BDL, below limit detection. (BLD for phytic acid: 139 mg/100 g; BLD for tannin: 35 mg/100 g catechin).

Rice bran and cupuaçu seed peel contained the highest amount of tannin (300 and 462 mg/100 g catechin, respectively). Levels of tannin in cucumber peel (189 mg/100 g catechin) were approximately 40% of cupuaçu seed peel samples. Jackfruit peel tannin levels were BLD (<35 mg/100 g catechin).

Cucumber peel presented the highest amount of protein and total fiber, and low concentration of lipids and carbohydrates. Pumpkin peel had the highest amount of carbohydrates, and low concentration of total fiber. Levels of dietary fiber varied between 50 and 24 g/100 g of sample; Jackfruit peel and cucumber peel had the highest amounts (50 and 46 g/100 g, respectively), followed by cupuaçu seed peel and rice bran (31 and 29 g/100 g), respectively). Pumpkin peel presented the lowest value (24 g/100 g), just 48% of the total fiber present in jackfruit peel sample.

3.4. Influence of Phytic Acid, Tannins and Total Iron Content on Ferritin Formation

The correlation between concentrations of phytic acid, tannins and total iron versus ferritin formation by Caco-2 cells, in Experiment I (no added iron) and II (addition of 25 μg Fe) can be observed in Figure 2; R^2 for the regression is shown for each individual inhibitor with or without added iron. Statistical significance is designated by an asterix.

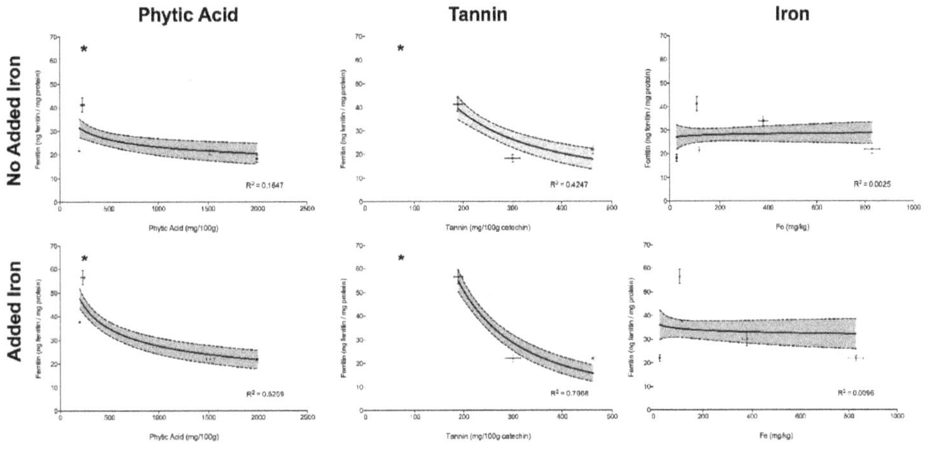

Figure 2. Correlation between phytic acid, tannins and total iron content versus ferritin formation in samples alone, and with added iron; R^2 for the regression is shown for each individual inhibitor with or without added iron. Phytic acid and tannins concentrations were significantly correlated with ferritin formation in both experiments (i.e., in the absence, and presence, of added extrinsic Fe). The total iron content was not correlated with ferritin formation. Values are presented as the mean ± SEM (n = 18 for ferritin; n = 3 for phytic acid, tannin and iron). Asterisks show statistically significant differences ($p < 0.05$).

Phytic acid and tannin concentrations showed an inverse correlation with ferritin formation in Experiments I, where no extrinsic iron had been added ($p < 0.05$) (i.e., the ferritin formation by Caco-2 cells was lower when phytic acid and/or tannin concentrations were higher). This effect was more pronounced when extrinsic iron was added, as in Experiment II ($p < 0.05$). The amount of total iron was not correlated with ferritin formation in either Experiment I or Experiment II ($p > 0.05$), demonstrating that high amounts of iron may not predict high iron bioavailability.

4. Discussion

The problem of by-product generation by agro-industries is currently of great concern, especially in a country as large as Brazil, where the agro-industry is responsible for about 6% of the Gross Domestic Product (GDP). The use of these by-products as an iron source could thus potentially reduce waste generation, contribute to iron intake in populations at risk of ID/IDA and be an alternative source of food for the growing population.

In this study, five pre-selected food-based by-products from Brazilian agro-industry were analyzed as a potential source of iron. These by-products were specifically selected because they had high iron content (≥9.7 mg/100 g), analyzed by NAA, as can be observed in Table 1. The amount of total iron in the by-product samples is similar (or higher) to plant-based foods usually recommended as sources of iron, such as green leafy vegetables (spinach: 36 mg/100 g, cauliflower: 67 mg/100 g) and beans (5 mg/100 g) [31,32]. In all these cases, it is higher than the edible part (pulp and grain), when compared with the numbers reported in the literature [33]. In similar studies, where iron concentration of several fruit peels was determined, the iron concentration was higher in the peel than in the pulp [9,34].

Although the iron content is high in these agro by-products, it is well-established that total iron levels cannot be used to predict iron bioavailability [35]. As can be observed in Table 1, the percentage of dialyzable iron is low (less than 20%), as expected for plant-based foods [36,37]. ICP-OES rather than neutron activation analysis (NAA) was used to measure iron in digestas as NAA can't be used for liquid sample analysis, without a sample concentration step; the research literature supports the relative accuracy of these methods both in general, and in comparison with each other [38]. Iron dialyzability studies do not provide accurate information about the strength of the effect of iron inhibitors and enhancers [39]. In addition, they usually markedly underestimate iron available for absorption from large intact iron-protein complexes such as ferritin, for which there is evidence that physiological absorption does occur [40]. Indeed, ferritin may provide significant amounts of iron from plant based sources, such as the tested food by-products evaluated in this study.

In Experiment I, ferritin formation by Caco-2 cells was measured after treatment with the 5 agro food by-products on a weight per weight basis. Despite the high amount of absolute and dialyzable iron in cupuaçu seed peel when compared to pumpkin peel and rice bran, Caco-2 cells produced similar amounts of ferritin in response to cupuaçu seed peel, pumpkin peel and rice bran, corroborating that a high amount of iron does not always predict high iron absorption (Figure 2).

In Experiment II, 25 μg of Fe were added to by-product samples to assess the effects of inhibitors or enhancers in the by-products. The addition of iron to pumpkin peel increased ferritin formation by approximately 75% ($p < 0.0001$), indicating that the Fe added (or part of it) was in a soluble form and could be absorbed; this may be related to low levels of inhibitors, or the presence of enhancers such as ascorbate, or fructose that would be expected to be found in pumpkin peels. In contrast, when Fe was added to the samples of cupuaçu seed peel, jackfruit peel and rice bran, no increase in Caco-2 cell ferritin formation was observed, suggesting that there are some compounds in these samples that inhibit iron absorption.

There are several dietary factors that can interfere with iron absorption in plant-based diets. The main inhibitor of iron absorption in general diets is phytic acid. In this study, phytic acid concentrations in by-products were between 201 and 1994 mg/100 g (Table 2). These figures are consistent with findings reported by others measuring phytic acid in plant-based food, including Greiner and Konietzny [41] who found 840–1210 mg/100 g of phytic acid in oat flakes, 850–1730 mg/100 g in cooked black beans and 1270–2160 mg/100 g in cooked wild rice. The high amount of phytic acid in the rice bran (1994 mg/100 g) was expected as, in cereals, phytate is more concentrated in the bran. Others studies have found even higher levels of phytic acid in rice bran (3650 and 5800 mg/100 g) [42,43]. Consistent with the described inhibitory effects of phytates on iron bioavailability ferritin formation from rice bran was low and stayed low even when exogenous iron was added to the samples (Figure 2). Thus, rice bran-based iron supplements or fortificants would not be predicted to be good sources of additional dietary iron.

Plant foods and beverages, such as vegetables, fruits, tea, coffee and wine, are also rich in polyphenols that can act as powerful iron absorption inhibitors [26,44,45]. In cereals and legumes, polyphenols add to the inhibitory effect of phytate [16]. Tannin (a polyphenol with a high molecular weight) levels were analyzed in this study. The high concentration of both phytic acid and tannin in the cupuaçu seed peel and rice bran can explain Caco-2 cell low ferritin formation from these samples, since tannins are powerful inhibitors of iron absorption (Figure 2). Cupuaçu seed peel would therefore probably not be a good source of supplemental iron.

Interestingly, although jackfruit peel tannins levels were below the limit of detection of our assay and phytic acid levels were also low, and iron levels were moderate, iron bioavailability (as measured by ferritin) was low in comparison with other samples and positive controls (Figure 2). The high amount of fiber found in the jackfruit peel (50.4 g/100 g) (Table 2) may explain this particular result. Some studies have found a correlation between fiber content and iron binding [46,47]. However, the effect of fiber on mineral absorption is not well described [48]. Jackfruit peel and cucumber peel contained similar amounts of fiber, but when the iron was added in the Experiment II, only jackfruit peel + Fe ferritin formation was compromised, being 47% lower than cucumber peel + Fe ferritin formation ($p = 0.0013$). This contradictory result may be due to other, unmeasured, inhibitory factors present in jackfruit peel, or unmeasured enhancing factors in the cucumber peel samples.

One of the limitations of our study was that we did not measure levels of known enhancers of iron bioavailability. Established dietary enhancers of non-heme iron absorption include ascorbic acid, meat, poultry, and fish. In vitro experiments suggest fructose may also enhance non-heme iron bioavailability [30]. Levels of these substances would be predicted to vary amongst these different agro-industrial food by-products.

Additionally, iron concentrations varied between digestas (samples that had undergone in vitro digestion), thus ferritin levels reflect the weight per weight iron bioavailability of the tested products irrespective of iron content of the raw material. The findings from Experiment II, in which a known and identical amount of exogenous iron was added to all samples, are illuminating in this respect; it would be beneficial to use food processing by-products that when fortified with iron did lead to increased bioavailability, such as cucumber peel.

In conclusion, with the fast increase of the world population and the imminent decrease of natural resources, the use of by-products as an alternative source of nutrients and calories in both developing and developed countries may contribute to global food security. Some by-products, in particular cucumber and pumpkin peels, may contribute significantly to iron intake and thus potentially reduce ID/IDA in at-risk populations of Brazil and other low and middle-income countries. In addition, they might be useful as an alternative source of proteins, carbohydrates and fiber. However, the absolute amount of iron ingested does not necessarily correlate with the fraction absorbed, as indicated by our results; rather, iron bioavailability reflects the balance between iron absorption inhibitors and enhancers. We encourage the search for new by-products that can be used as alternative and inexpensive iron sources, and research in the development of new products based on cucumber and pumpkin peel. Further research, including in vivo studies to confirm our results, warrants investigation.

Author Contributions: All authors were involved in the experimental design. E.A.D.N.F. conceived the total iron and iron absorption inhibitors analysis and T.C. designed the in vitro digestion/Caco-2 studies. E.A.D.N.F. contributed reagents, materials and analysis tools. G.M.C. performed the experiments; G.M.C. and T.C. analyzed the data and wrote the first draft; S.F.-T. and A.A.W. oversaw and edited all draft versions. All authors read and approved the final version submitted for peer review and publication.

Acknowledgments: This work was supported by "Conselho Nacional de Desenvolvimento Científico e Tecnológico" (CNPq—grant number 559710/2010-0). Gabriela M. Chiocchetti received a personal scholarship from "Fundação de Amparo à Pesquisa do Estado de São Paulo" (FAPESP—grant number 10/14566-8 and 12/03573-9) to develop this work. The authors gratefully acknowledge the financial support that has made this work possible. We are also grateful to the laboratory of Professor Paul Sharp (Mineral Metabolism Group, King's College London) for sharing the TC7 Caco-2 cell clone with us, and the companies that provided us with the samples: Cupuama (Careiro—AM), Dimas Ometto Beneficiadora de Arroz (Piracicaba—SP), Já-já (Iperó—SP), Nutri e Vegetais (Estiva Gérbi—SP), Ricaeli (Cabreúva—SP). Finally, we would like to thank Márcio A. Bacchi and Silvana R. V. Sarriés for the support on the total and dialyzable iron analysis and David S. Ganis for his development of the Iron Data Manger Excel software for analysis of ferritin levels in Caco-2 cells.

Conflicts of Interest: The authors declare no conflict of interest.

References

1. Cilla, A.; López-García, G.; Barberá, R. In vitro bioavailability of iron and calcium in cereals and derivatives: A review. *Food Rev. Int.* **2016**, *34*, 1–33. [CrossRef]
2. Otten, J.J.; Hellwig, J.P.; Meyers, L.D. *Dietary Reference Intakes (DRI)—The Essential Guide to Nutrient Requirements*; The National Academies Press: Washington, DC, USA, 2006; p. 543.
3. Miller, J.L. Iron deficiency anemia: A common and curable disease. *Cold Spring Harb. Perspect. Med.* **2013**, *3*, a011866. [CrossRef] [PubMed]
4. World Health Organization. *Global Database on Anemia*; World Health Organization: Geneva, Switzerland, 2008.
5. Saúde, M.D. (Ed.) *Política Nacional de Alimentação e Nutrição*; Departamento de Atenção Básica: Rio de Janeiro, Brazil, 2004.
6. Dos Santos, M.E.C.; Scherer, P.T. Política alimentar brasileira: Fome e obesidade, uma história de carências. *Textos Context.* **2012**, *11*, 92–105.
7. Velloso, K. Comida é que não falta. *Superinteressante* **2002**, *174*, 47–51.
8. Cheok, C.Y.; Adzahan, N.M.; Rahman, R.A.; Abedin, N.H.; Hussain, N.; Sulaiman, R.; Chong, G.H. Current trends of tropical fruit waste utilization. *Crit. Rev. Food Sci. Nutr.* **2018**, *58*, 335–361. [CrossRef] [PubMed]
9. Felipe, E.M.F.; Costa, J.M.C.; Maia, G.A.; Hernandez, F.F.H. Avaliação da qualidade de parâmetros minerais de pós-alimentícios obtidos de casca de manga e maracujá. *Alimentos e Nutrição Araraquara* **2006**, *17*, 79–83.
10. Ishimoto, F.Y.; Harada, A.I.; Branco, I.G.; Conceição, W.A.S. Aproveitamento alternativo da casca do maracujá-amarelo para produção de biscoitos. *Revista Ciências Exatas e Naturais* **2007**, *9*, 279–292.
11. Abud, A.K.S.; Narain, N. Incorporação da farinha de resíduo do processamento de polpa de fruta em biscoitos: Um alternativa de combate ao desperdício. *Braz. J. Food Technol.* **2009**, *12*, 257–265. [CrossRef]
12. Staichok, A.C.B.; Mendonça, K.R.B.; dos Santos, P.G.A.; Garcia, L.G.C.; Damiani, C. Pumpkin peel flour (*Cucurbita máxima* L.)—Characterization and techological applicability. *J. Food Nutr. Res.* **2016**, *4*, 327–333.
13. Pereira, G.I.S.; Pereira, R.G.F.A.; Barcelos, M.F.P.; Morais, A.R. Avaliação química da folha de cenoura visando ao seu aproveitamento na alimentação humana. *Ciência e Agrotecnologia* **2003**, *27*, 852–857. [CrossRef]
14. Chiocchetti, G.M.; De Nadai Fernandes, E.A.; Bacchi, M.A.; Pazim, R.A.; Sarriés, S.R.V.; Tomé, T.M. Mineral composition of fruit by-products evaluated by neutron activation analysis. *J. Radioanal. Nucl. Chem.* **2013**, *297*, 399–404. [CrossRef]
15. Collings, R.; Harvey, L.J.; Hooper, L.; Hurst, R.; Brown, T.J.; Ansett, J.; King, M.; Fairweather-Tait, S.J. The absorption of iron from whole diets: A systematic review. *Am. J. Clin. Nutr.* **2013**, *98*, 65–81. [CrossRef] [PubMed]
16. Hurrell, R.; Egli, I. Iron bioavailability and dietary reference values. *Am. J. Clin. Nutr.* **2010**, *91*, 1461S–1467S. [CrossRef] [PubMed]
17. Glahn, R.P.; Lai, C.; Hsu, J.; Thompson, J.F.; Guo, M.; Van Campen, D.R. Decreased citrate improves iron availability from infant formula: Application of an in vitro digestion/Caco-2 cell culture model. *J. Nutr.* **1998**, *128*, 257–264. [CrossRef] [PubMed]
18. Caetano-Silva, M.E.; Cilla, A.; Bertoldo-Pacheco, M.T.; Netto, F.M.; Alegría, A. Evaluation of in vitro iron bioavailability in free form and as whey peptide-iron complexes. *J. Food Compos. Anal.* **2018**, *68*, 95–100. [CrossRef]

19. Christides, T.; Amagloh, F.K.; Coad, J. Iron bioavailability and provitamin a from sweet potato- and cereal-based complementary foods. *Foods* **2015**, *4*, 463–476. [CrossRef] [PubMed]
20. Wawer, A.A.; Harvey, L.J.; Dainty, J.R.; Perez-Moral, N.; Sharp, P.; Fairweather-Tait, S.J. Alginate inhibits iron absorption from ferrous gluconate in a randomized controlled trial and reduces iron uptake into Caco-2 cells. *PLoS ONE* **2014**, *9*, e112144. [CrossRef] [PubMed]
21. Greenberg, R.R.; Bode, P.; De Nadai Fernandes, E.A. Neutron activation analysis: A primary method of measurement. *Spectrochim. Acta Part B* **2011**, *66*, 193–241. [CrossRef]
22. França, E.; Fernandes, E.A.N.; Bacchi, M.A. Ni-Cr alloy as neutron flux monitor: Composition and homogeneity assessment by naa. *J. Radioanal. Nucl. Chem.* **2003**, *257*, 113–115. [CrossRef]
23. Bacchi, M.A.; Fernandes, E.A.N. Quantu-design and development of a software: Package dedicated to k_0-standardized INAA. *J. Radioanal. Nucl. Chem.* **2001**, *257*, 577–582. [CrossRef]
24. Whittaker, P.; Fox, M.R.S.; Forbes, A.L. In vitro prediction of iron bioavailability for food fortification. *Nutr. Rep. Int.* **1989**, *39*, 1205–1215.
25. Glahn, R.P.; Lee, O.A.; Yeung, A.; Goldman, M.I.; Miller, D.D. Caco-2 cell ferritin formation predicts nonradiolabeled food iron availability in an in vitro digestion/Caco-2 culture model. *J. Nutr.* **1998**, *128*, 1555–1561. [CrossRef] [PubMed]
26. Boato, F.; Wortley, G.M.; Liu, R.H.; Glahn, R.P. Red grape juice inhibits iron availability: Application of an in vitro digestion/Caco-2 cell model. *J. Agric. Food Chem.* **2002**, *50*, 6935–6938. [CrossRef] [PubMed]
27. Grynspan, F.; Cheryan, M. Phytate-calcium interactions with soy protein. *J. Am. Oil Chem. Soc.* **1989**, *66*, 93–97. [CrossRef]
28. Price, M.L.; Hagerman, A.E.; Butler, L.G. Tannin content of cowpeas, chickpeas, pigeon peas and mung beans. *J. Agric. Food Chem.* **1980**, *28*, 459–461. [CrossRef] [PubMed]
29. Dorfman, R. A note on the delta-method for finding variance formulae. *Biom. Bull.* **1938**, *1*, 129–137.
30. Christides, T.; Sharp, P. Sugars increase non-heme iron bioavailability in human epithelial intestinal and liver cells. *PLoS ONE* **2013**, *8*, e83031. [CrossRef] [PubMed]
31. Singh, G.; Kawatra, A.; Sehgal, S. Nutritional composition of selected green leafy vegetables, herbs and carrots. *Plant. Foods Hum. Nutr.* **2001**, *56*, 359–364. [CrossRef] [PubMed]
32. Brigide, P.; Ataide Tda, R.; Canniatti-Brazaca, S.G.; Baptista, A.S.; Abdalla, A.L.; Filho, V.F.; Piedade, S.M.; Bueno, N.B.; Sant'Ana, A.E. Iron bioavailability of common beans (*Phaseolus vulgaris* L.) intrinsically labeled with (59)fe. *J. Trace Elem. Med. Biol.* **2014**, *28*, 260–265. [CrossRef] [PubMed]
33. Lima, D.M. *Tabela Brasileira de Composição de Alimentos (TACO)*, 4th ed.; NEPA-Unicamp: Campinas, Brazil, 2011.
34. De Souza Sabino, L.B.; de Lima, A.C.S.; Soares, D.J.; da Silva, L.M.R.; de Oliveira, L.S.; de Figueiredo, R.W.; de Sousa, P.H.M. Composição mineral de farinhas obtidas a partir de cascas de frutos tropicais baseado na ingestão diária recomendada. *Braz. J. Food Res.* **2017**, *8*, 102–111. [CrossRef]
35. Fairweather-Tait, S.J. Bioavailability of trace elements. *Food Chem.* **1992**, *43*, 213–217. [CrossRef]
36. Cámara, F.; Amaro, M.A.; Barberá, R.; Clemente, G. Bioaccessibility of minerals in school meals: Comparision between dialysis and solubility methods. *Food Chem.* **2005**, *92*, 481–489. [CrossRef]
37. Hurrell, R.F.; Lynch, S.R.; Trinidad, T.P.; Dassenko, S.A.; Cook, J.D. Iron absorption in humans as influenced by bovine milk proteins. *Am. J. Clin. Nutr.* **1989**, *49*, 546–552. [CrossRef] [PubMed]
38. Moens, L.; Dams, R. NAA and ICP-MS: A comparison between two methods for trace and ultra-trace elements analysis. *J. Radioanal. Nucl. Chem.* **1995**, *192*, 29–38. [CrossRef]
39. Wienk, K.J.H.; Marx, J.J.M.; Beynen, A.C. The concept of iron bioavailability and its assessment. *Eur. J. Nutr.* **1999**, *38*, 51–75. [CrossRef] [PubMed]
40. Lönnerdal, B.; Bryant, A.; Liu, X.; Theil, E.C. Iron absorption from soybean ferritin in nonanemic women. *Am. J. Clin. Nutr.* **2006**, *83*, 103–107. [CrossRef] [PubMed]
41. Greiner, R.; Konietzny, U. Phytase fof foor application. *Food Technol. Biotechol.* **2006**, *44*, 125–140.
42. García-Estepa, R.M.; Guerra-Hernández, E.; García-Villanova, B. Phytic acid content in milled cereal products and breads. *Food Res. Int.* **1999**, *32*, 217–221. [CrossRef]
43. Ravindran, V.; Ravindran, G.; Sivalogan, S. Total and phytate phosphorus contents of various foods and feedstuffs of plant origin. *Food Chem.* **1994**, *50*, 133–136. [CrossRef]

44. Ma, Q.; Kim, E.Y.; Lindsay, E.A.; Han, O. Bioactive dietary polyphenols inhibit heme iron absorption in a dose-dependent manner in human intestinal caco-2 cells. *J. Food Sci.* **2011**, *76*, H143–H150. [CrossRef] [PubMed]
45. Ma, Q.; Kim, E.Y.; Han, O. Bioactive dietary polyphenols decrease heme iron absorption by decreasing basolateral iron release in human intestinal caco-2 cells. *J. Nutr.* **2010**, *140*, 1117–1121. [CrossRef] [PubMed]
46. Bosscher, D.; Van Caillie-Bertrand, M.; Van Cauwenbergh, R.; Deelstra, H. Availabilities of calcium, iron, and zinc from dairy infant formulas is affected by soluble dietary fibers and modified starch fractions. *Nutrition* **2003**, *19*, 641–645. [CrossRef]
47. Debon, S.J.J.; Tester, R.F. In vitro binding of calcium, iron and zinc by non-atarch polyssacharides. *Food Chem.* **2001**, *73*, 401–410. [CrossRef]
48. Baye, K.; Guyot, J.P.; Mouquet-Rivier, C. The unresolved role of dietary fibers on mineral absorption. *Crit. Rev. Food Sci. Nutr.* **2017**, *57*, 949–957. [CrossRef] [PubMed]

medicines MDPI

Article

Antiproliferative and Antioxidant Activities of Two Extracts of the Plant Species *Euphorbia dendroides* L.

Agena Ghout [1], Amar Zellagui [1], Noureddine Gherraf [2], Ibrahim Demirtas [3], Yaglioglu Ayse Sahin [3], Meriem Boukhenaf [4], Mesbah Lahouel [5], Gema Nieto [6] and Salah Akkal [7,*]

1 Laboratory of Biomolecules and Plant Breeding, Life Science and Nature Department, Faculty of Exact Science and Life Science and Nature, University of Larbi Ben Mhidi, Oum El Bouaghi 04000, Algeria; agenaghout@yahoo.fr (A.G.); zellaguia@yahoo.com (A.Z.)
2 Department of Chemistry, Faculty of Exact Science and Life Science and Nature, University of Larbi Ben, Mhidi Oum El Bouaghi 04000, Algeria; ngherraf@yahoo.com
3 Laboratory of Plant Research, Department of Chemistry, Faculty of Science, Uluyazi Campus, Cankiri Karatekin University, Cankiri 18100, Turkey; ibdemirtas@gmail.com (I.D.); aysesahin1@gmail.com (Y.A.S.)
4 Department of Pathological Anatomy, University Hospital Center of Constantine, Constantine 25000, Algeria; Boukhenaf.Meriem@gmail.com
5 Laboratory of Molecular Toxicology, University of Jijel, Jijel 18000, Algeria, lahouelmesbah@yahoo.fr
6 Department of Food Technology, Nutrition and Food Science, Faculty of Veterinary Sciences, University of Murcia, Campus de Espinardo, Espinardo, Murcia 30100, Spain; gnieto@um.es
7 Laboratoire de Phytochimie et Analyses Physico-Chimiques et Biologiques, Université Mentouri de Constantine, Route de Aïn El Bey, Constantine 25000, Algeria
* Correspondence: salah4dz@yahoo.fr or salah.akkal@umc.edu.dz; Tel./Fax: +21-33181-1102

Received: 28 February 2018; Accepted: 13 April 2018; Published: 20 April 2018

Abstract: Background: These days, the desire for naturally occurring antioxidants has significantly increased, especially for use in foodstuffs, cosmetics, and pharmaceutical products, to replace synthetic antioxidants that are regularly constrained due to their carcinogenicity. **Methods:** The study in hand aimed to appraise the antioxidant effect of two *Euphorbia dendroides* extracts using reducing power, anti-peroxidation, and DPPH (1,1 Diphenyl 2 Pycril Hydrazil) scavenging essays, in addition to the anticancer activity against two tumor cell lines, namely C6 (rat brain tumor)cells, and Hela (human uterus carcinoma)cell lines. **Results:** The results indicated that the ethyl acetate extract exhibited antiradical activity of 29.49%, higher than that of *n*-butanol extract (18.06%) at 100 μg/mL but much lower than that of gallic acid (78.21%).The ethyl acetate extract exhibits better reducing capacity and lipid peroxidation inhibitory activity compared to *n*-butanol extract but less than all tested standards. Moreover, the ethyl acetate extract was found to have an antiproliferative activity of more than 5-FU (5-fluoro-Uracil) against C6 cells at 250 μg/mL with IC_{50} and IC_{75} of 113.97, 119.49 μg/mL, respectively, and good cytotoxic activity against the Hela cell lines at the same concentration. The HPLC-TOF-MS (high performance liquid chromatography-Time-of-flight-Mass Spectrometry) analyses exposed the presence of various compounds, among which Gallic and Chlorogenic acids functioned as major compounds. **Conclusions:** The two extracts exhibited moderate anticancer abilities and behaved somewhat as average antioxidant agents. Based on the total phenolics and flavonoids contents, as well as HPLC results, it could be concluded that antiproliferative and antioxidant activities depend upon the content of different phenolics and flavonoids.

Keywords: *Euphorbia dendroides*; phenolic compounds; HPLC; antioxidant activity; antiproliferative activity

1. Introduction

The free radicals are chemical compounds, which involve in their structure one or more impaired electrons, making them extremely unstable and hence predisposing them to extract electrons from other compounds to reach stability. Oxidative stress refers to an imbalance between the production of the free radicals and the antioxidant defense system. Oxidative stress is regarded as substantial in the initiation and expansion of many recent ailments including irritation, cataracts, tumors, and autoimmune and neurodegenerative disorders [1–3].

At present, the interest in naturally antioxidants has noticeably increased for use in foodstuffs and cosmetic and pharmaceutical ingredients as a substitute for artificial antioxidants that are steadily limited due to their suspicious carcinogenic effect [4,5]. Plants are viewed as a prospective source of natural antioxidants, especially the secondary metabolites such as phenolics, flavonoids, and terpenes, which are formed by plants to support growth under unfavorable conditions [6]. These herbs represent crucial ingredients of folk medicine applied throughout the world owing to their low price, effortless access, and inherited practice [7]. Lately, phenolics have received extensive awareness because of their physiological role, including as antioxidants and in antimutagenic and antitumor activities [8]. *Euphorbia,* one of the most various genus of flowering plants and the largest genus of the *Euphorbiaceae,* comprises about 2000 species [9,10]. The frequent name "spurge" derives from the French word espurgier (latinexpurgare), which denotes "to purge" due to the use of Euphorbia latex as purgative. The Botanical name Euphorbia derives from the Greek *Euphorbus* [11]. The compounds extracted from this genus comprise flavonoids, triterpenoids, amino acids, and alkaloids [12]. *Euphorbia* is reported to possess inflammatory, antiarthritic, antiamoebic, spasmolytic, antiviral, hapatoprotective, and antitumor activity [13–16]. Some species are used in folk medicine to treat skin diseases, gonorrhea, migraines, intestinal vermins, and warts [17,18].

Euphorbia dendroides encloses rich ethnopharmacological properties already documented in the old medical literature; it was used to remove warts and as a fish poison [19]. It was reported as well to contain many bioactive chemical compounds such as Jatrophane Esters [20].

The study in hand aims to assess the in vitro antioxidant and antiproliferative effects of the ethyl acetate and *n*-butanol extracts of the aerial parts of *Euphorbia dendroides* grown in Algeria.

2. Materials and Methods

2.1. Chemicals

Folin-ciocalteu reagent, anhydrous sodium carbonate (Na_2CO_3), Gallic acid, Ascorbic acid, Aluminum chloride ($AlCl_3$), 2,2-diphenyl-1-picrylhydrazyl radical (DPPH), quercetin, potassium ferric cyanide ($K_3Fe(CN)_6$), iron (III) chloride ($FeCl_3$), methanol, ethyl acetate, *n*-hexane, *n*-butanol, ethanol, trichloroacetic acid(TCA), thiobarbituric acid (TBA), HCl, NaOH, $FeSO_4$, Tween 20, phosphate buffer, and BrdU Cell Proliferation ELISA assay reagent were provided by Roche, Berlin, Germany. Dulbecco's modified eagle's medium was purchased from DMEM, Sigma, Munich, Germany. Fetal bovine serum, PenStrep solution, and 5-fluorouracil were purchased from Sigma, Munich, Germany.

2.2. Plant Material

The above ground part of the plant was collected from Bejaia (Cap-Carbon) during May 2013 (flowering stage). Dr. Rebbas from the Department of botany, M'sila, Algeria identified the plant. A voucher sample was deposited in the Laboratory of Biomolecules and Plant Breeding, University of Larbi Ben M'hidi Oum El Bouaghi, Algeria under the voucher number ZA 140.

2.3. Extraction

The extraction process was carried out according to the method of Wang [21]. The plant was air-dried and preserved at ambient temperature and then crushed into powder. 200 g of plant was soaked in 500 mL of 70% methanol-water for 1 week at room temperature and filtered using Whatman paper N°1. The extraction process was repeated three times and the hydroalcoholic solutions were collected, filtered, and dried under vacuum. The residue was suspended in 200 mL of distilled water and partitioned in ethyl acetate (3 × 150 mL) and *n*-butanol (3 × 150 mL). The resulting solutions were concentrated in vacuum, to yield the following fractions: EtOAc (0.84 g), *n*-butanol (4.5 g). The fractions were kept at 4 °C in the dark until further analysis.

2.4. HPLC-TOF/MS Analysis

Phenolic content of the plant extract was determined using Agilent Technology of 1260 Infinity HPLC System (Agilent Technologies, Santa Clara, CA, USA)joined with 6210 Time of Flight (TOF) LC/MS detector (Agilent Technologies, Santa Clara, CA, USA) and ZORBAX SB-C18 (4.6 × 100 mm, 3.5 µm) column (Agilent Technologies, Santa Clara, CA, USA). Mobile phases A and B were ultra-pure water with 0.1% formic acid and acetonitrile, respectively. Flow rate was 0.6 mL min^{-1}, and column temperature was 35 °C. Injection volume was 10 µL. The solvent rate was 0–1 min 10% B, 1–20 min 50% B, 20–23 min 80% B, 23–25 min 10% B, and 25–30 min 10% B. Determination of the phenolic compounds was performed by comparison of the standard compounds with the samples in terms of retention times and m/z values. Ionization mode of HPLC-TOF/MS instrument was negative and operated with a nitrogen gas temperature of 325 °C, nitrogen gas flow of 10.0 L min^{-1}, nebulizer of 40 psi, capillary voltage of 4000 V, and, finally, fragmentor voltage of 175 V. For sample analysis, dried crude extracts (200 ppm) were dissolved in methanol at room temperature. Samples were filtered passing through a PTFE (0.45 µm) filter by an injector to remove particulates.

2.5. Phenolic Contents Analysis

2.5.1. Total Phenolic Content (TPC)

The Total phenolic content (TPC) of both extracts was determined using the Folin-Ciocalteau Reagent (FCR) according to the method of Singleton [22] and external calibration with Gallic acid. Briefly, 0.5 mL of the diluted solution of each extract in methanol was added to 2.5 mL of FCR (diluted 1/10 with distilled water) and mixed. After 5 min, 2 mL of sodium carbonate aqueous solution Na_2CO_3 (75 g/L) was added to the mixture and incubated at 40 °C for 30 min. The absorbance was measured at 760 nm. Results are presented as mg of Gallic acid equivalent (GAE)/g of dry extract using Gallic acid calibration curve. All experiments were performed in triplicate, and the results were averaged.

2.5.2. Total Flavonoids Content (TFC)

Flavonoids as among the most varied and prevalent group of natural compounds are probably the most important natural phenolics [23]. In this study, total flavonoids content of the two extracts was assessed following the aluminum Chloride colorimetric method [5].This method stands on the formation of a flavonoid-aluminum complex having λ_{max} at 430 nm. 1 mL of methanol extract was mixed with 1 mL of 2% $AlCl_3$ methanol solution, and then the absorbance was determined at 430 nm using UV-VIS spectrophotometer. Total flavonoids content was expressed as mg quercetin equivalent (QE) per g of dry extract. All tests were done in triplicates.

2.6. Determination of Antioxidant Activity

2.6.1. DPPH Radical Scavenging Assay

The radical scavenging activity of the two extracts was measured against DPPH (2,2-Diphenyl-1-picryl hydrasyl radical was measured according to the method of Masuda [24]). DPPH is a stable free radical, which on reaction with an antioxidant reduces from a violet color to the yellow-colored diphenyl-picryl-hydrazine. The free radical DPPH absorbs at 517 nm, but after reduction by an antioxidant the absorption decreases. Briefly, 20 µL of each extract (different concentrations, w/v) was mixed with 2 mL of methanol solution of DPPH radical (10^{-4} M). The mixture was shaken vigorously, and the absorbance values were read at 517 nm after incubation for 20 min in dark at room temperature.

The radical scavenging activity was calculated using the following formula:

$$\% \text{ inhibition} = \{[A_b - A_a]/A_b\} \times 100$$

Quercetin, gallic acid, and ascorbic acid were used as the positive control. The experiment was performed in triplicate.

2.6.2. Reducing Power Assay

In this test, the yellow color of the test solution shifts to green reflecting the reducing power of the sample. The reducing agents in the solution initiate the reduction of the Fe^{3+}/ferricyanide complex to the ferrous structure. Therefore, Fe^{2+} can be observed by measurement of the absorbance at 700 nm [25].

The reducing power of both extracts was determined according to the method of Oyaizu [26]. Briefly, 1mL of serial concentrations of the extract (20–100 μg/mL) was mixed with 1 mL of sodium phosphate buffer (0.2 mol dm^{-3}, pH = 6.6) and 1 mL of potassium ferricyanide (1%). Reaction mixture was incubated at 50 °C for 20 min, and then 1 mL of trichloro-acetic acid (10%) was added and centrifuged for 10 min. From the upper layer, 1 mL was mixed with 1 mL of distilled water and 0.3 mL of $FeCl_3$ (0.1%). Absorbance of resulting solution was measured at 700 nm. Quercetin, gallic acid, and ascorbic acid were used as standards. Values are presented as mg quercetin equivalent per g of extract.

2.6.3. The Inhibition of Linoleic Acid Peroxidation

The antiperoxidation test of both extracts was realized using thiobarbituric acid (TBA) method, which is based on inhibition of linoleic acid peroxidation in accordance with the method of Choi [27].

This method was adopted for the lipid peroxidation test, with linoleic acid as the source of linoleic acid in an oxidation system catalysed by Fe-ascorbate. The samples (50–500 μg/mL) were mixed with linoleic acid solution (0.28 mg of linoleic acid and 0.28 mg of tween-20) in 100 μM phosphate buffer (500 mL of phosphate buffer (100 μM, pH = 7.4) and 150 μL of ascorbic acid (10 μM). The mixture was stirred and sonicated to give a homogeneous suspension solution. The linoleic acid peroxidation test started with the addition of 0.1 mL $FeSO_4$ (10 μM) and was incubated at 37 °C for 60 min. The reaction mixture was cooled and added to 1.5 mL of trichloroacetic acid (10% in 0.5% HCl). Then, 3 mL TBA (1%, in 50 mM NaOH) was added. The reaction mixture and TBA solution were heated in the water bath at 90 °C for 60 min. After cooling down, 2 mL aliquots were taken from each sample and mixed with 2 mL of *n*-butanol and centrifuged at 1000×*g* for 30 min. The upper layer solution was separated for the spectroscopic measurement, and the absorbance of thiobarbituric acid-reacting substances (TBARS) in the supernatant were read at 532 nm and converted into the percentage of antioxidant activity.

The percentage of linoleic acid peroxidation inhibition was defined as (%) = $[(A_o - A_1)/A_o] \times 100$, in which A_o is the absorbance of control reaction (containing all reagents except the sample) and A_1 is the absorbance of the sample or the standard.

2.7. Determination of In Vitro Antiproliferative Activity

Antiproliferative activity was evaluated by estimation of the inhibitory effect of the phenolics on the growth of cells on C6 (rat brain tumor) using proliferation BrdU ELISA assay, and was tested for HeLa cell lines using a real-time cell analyzer (xCELLigence) [28,29].

2.7.1. Cell Culture

The cells were developed in Dulbecco's modified eagle's medium (DMEM, Sigma, Munich, Germany), complemented with 10% (*v*/*v*) fetal bovine serum (Sigma, Munich, Germany) and PenStrep solution (Sigma, Munich, Germany) at 37 °C in a 5% CO_2 humidified atmosphere.

2.7.2. Cell Proliferation Assays

- *ELISA Assay*

The cells were laminated in 96-well culture plates (COSTAR, Corning, Oneonta, NY, USA) at a density of 30,000 cells per well. The samples activities were investigated at 250, 100, and 50 μg/mL. 5-FU was used as standard. Afterwards, the cells were incubated all night before applying the BrdU Cell Proliferation ELISA assay reagent (Roche, Berlin, Germany) in accordance with the manufacturer's method. The quantity of cell proliferation was read at 450 nm using a microplate reader (Awareness Chromate, Ramsey, MN, USA).

Results were given as percentage of the inhibition, in which the optical density measured from vehicle-treated cells was considered to be 100% of proliferation. The stock solution of the extracts was prepared in dimethyl-sulfoxide (DMSO) and diluted with DMEM. DMSO final concentration is below 0.1% in all tests. 5-FU was used as standard compounds. Percentage of inhibition of cell proliferation was calculated as follows: inhibition percentage = $[1 - (A_{treatments}/A_{vehicle\ control})] \times 100$.

The half-inhibitory concentration (IC_{50}) is a measure of the effectiveness of a compound in inhibiting a biological function. In this paper, IC_{50} and IC_{75} values were determined using ED_{50} in addition to V1.0.

- *Xcelligence Assay*

A real-time cell analyzer–single plate (RTCA-SP) instrument (Roche Applied Science, Basel, Switzerland) was used to analyze the ability of extracts to induce cell growth of HeLa cell line. A newly developed electronic cell sensor array, the xCELLigence RTCA, was used with a recently published literature method at concentrations of 250, 100, and 50 μg/mL. All the measurements were done in 10 min intervals and triplicated [30].

- *Statistical analysis*

The in vitro results of anticancer activity are means ± SD of six measurements. Differences between groups were tested with ANOVA. p values of <0.01 were considered as significant and analyzed by SPSS (version 11.5 for Windows 2000, SPSS Inc., Chicago, IL, USA).

The results of scavenging activity and total phenolic compounds were performed from the samples reading mean ±SD (standard deviation) using EXEL 2003. All analyses were carried out in triplicates.

3. Results and Discussion

3.1. Extraction Yield

The yield of the two crude extracts was calculated and presented in Table 1 and expressed as the ratio of the dry weight of plant extract to the dry weight of the plant material. The extraction yield varies depending on the nature of the used solvent. The higher yield is obtained with *n*-butanol extract (2.12%) followed by ethyl acetate extract (0.42%).

Table 1. Extractive values of *Euphorbia dendroides* extracts.

Extract	Yield (%)
Ethyl acetate extract	0.42%
n-Butanol extract	2.12%

3.2. Total Phenolic Compounds and Total Flavonoids

A number of modern studies are evidence for phenolics as the most dominant antioxidant compounds [31]. Therefore, the amount of total phenolic compounds and flavonoids in the two extracts were evaluated (Table 2).

The total phenolics of the plant extracts measured by the folin-ciocalteu method are presented as gallic acid equivalent in milligrams per gram of extract (mg GAE/g). Total phenolic content was found to range from 164.25 to 929.51 mg GAE/g.

The extraction of phenolics in plant material is affected by their chemical environment, the extraction process, particle size, period, and conditions of storage, as well as the presence of intrusive substances [32], in addition to solvent polarity, which has diverse effects on total phenolics and antioxidant activities [33,34].

The peak amount of total flavonoids was obtained in ethyl acetate extract (26.04 mg QE/g) followed by *n*-butanol extract (12.16 mg QE/g), signifying that the extracts are very complex and hold many other polyphenols, or that the polymerization degree of the polyphenols in the samples is important.

Table 2. Phenolic compounds of *Euphorbia dendroides* extracts.

Extract	TPC(mg GAE/g of Extract)	TF(mg QE/g of Extract)
Ethyl acetate	929.51 ± 20.1	26.04 ± 0.32
n-Butanol	164.25 ± 16.40	12.16 ± 0.2

TPC: total phenolic compounds, TF: total flavonoids.

3.3. *High Performance Liquid Chromatography Analysis*

The phenolic composition of the two extracts was performed using HPLC analysis. Ten compounds were detected in ethyl acetate extract including Gallic and Chlorogenic acids as major components representing 614.12 and 642.01 mg/kg of plant, respectively. *N*-butanol extract, in turn, contains fourteen compounds, among which Gallic and Chlorogenic acids represent, as well, the major components with 481.94 and 4505.78 mg/kg of plant, respectively. The compounds were identified by comparing their chromatographic characteristics (retention time (t_R), mass spectra) with reference standards (Table 3).

The HPLC revealed the presence Rutin only in Ethyl acetate extract. On the contrary, Resveratrol, Hesperidin, Salicylic acid, 4-hydroxybenzoic acid, and Cinnamic acid were detected only in *n*-Butanol extract.

Table 3. Composition of ethyl acetate and *n*-butanol extracts determined by HPLC-TOF/MS (mg of phenolic compound/kg plant).

Compounds	RT	EtOAc	*n*-Butanol
Gallic acid	2.831	614.12	481.94
Gentisic acid	4.358	33.61	1.25
4-hydroxybenzoic acid	5.531		9.35
chlorogenic acid	5.984	642.01	4505.78
protocatechuic acid	6.959	7.74	3.08
caffeic acid	7.623	67.79	2.51
Vanillic acid	7.796	10.88	4.05
Rutin	9.081	0.03	-
P-coumaric acid	9.917	11.64	10.07
chicoric acid	10.982	1.02	3.22
Ferulic acid	11.082	8.81	6.84
Hesperidin	12.284	-	1.49
Salicylic acid	13.284	--	9.70
Resveratrol	14.682	-	42.31
Cinnamic acid	15.779	--	10.70

3.4. Antioxidant Activity

3.4.1. DPPH Radical Assay

The DPPH assay has been broadly used to estimate the free radical scavenging ability of natural compounds [35].In the presence of an antioxidant, DPPH radical obtains 1 more electron, and the absorbance decreases [36]. The degree of reduction in absorbance measurement is indicative of the radical scavenging strength of the extract. The two extracts of *Euphorbia dendroides* at different concentrations (100–1000 μg/mL) and the standards were tested for the scavenging effect on DPPH radical, and the inhibition percentage was balanced with those of quercetin, gallic acid, and ascorbic acid when used as standards. In this test, the two extracts of *E. dendroides* exhibited dose-dependent activities (Figures 1 and 2).

Gallic acid expressed the best antiradical activity (78.21%) compared to quercetin (39.45%) and ascorbic acid (58.41) at 100 μg/mL (Figure 1).

The Ethyl acetate extract demonstrated a moderate scavenger effect with inhibition rate of 29.49% at 100 μg/mL. In brief, the two extracts showed a lower antiradical activity than those exerted by positive controls (Figure 3).

Numeral reports on flavonoids, triterpenoids, and polyphenols designated that they acquire antioxidant and free radical scavenging activity [37]. Therefore, the presence of flavonoids and phenolics in the two extracts is probably responsible for the scavenging effects observed in this study.

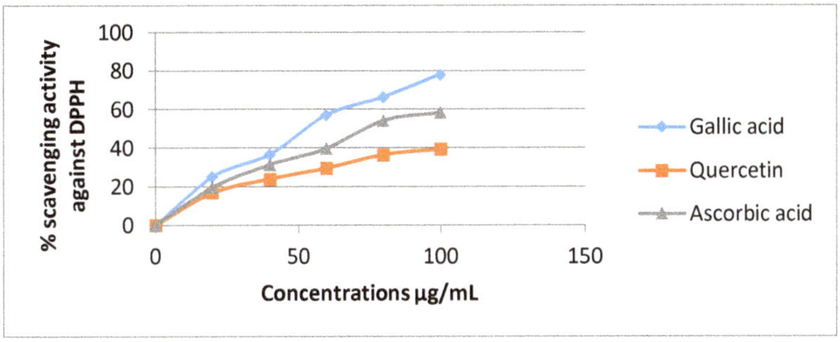

Figure 1. Inhibition of DPPH radical by the standards at different concentrations.

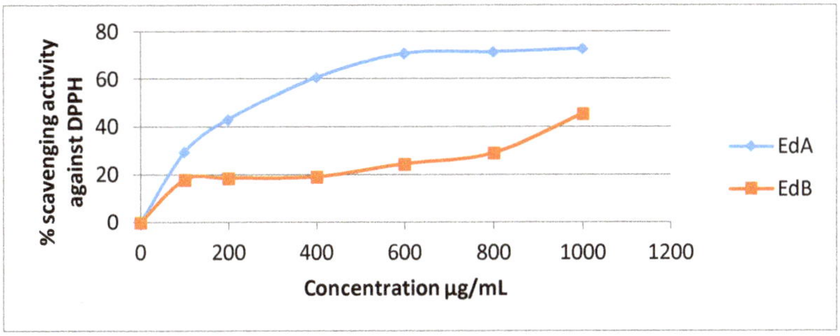

Figure 2. Inhibition of DPPH radical by the two extracts of *E. dendroides* at different concentrations.

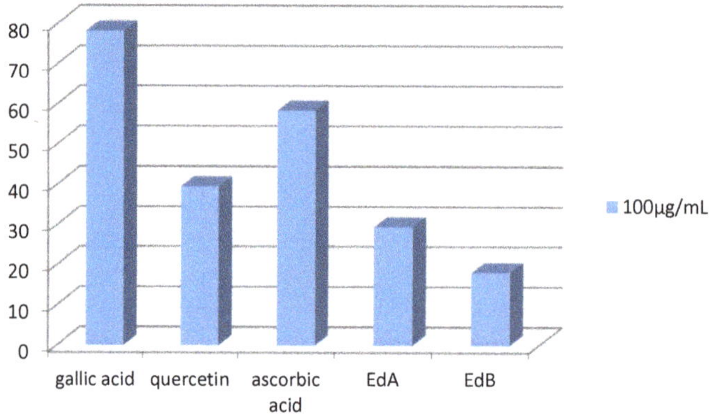

Figure 3. Comparison of DPPH inhibition between standards and both extracts at the same concentrations.

3.4.2. Reducing Power Assay

Antioxidant activity was reported to be the development associated with reducing power [38]. Antioxidants decrease reactive radicals to stable species by producing electrons [21]. The reducing effect is a key parameter for estimation of antioxidant activity. The ferric reducing assay is simple, fast, and responsive for the antioxidant screening.

The antioxidant activity of both extracts was evaluated by reducing power assay, based on the reduction of Fe^{3+}/ferricyanide complex to the ferrous form in presence of antioxidants, over a concentration range of 20–100 µg/mL (Figure 4).A high absorbance value reveals that the sample has a stronger antioxidant activity [39].

The reducing power of the two extracts and standards on Fe^{3+} was found to be concentration-dependent. The two extracts exhibited varying reduction capacities. Ethyl acetate extract showed a higher reduction capacity with a value of 471.82 mg QE/g of extract. Both extracts had lower antioxidant activities than quercetin, gallic acid, and ascorbic acid when used as standards. The order of reducing capacity at 100 µg/mL is as follows: quercetin > ascorbic acid > gallic acid > ethyl acetate extract > *n*-butanol extract.

The antioxidant activities of many plant extracts increase with polyphenols content [39]. The reducing power activity follows the same order of the total flavonoids and total phenolics. The results of the antioxidant capacity of an extract depend greatly on the adopted methodology. Therefore, it is essential to compare diverse analytical methods varying in their oxidation initiators and targets in order to understand the biological activity of an oxidant [40–43].

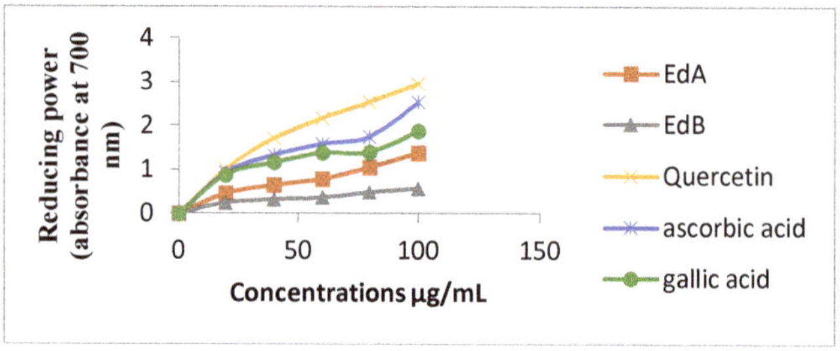

Figure 4. Reducing power of *E. dendroides* extracts and the standards at different concentrations.

3.4.3. The Inhibition of Linoleic Acid Peroxidation

Lipid peroxidation is the oxidative degeneration of polyunsaturated lipids to make radical intermediates that cause oxidative damage. Lipid peroxidation (LP) acts as main agent in carcinogenesis [43]. Many cytolytic compounds such as reactive aldehyde products, including malondialdehyde (MDA), 4-hydroxy-2-nonenal (HNE), 4-hydroxy-2-hexenal (4-HHE), and acrolein are produced as metabolites of lipid peroxidation [44]. MDA has been frequently used as a suitable biomarker for lipid peroxidation. The thiobarbituric method establishes the amount of peroxide in the reaction medium, as peroxide is the major product generated in lipid peroxidation. This assay provides information about the aptitude of phenolics to make complex with Fe^{++} or antagonizes linoleic acid. The inhibition of linoleic acid is found to be dose dependent.

The standard BHT used in this assay exhibited the highest potency against non-enzymatic linoleic acid's peroxidation with inhibition value of 86.65% at 500 μg/mL.

The Ethyl acetate extract illustrates good Lipid peroxidation inhibitory action (73.11% at 500 μg/mL) and *n*-butanol extract has the least potency (37.12% at 500 μg/mL) (Figure 5).

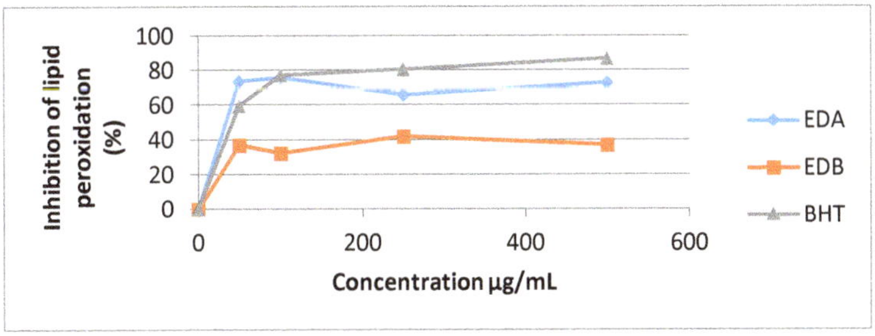

Figure 5. Percentage inhibition of linoleic acid peroxidation of the two *E. dendroides* extracts.

3.5. Antiproliferative Activity

The discovery of new anticancer substances from nature is a current research tendency because of the minor toxicity of natural compounds [45]. Herbal medicine is being increasingly employed in the supervision of many cancer cures [46].

Antiproliferative assays of the two extracts and 5-FU were investigated on C6 cell lines using proliferation BrdU ELISA test and against HeLa cell lines using xCELLigence RTCA instrument at 250 μg/mL, 100 μg/mL, and 50 μg/mL. The antiproliferative effect increased with increasing dose against C6 cells (Figure 6) and Hela cells (Figures 7 and 8). The IC_{50} and IC_{75} values are given in Table 4. The Ethyl acetate extract exhibits higher antiproliferative activities than 5-FU against C6 cells at 250 μg/mL (Figure 6). *N-butanol* extract, in turn, has a remarkable antiproliferative activity compared with the standard at 250 μg/mL.

Some studies on the antiproliferative effect of *E. helioscopia* on five human cancer cell lines (human hepatocellular carcinoma cell lines SMMC-7721, BEL-7402, HepG2, gastric carcinoma cell line SGC-7901, and colorectal cancer cell line SW480) were reported by Wang and revealed that *n*-butanol extract exerted no inhibitory effects on all cells. Nevertheless, ethyl acetate extract was very active at 200 μg/mL on SMMC-7721 cells for 72 h by exerting an inhibition rate of 80.91% on cell growth [36].

Table 4. IC_{50} and IC_{75} values of the extracts against C6 cell.

Inhibition Concentration	Ethyl Acetate	*N*-Butanol
IC_{50} (μg/mL)	119.49	151.18
IC_{75} (μg/mL)	185.74	200.62

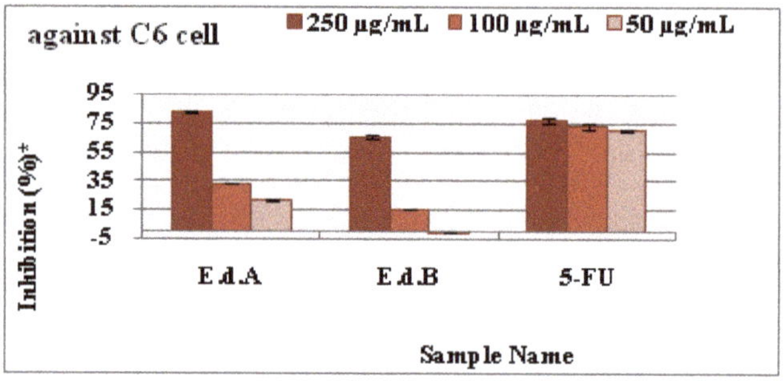

Figure 6. The antiproliferative activities of the two extracts against C6 cells. Each substance was tested twice in triplicates against cell lines. Data show average of two individual experiments ($p < 0.01$).

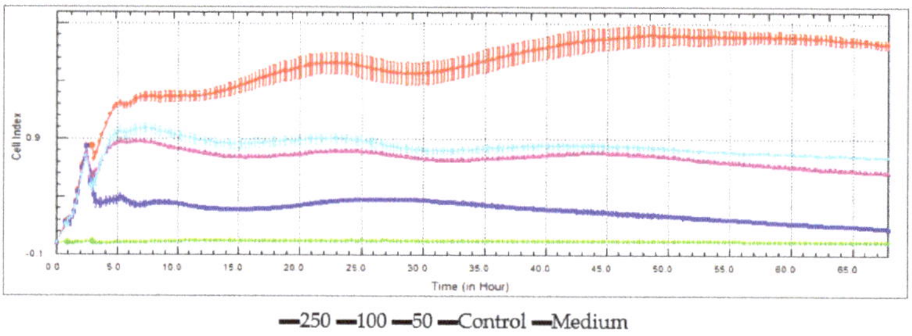

Figure 7. Antiproliferative activity against the Hela cell lines of ethyl acetate extract.

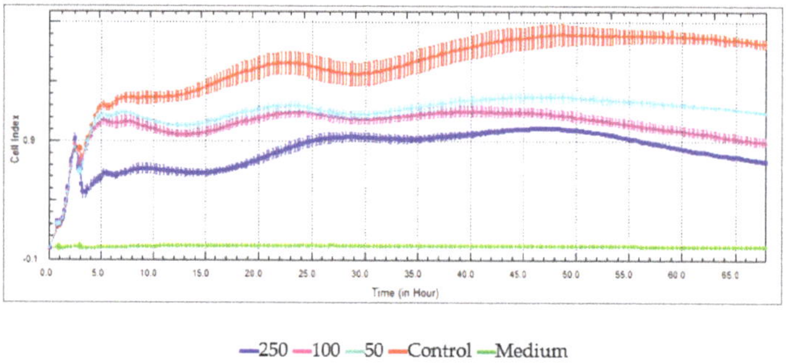

Figure 8. Antiproliferative activity against the Hela cell lines of *n*-butanol extract.

4. Conclusions

In light of the results obtained, it is concluded that the two extracts of *E. dendroides* display important antiradical, reducing capacity, and lipid peroxidation inhibition activities. Antiproliferative activity carried out against two cancer lines revealed that the ethyl acetate extract is more potent than the *n*-butanol extract. Based on the HPLC results, the two extracts were found to contain many important phenolic compounds that contribute to enhancing the studied activities. More studies are required to perform in vivo assays.

Acknowledgments: The authors gratefully acknowledge the Ministry of Higher Education and Scientific Research, Algeria, for financial support.

Author Contributions: Agena Ghout, and Noureddine Gherraf conceived and designed the experiments; Ibrahim Demirtas and Yaglioglu Ayse Sahin contributed to the data handling; Amar Zellagui, Meriem Boukhenaf and Mesbah Lahouel contributed to the antiproliferative and antioxidant activities; Gema Nieto and Salah Akkal contributed for the writing of the paper.

Conflicts of Interest: The authors declare no conflict of interest.

References

1. Lobo, V.; Patil, A.; Phatak, A.; Chandra, N. Free radicals, antioxidants and functional foods: Impact on human health. *Pharmacogn. Rev.* **2010**, *4*, 118–126. [CrossRef] [PubMed]
2. Pham-Huy, L.A.; He, H.; Pham-Huy, C. Free Radicals, Antioxidants in Disease and Health. *Int. J. Biomed. Sci.* **2008**, *4*, 89–96. [PubMed]
3. Rahman, K. Studies on free radicals, antioxidants, and co-factors. *Clin. Interv. Aging* **2007**, *2*, 219–236. [PubMed]
4. Kumar, S. The importance of antioxidant and their role in pharmaceutical science—A review. *Asian J. Res. Chem. Pharm. Sci.* **2014**, *1*, 27–44.
5. Carocho, M.; Barreiro, M.F.K.; Morales, P.; Ferreira Isabel, C.F.R. Adding Molecules to Food, Pros and Cons: A Review on Synthetic and Natural Food Additives. *Compr. Rev. Food Sci. Food Saf.* **2014**, *13*, 377–399. [CrossRef]
6. Ksouri, R.; Ksouri, W.M.; Jallali, I.; Debez, A.; Magné, C.; Hiroko, I. Medicinal halophytes: Potent source of health promoting biomolecules with medical, nutraceutical and food applications. *Crit. Rev. Biotechnol.* **2012**, *32*, 289–326. [CrossRef] [PubMed]
7. Martin-Bettolo, G.B. Present aspects of the use of medicinal plants in traditional medicine. *J. Ethnopharmacol.* **1980**, *2*, 5–7. [CrossRef]
8. Othman, A.; Ismail, A.; Ghani, N.A.; Adenan, I. Antioxidant capacity and phenolic content of cocoa beans. *Food Chem.* **2007**, *100*, 1523–1530. [CrossRef]
9. Gómez, C.; Espadaler, X. Curva de dispersión de semillasporhormigas en *Euphorbiacharacias* L. y Euphorbianicaeensis All. (Euphorbiaceae). *Ecol. Mediterr.* **1994**, *20*, 51–59.
10. Rechinger, K.H.; Schiman-Czeika, H. Euphorbiaceae. In *Flora Iranica*; AkademischeDruck- und Verlagsanstalt: Graz, Austria, 1964; Volume 6, pp. 1–48. ISBN 978-3-201-00728-3.
11. Appendino, G.; Szallasi, A. Euphorbium: Modern research on its active principle, resiniferatoxin, revives an ancient medicine. *Life Sci. J.* **1997**, *60*, 681–696. [CrossRef]
12. Singla, A.K.; Pathak, K. Phytoconstituents of *Euphorbia* species. *Fitoterapia* **1990**, *61*, 483–516.
13. Bani, S.; Kaul, A.; Jaggi, B.S.; Suri, K.A.; Suri, O.P.; Sharma, O.P. Anti-inflammatory activity of the hydrosoluble fraction of *Euphorbia royleana* latex. *Fitoterapia* **2000**, *71*, 655–662. [CrossRef]
14. Tona, L.; Kambu, K.; Ngimbi, N.; Meisa, K.; Penge, O.; Lusakibanza, M.; Cimanga, K.; de Bruyne, T.; Apers, S.; Totté, J.; et al. Antiamoebic and spasmolytic activities of extracts from some amtidiarrhoeal traditional preparations used in Kinshasa, Congo. *Phytomedicine* **2000**, *7*, 31–38. [CrossRef]
15. Semple, S.J.; Reynolds, G.D.; O'Leary, M.C.; Flower, R.L. Screening of Australian medicinal plants for antiviral activity. *J. Ethnopharmacol.* **1998**, *60*, 163–172. [CrossRef]
16. Shimura, H.; Watanabe, N.; Tamai, M.; Hanada, K.; Takahashi, A.; Tanaka, Y.; Arai, K.; Zhang, P.L.; Chang, R. Hepatoprotective compounds from *Canarium album* and *Euphorbia nematocypha*. *Chem. Pharm. Bull. (Tokyo)* **1990**, *38*, 2201–2203.
17. Ernst, M.; Grace, O.M.; Saslis-Lagoudakis, C.H.; Nilsson, N.; Simonsen, H.T.; Rønsted, N. Global medicinal uses of *Euphorbia* L. (Euphorbiaceae). *J. Ethnopharmacol.* **2015**, *176*, 90–101. [CrossRef] [PubMed]
18. Özbilgin, S.; Citoğlu, G.S.T. Uses of Some *Euphorbia* Species in Traditional Medicine in Turkey and Their Biological Activities. *Turk. J. Pharm. Sci.* **2012**, *9*, 241–256.
19. Brussell, D.E. Medicinal plants of Mt. Pelion, Greece. *Econ. Bot. Spec. Sect. Med. Plants* **2004**, *58*, S174–S202. [CrossRef]
20. Esposito, M.; Nothias, L.F.; Nedev, H.; Gallard, J.F.; Leyssen, P.; Retailleau, P.; Costa, J.; Roussi, F.; Iorga, B.I.; Paolini, J.; et al. *Euphorbia dendroides* Latex as a Source of Jatrophane Esters: Isolation, Structural Analysis, Conformational Study, and Anti-CHIKV Activity. *J. Nat. Prod.* **2016**, *79*, 2873–2882. [CrossRef] [PubMed]

21. Wang, L.; Weller, C.L. Recent Advances in Extraction of Nutraceuticals from Plants. *Trends Food Sci. Technol.* **2006**, *17*, 300–312. [CrossRef]
22. Singleton, V.L.; Rossi, J.A. Colorimetry of total phenolics with phosphomolybdic-phosphotungstic acid reagents. *Am. J. Enol. Vitic.* **1965**, *16*, 144–158.
23. Aruoma, O.I. Free radicals, oxidative stress and antioxidants in human health and disease. *J. Am. Oil Chem. Soc.* **1989**, *75*, 199–212. [CrossRef]
24. Masuda, T.; Yonemory, S.; Ouyama, Y.; Takeda, Y.; Tanaka, T.; Andoh, T. Evaluation of the antioxidant activity of environmental plants: Activity of the leaf extracts from seashore plants. *J. Agric. Food Chem.* **1999**, *47*, 1749–1754. [CrossRef] [PubMed]
25. Zou, Y.P.; Lu, Y.H.; Wei, D.Z. Antioxidant activity of a flavonoid-rich extract of *Hypericum perforatum* L. in vitro. *J. Agric. Food Chem.* **2004**, *52*, 5032–5039. [CrossRef] [PubMed]
26. Oyaizu, M. Studies on products of the browning reaction prepared from glucose amine. *Jpn. J. Nutr.* **1986**, *44*, 307–315. [CrossRef]
27. Choi, C.W.; Kim, S.C.; Hwang, S.S.; Choi, B.K.; Ahn, H.J.; Lee, M.Y.; Park, S.H.; Kim, S.K. Antioxidant activity and free radical scavenging capacity between Korean medicinal plants and flavonoids by assay-guided comparison. *Plant Sci.* **2002**, *163*, 1161–1168. [CrossRef]
28. Yaglioglu, A.S.; Demirtas, I.; Goren, N. Bioactivity-guided isolation of antiproliferative compounds from *Centaurea carduiformis* DC. *Phytochem. Lett.* **2014**, *8*, 213–219. [CrossRef]
29. Demirtas, I.; Yaglioglu, A.S. Bioactive Volatile Content of the Stem and Root of *Centaurea carduiformis* DC. subsp. *carduiformis* var. *carduiformis*. *J. Chem.* **2012**, *2013*. [CrossRef]
30. Koldaş, S.; Demirtas, I.; Ozen, T.; Demirci, M.A.; Behçet, L. Phytochemical screening, anticancer and antioxidant activities of *Origanum vulgare* L. ssp. viride (Boiss.) Hayek, a plant of traditional usage. *J. Sci. Food Agric.* **2015**, *95*, 786–1482. [CrossRef] [PubMed]
31. Maisuthisakul, P.; Suttajit, M.; Pongsawatmanit, R. Assessment of phenolic content and free radical-scavenging capacity of some Thai indigenous plants. *Food Chem.* **2007**, *4*, 1409–1418. [CrossRef]
32. Prior, R.L.; Cao, G.H. In vivo total antioxidant capacity: Comparison of different analytical methods. *Free Radic. Biol. Med.* **1999**, *27*, 1173–1181. [CrossRef]
33. Xu, B.J.; Chang, S.K. A comparative study on phenolic profiles and antioxidant activities of legumes as affected by extraction solvents. *J. Food Sci.* **2007**, *72*, S159–S166. [CrossRef] [PubMed]
34. Hodgson, J.M.; Croft, K.D. Tea flavonoids and cardiovascular health. *Mol. Asp. Med.* **2010**, *31*, 495–502. [CrossRef] [PubMed]
35. Kanatt, S.R.; Chander, R.; Radhakrishna, P.; Sharma, A. Potato peel extract—A natural antioxidant for retarding lipid peroxidation in radiation processed lamb meat. *J. Agric. Food Chem.* **2005**, *53*, 1499–1504. [CrossRef] [PubMed]
36. Wang, Z.Y.; Liu, H.P.; Zhang, Y.C.; Guo, L.Q.; Li, Z.X.; Shi, X.F. Anticancer potential of *Euphorbia helioscopia* L extracts against human cancer cells. *Anat. Rec. (Hoboken)* **2012**, *295*, 223–233. [CrossRef] [PubMed]
37. Frankel, E. Nutritional benefits of flavonoids. In Proceedings of the International Conference on Food Factors: Chemistry and Cancer Prevention, Hamamatsu, Japan, 10–15 December 1995.
38. Yildrim, A.; Mavi, A.; Oktay, M.; Kara, A.A.; Algur, F.; Bilaloglu, V. Comparison of antioxidant and antimicrobial activities of tilia (TiliaargenteaDesf ex DC), sage (*Salvia triloba* L.), and black tea (*Camellia sinensis*) extracts. *J. Agric. Food Chem.* **2000**, *48*, 5030. [CrossRef]
39. Aktumsek, A.; Zengin, G.; Guler, G.O.; Cakmak, Y.S.; Duran, A. Antioxidant potentials and anticholinesterase activities of methanolic and aqueous extracts of three endemic *Centaurea* L. species. *Food Chem. Toxicol.* **2013**, *55*, 290–296. [CrossRef] [PubMed]
40. Sarikurkcu, C.; Tepe, B.; Semiz, D.K.; Solak, M.H. Evaluation of metal concentration and antioxidant activity of three edible mushrooms from Mugla, Turkey. *Food Chem. Toxicol.* **2010**, *48*, 1230–1233. [CrossRef] [PubMed]
41. Katsube, T.; Tabata, H.; Ohta, Y.; Yamasaki, Y.; Anuurad, E.; Shiwaku, K.; Yamane, Y. Screening for antioxidant activity in edible plant products: Comparison of low-density lipoprotein oxidation assay, DPPH radical scavenging assay, and Folin-Ciocalteu assay. *J. Agric. Food Chem.* **2004**, *52*, 2391–2396. [CrossRef] [PubMed]
42. Cao, G.H.; Prior, R.L. Comparison of different analytical methods for assessing total antioxidant capacity of human serum. *Clin. Chem.* **1998**, *44*, 1309–1315. [PubMed]

43. Banakar, M.C.; Paramasivan, S.K.; Chattopadhyay, M.B.; Datta, S.; Chakraborty, P.; Chatterjee, M.; Kannan, K.; Thygarajan, E. 1-alpha, 25-dihydroxyvitamin D3 prevents DNA damage and restores antioxidant enzymes in rat hepatocarcinogenesis induced by diethylnitrosamine and promoted by phenobarbital. *World J. Gastroenterol.* **2004**, *10*, 1268–1275. [CrossRef] [PubMed]
44. Esterbauer, H.; Chaur, R.J.; Zollner, H. Chemistry and biochemistry of 4-hydroxynonenal, malonaldehyde and related aldehydes. *Free Radic. Biol. Med.* **1991**, *11*, 81–128. [CrossRef]
45. Miyoshi, N.; Nakamura, Y.; Ueda, Y.; Abe, M.; Ozawa, Y.; Uchida, K.; Osawa, T. Dietary ginger constituents, galanals A and B, are potent apoptosis inducers in Human T lymphoma Jurkat cells. *Cancer Lett.* **2003**, *199*, 113–119. [CrossRef]
46. Wang, J.L.; Liu, K.; Gong, W.Z.; Wang, Q.; Xu, D.T.; Liu, M.F.; Bi, K.L.; Song, Y.F. Anticancer, antioxidant, and antimicrobial activities of anemone (*Anemone cathayensis*). *Food Sci. Biotechnol.* **2012**, *21*, 551–557. [CrossRef]

medicines MDPI

Article

Antioxidant Potential of Extracts Obtained from Macro- (*Ascophyllum nodosum*, *Fucus vesiculosus* and *Bifurcaria bifurcata*) and Micro-Algae (*Chlorella vulgaris* and *Spirulina platensis*) Assisted by Ultrasound

Rubén Agregán [1], Paulo E. S. Munekata [2], Daniel Franco [1], Javier Carballo [3], Francisco J. Barba [4] and José M. Lorenzo [1,*]

[1] Centro Tecnológico de la Carne de Galicia, Adva. Galicia No. 4, Parque Tecnológico de Galicia, San Cibrao das Viñas, 32900 Ourense, Spain; rubenagregan@ceteca.net (R.A.); danielfranco@ceteca.net (D.F.)

[2] Department of Food Engineering, Faculty of Animal Science and Food Engineering, University of São Paulo, 225 Duque de Caxias Norte Ave, Jardim Elite, Pirassununga 13635-900, São Paulo, Brazil; pmunekata@gmail.com

[3] Area de Tecnologia de los Alimentos, Facultad de Ciencias de Ourense, Universidad de Vigo, 32004 Ourense, Spain; carbatec@uvigo.es

[4] Nutrition and Food Science Area, Preventive Medicine and Public Health, Food Science, Toxicology and Forensic Medicine Department, Universitat de València, Avda. Vicent Andrés Estellés, s/n, Burjassot, 46100 València, Spain; francisco.barba@uv.es

* Correspondence: jmlorenzo@ceteca.net; Tel.: +34-988-548-277

Received: 15 March 2018; Accepted: 9 April 2018; Published: 10 April 2018

Abstract: Background: Natural antioxidants, which can replace synthetic ones due to their potential implications for health problems in children, have gained significant popularity. Therefore, the antioxidant potential of extracts obtained from three brown macroalgae (*Ascophyllum nodosum*, *Fucus vesiculosus* and *Bifurcaria bifurcata*) and two microalgae (*Chlorella vulgaris* and *Spirulina platensis*) using ultrasound-extraction as an innovative and green approach was evaluated. **Methods:** Algal extracts were obtained by ultrasound-assisted extraction using water/ethanol (50:50, *v:v*) as the extraction solvent. The different extracts were compared based on their antioxidant potential, measuring the extraction yield, the total phenolic content (TPC) and the antioxidant activity. **Results:** Extracts from *Ascophyllum nodosum* (AN) and *Bifurcaria bifurcata* (BB) showed the highest antioxidant potential compared to the rest of the samples. In particular, BB extract presented the highest extraction (35.85 g extract/100 g dry weight (DW)) and total phenolic compounds (TPC) (5.74 g phloroglucinol equivalents (PGE)/100 g DW) yields. Regarding the antioxidant activity, macroalgae showed again higher values than microalgae. BB extract had the highest antioxidant activity in the ORAC, DPPH and FRAP assays, with 556.20, 144.65 and 66.50 μmol Trolox equivalents (TE)/g DW, respectively. In addition, a correlation among the antioxidant activity and the TPC was noted. **Conclusions:** Within the obtained extracts, macroalgae, and in particular BB, are more suitable to be used as sources of phenolic antioxidants to be included in products for human consumption. The relatively low antioxidant potential, in terms of polyphenols, of the microalgae extracts studied in the present work makes them useless for possible industrial applications compared to macroalgae, although further in vivo studies evaluating the real impact of antioxidants from both macro- and micro-algae at the cellular level should be conducted.

Keywords: macroalgae; microalgae; extraction yield; total phenolic content; antioxidant activity

1. Introduction

Free radicals may produce damage to lipids, proteins, cell membranes and nucleic acids, thus promoting the development of noncommunicable diseases [1]. Therefore, an increased interest in natural antioxidants to fight against free radicals has been shown. Consumers are particularly interested in natural antioxidants rather than synthetics [2] due to the problems of toxicity and carcinogenic effects that these may cause [3,4].

Brown seaweed species are rich in antioxidant polyphenols (from 1–14% dry solid), *Ascophyllum* and *Fucus* being two genera with the highest content [5]. Polyphenols are reported to possess benefits for heath, such as anticancer, antimicrobial, anti-inflammatory and antidiabetic activities [6]. Brown algae are rich in phlorotannins [5], polyphenols with multiple phenolic groups, which provide good antioxidant activities [7]. These compounds are exclusively from brown algae species [8,9].

In the same way as macroalgae, microalgae could represent an important source of antioxidant compounds [10,11]. They are a rich source of natural pigments with antioxidant properties, such as chlorophylls and carotenoids, thus giving an added value from a commercial point of view [12]. Moreover, their biodiversity, ease of cultivation and modulation of growth conditions has resulted in microalgae becoming among the most important resources in nature having antioxidant properties [13].

Conventional extraction has been traditionally used to recover antioxidants from algae. However, this presents some important drawbacks such long extraction time, high cost and degradation of product quality. In addition, the use of organic solvents as extractive compounds should be minimized since they may be harmful from a health and environmental point of view [14,15]. For this reason, non-conventional extraction methods were employed to recover bioactives in food and pharmaceutical applications, providing satisfactory results, such as reducing process time and cost and increasing yield [16,17]. Ultrasound-assisted extraction (UAE) is an innovative extraction approach, which is based on sound wave migration, thus promoting cavitation phenomena and leading to a disruption of cell walls and the subsequent release of intracellular compounds [18]. This extraction method offers many advantages, such as a better solvent penetration into cellular material, higher product yields and reproducibility, lower solvent consumption and higher processing throughput compared to the conventional extraction methods [19]. Actually, UAE is very often used in the extraction of natural antioxidant compounds [20]. It has been employed in the extraction of antioxidant compounds from seaweeds with satisfactory results [21–23]. Therefore, the aim of this work was to evaluate the potential use of *Ascophyllum nodosum* (AN), *Fucus vesiculosus* (FV) and *Bifurcaria bifurcata* (BB) macroalgae extracts and *Chlorella vulgaris* (CV) and *Spirulina platensis* (SP) microalgae extracts as antioxidants for the possible application in products intended to be used for human consumption. For this purpose, UAE will be used as the extraction technology to recover the antioxidant bioactive compounds.

2. Materials and Methods

2.1. Algal Material

Brown macroalgae, *Ascophyllum nodosum* (AN), *Fucus vesiculosus* (FV) and *Bifurcaria bifurcata* (BB) (Chromista, Ochrophyta, Phaeophyceae, Fucales), were purchased to Portomuiños company (A Coruña, Spain). The collection was carried out in the Atlantic Ocean near the Camariñas area (A Coruña, Spain). Microalgae, *Chlorella vulgaris* (CV) (Plantae, Chlorophyta, Trebouxiophyceae, Chlorellales) and *Spirulina platensis* (SP) (Eubacteria, Cyanobacteria, Cyanophyceae, Spirulinales) were provided by AlgaEnergy (Madrid, Spain). Macroalgae samples were ground obtaining particles lower than 0.8 mm, by a conventional mincer. Then, algae were stored under vacuum (75%) at −20 °C until further use.

2.2. Obtaining Extracts from Macroalgae and Microalgae by UAE Method

Each of the algae (5 g) was extracted using a mixture consisting of water/ethanol (50:50, *v:v*) (50 mL) in glass bottles. The extraction was performed in an ultrasonic bath (Branson ultrasonic

M3800-E, Dietzenbach, Germany) at room temperature for 30 min. After extraction, the solvent was separated from the alga by centrifuging at 3000× *g* for 10 min at 4 °C and filtering with filter paper using a vacuum to remove the algal material. The supernatant was stored at −20 °C until analysis. Extraction yield, total phenolic content (TPC) and antioxidant activity (ORAC, ABTS, DPPH and FRAP assays) were evaluated for the obtained extracts, as described below. All experiments were performed in duplicate.

2.3. *Measurement of the Extraction Yield*

Five milliliters of each extract were taken and evaporated in a drying oven at 100 °C overnight. The weight of the final residue was used to calculate the extraction yield by gravimetry. Results were expressed as g extract/100 g dry weight of algae (DW). The DW of each alga was calculated subtracting its moisture content to total weight of the algae. Moisture content was measured according to the method previously reported in the ISO recommendation [24].

2.4. *Determination of the Total Phenolic Compounds*

TPC determination was based on a method described by Medina-Remón et al. [25]. Fifteen microliters of sample were mixed with 170 μL of Milli-Q water, adding later 12 μL of Folin-Ciocalteu reagent and 30 μL of sodium carbonate. The mixtures were incubated for 1 h at room temperature under darkness. Once the reaction was over, 73 μL of Milli-Q water were added with a multichannel pipette. The absorbance measurement was performed at 765 nm. TPC was expressed as g of phloroglucinol equivalents (PGE)/100 g extract and as g PGE/100 g DW.

2.5. *Determination of the Antioxidant Activity*

2.5.1. Oxygen Radical Absorbance Capacity Assay

The original method of Ou et al. [26] modified by Dávalos et al. [27] was used. The reaction was carried out in 75 mM phosphate buffer (pH 7.4), 200 μL being the final reaction mixture. The mixture with antioxidant (20 μL) and fluorescein (120 mL; 70 nM final concentration) was pre-incubated for 15 min at 37 °C. AAPH (2,20-azobis (2-methylpropionamidine) dihydrochloride) solution (60 mL; 12 mM, final concentration) was added rapidly using a multichannel pipette. The plate was immediately placed in the reader, and the fluorescence was recorded every minute for 120 min (excitation wavelength 485 nm, emission wavelength 520 nm). Samples were stirred prior to each reading. Eight calibration solutions using Trolox as the antioxidant were used in each assay, and phosphate buffer was used as blank. Results were calculated on the basis of the differences in areas under the fluorescein decay curve between the blank and the sample and were expressed as μmol Trolox equivalents (TE)/g DW.

2.5.2. ABTS Radical Cation Decolorization Assay

The method of Re et al. [28] was adapted to the use of a plate reader. $ABTS^{\bullet+}$ was produced by mixing 7 mM ABTS stock solution with 2.45 mM potassium persulfate (final concentration) leaving the mixture in the dark at room temperature for 12–16 h before use. In the following step, $ABTS^{\bullet+}$ solution was diluted with PBS (pH 7.4) to get an absorbance of 0.70 at 734 nm, being equilibrated at 30 °C. The working solution of $ABTS^{\bullet+}$ (sample: ABTS solution relation, 1:100) was added to an aliquot of each sample (with appropriate dilution). The decrease in absorbance was measured after 6 min at 734 nm in a microplate spectrophotometer reader. Trolox was used as the reference standard, and the results were expressed as μmol TE/g DW.

2.5.3. DPPH Radical Scavenging Assay

The $DPPH^{\bullet}$ scavenging method was performed with some modifications according to the procedure previously described by Brand-Williams et al. [29]. Five microliters of samples (previously diluted) were added to 195 μL of DPPH solution (6×10^{-5} M in methanol) in 96-well plates. The mixture was lightly shaken and left at room temperature for 30 min. Then, the absorbance at 515 nm was measured against methanol using a microplate reader. The DPPH$^{\bullet}$ scavenging activity of extracts was determined using the standard curve of Trolox and expressed as μmol TE/g DW.

2.5.4. Ferric Reducing Antioxidant Power

Ferric reducing antioxidant power was determined using the method described by Benzie and Strain [30]. The FRAP reagent was freshly prepared from 300 mM acetate buffer, pH 3.6, 10 mM 2,4,6-tripyridyl-s-triazine (TPTZ) made up in 40 mM HCl and 20 mM $FeCl_3 \cdot 6H_2O$ solution. The three solutions were mixed together in the ratio of 10:1:1 (*v:v:v*). Three-hundred microliters of freshly-prepared FRAP reagent were mixed with 10 μL of properly diluted samples and 30 μL of distilled water in 96-well plates. The mixture was heated at 37 °C and left at this temperature during the reaction. After 8 min, the absorbance was measured using a microplate reader at 593 nm against reagent blank. The FRAP value was calculated and expressed as μmol TE/g DW based on a calibration curve plotted using Trolox as the standard.

3. Results and Discussion

3.1. Extraction Yield

Extraction yields from different algae are presented in Table 1. AN and BB macroalgae showed higher extraction yields compared to FV and microalgae species. Specifically, BB achieved the highest value (35.85 and 35.85 g extract/100 g DW). CV and SP microalgae presented lower extraction yields than macroalgae, SP being the one that had the lowest value (4.56 and 4.24 g extract/100 g DW). Farvin and Jacbsen [31] also found a lower extraction yield for FV compared to most of the algae used in their study when using water as the solvent. They attributed this fact to the important viscosity found in these extracts, which made the filtering process through filter paper difficult. On the other hand, other authors also reported significant differences in extraction yield among several seaweed species using different extraction solvents, such as water, ethanol or diethyl ether [31,32]. Matanjun et al. [32] found a positive correlation among yield and solvent polarity when extracting antioxidant bioactive compounds from eight seaweed species from north Borneo. At the same time, they found differences between algae using the solvents separately. According to them, the variation in the yields from several extracts may be due to the different polarities of the compounds found in plants [31]. Other factors that can explain the modifications in extraction yields are (i) the chemical composition of the raw material and (ii) the polarity of the solvents used [33]. For instance, different solvents, such as ethanol, water or aqueous solutions of organic solvents, were tested to obtain the optimal solvent for improving extraction yields, obtaining the best results when ethanol was used [31,34]. Thus, taking into account the extraction solvent used (ethanol:water 50:50, *v:v*), it could be said that BB and AN macroalgae are richer in polar compounds than FV and both microalgae species. The observed lower content of polar compounds found in CV and SP and their extracts may be related to the amount of carotenoids present in microalgae. Microalgae are a good source of carotenoids [35,36]. For instance, *Chlorella vulgaris* is reported to contain high amounts of carotenoids, such as lutein and β-carotene [37,38]. As is well known, carotenoids are lipophilic compounds [39], making their extraction difficult with polar solvents, such as ethanol, water or mixtures of both, as in our study. Therefore, the extraction yields from CV and SP microalgae were probably affected by the use of water/ethanol (50:50, *v:v*) as the extraction solvent.

Table 1. Extraction yields, TPCs and antioxidant activities from AN, FV, BB, CV and SP algae extracts obtained by the UAE method using water/ethanol (50:50, *v:v*) as the extraction solvent.

Algae	Extraction Yield		TPC				Antioxidant Activities							
							ORAC		ABTS		DPPH		FRAP	
	g/100 g DW		g PGE/100 g Extract		g PGE/100 g DW		µmol TE/g DW							
AN	25.86	25.86	18	18	4.66	4.66	297.19	300.29	565.66	542.38	50.69	50.69	4.66	4.40
FV	9.58	9.80	20	20	1.92	1.96	155.41	154.26	200.60	208.46	26.72	27.15	3.45	3.82
BB	35.85	35.85	16	16	5.74	5.74	537.38	575.02	537.74	549.21	143.04	146.27	67.40	65.60
CV	7.78	7.14	4.5	4.7	0.35	0.34	33.07	29.35	15.64	14.64	0.86	0.79	0.62	0.62
SP	4.56	4.24	4.3	4.6	0.20	0.19	12.30	12.12	6.74	6.53	1.00	0.89	1.00	1.02

Algae: AN, *Ascophyllum nodosum*; FV, *Fucus vesiculosus*; BB, *Bifurcaria bifurcata*; CV, *Chlorella vulgaris*; SP, *Spirulina platensis*. UAE, ultrasound–assisted extraction. TPC, total phenolic content. DW, dry weight of alga. PGE, phloroglucinol equivalents. TE, Trolox equivalents.

3.2. Total Phenolic Content

TPCs from the different algal extracts are presented in Table 1. As can be seen in the table, AN and BB macroalgae showed higher TPC contents compared to FV and both microalgae. BB presented the highest content (5.74 and 5.74 g PGE/100 g DW). It should be noted that microalgae presented lower TPCs than macroalgae, SP being the one that reached the lowest content (0.20 and 0.19 g PGE/100 g DW). The differences ($p < 0.05$) observed between TPC in macro- and micro-algae could be due to the high content of our three macroalgae in phlorotannins. As already mentioned above, brown algae genera are rich in these compounds [6], composed of units of phloroglucinol joined to form polymers [31]. In addition, phlorotannins are bi-polar in nature [40]; therefore, they are soluble in polar solvents such as in the aqueous solution at 50% ethanol used in this study, ensuring their presence in the extract and strengthening our hypothesis. These compounds could help algae in their struggle against oxidative stress, as well as participate in the defense against grazers such as marine herbivores thanks to their plasticity [41].

Chew et al. [42] found a much higher TPC content in the *Padina antillarum* brown alga than in the *Caulerpa racemosa* green alga and in the *Kappaphycus alvarezii* red alga. They also attributed this fact to the phlorotannin presence in the brown algae. On the other hand, we did not only find that macroalgae had different TPCs ($p < 0.05$) than microalgae, but that all algae studied showed different total content ($p < 0.05$) in phenolic compounds. Connan et al. [43] reported that external-environmental factors, such as light, depth or salinity, and intrinsic factors, such as age or length, may affect the phenolic metabolic expressions of algae, generating great differences in the phenolic content [43,44].

Observing the extraction yield data, a correlation between extraction yields and TPC was noted, since the highest extraction yield values corresponded to the highest TPC values, the order being increased in the following way: BB > AN > FV > CV > SP. This correlation is related to the percentage of TPC in the extracts. Moreover, this percentage, as can be expected, was very similar for both macroalgae (16–20 g PGE/100 g extract) and for microalgae (4.3–4.7 g PGE/100 g extract).

The differences observed for TPC in the different algae samples could be attributed to different factors, such as the period of the year or area in which they are collected. Hold and Kraan [6] reported that polyphenol content showed a correlation with the reproductive state of algae along time. Polyphenol content in *Ascophyllum nodosum* is minimum during May, the month with maximal fruit body shedding, and maximum in winter. However, March is the month in which the minimum of TPC was observed for *Fucus vesiculosus*, just before the period of maximum fertility [45]. On the other hand, *Porphyra umbilicalis* alga was affected by sun exposure and emersion. The authors noted that seaweeds exposed to air and water during the summer contained higher amounts of antioxidants than submerged seaweeds, submersion being a natural barrier for seaweeds against environmental stresses [46].

3.3. *Antioxidant Activity*

Antioxidant activities of the different algae extracts are presented in Table 1. Macroalgae showed higher antioxidant activities than microalgae for all the assays. As discussed above, brown algae are rich in phlorotannins showing high antioxidant activities. Ahn et al. [47] reported an interesting antioxidant capacity from three phlorotannins extracted from *Ecklonia cava* brown alga. Within macroalgae, BB had the highest values (537.38 and 575.02, 143.04 and 146.27, 67.40 and 65.60 μmol TE/g DW in the ORAC, DPPH and FRAP assays, respectively) and FV the lowest. This indicates that the BB algae are richer in compounds capable of scavenging free radicals. As expected, a positive correlation between TPC and antioxidant activity was noted. Thus, BB, which showed the highest TPC, also presented the highest antioxidant activity in almost all assays, followed by FV, AN and microalgae. The same correlation was reported by other authors after using the DPPH radical scavenging assay [42]. They found that when TPC content was higher, the IC_{50} decreased. According to these authors, the polyphenols present in seaweeds have the ability to scavenge free radicals. By using the DPPH assay, it was also found that seaweed extracts containing high levels of phenolic compounds also displayed potent antioxidant activities [31]. This correlation may mean that polyphenols are the compounds that contribute most to the antioxidant activity of our extracts. Other authors also came to the same conclusion with their extracts [31,42]. Focusing on microalgae, there are studies in which the results obtained were contradictory. On the one hand, it was found that the antioxidant capacity of microalgae is partly caused by polyphenols [48]. However, other authors did not find any correlation between the phenolic content and the antioxidant capacity of ethanolic extracts resulting from nine microalgae strains [49].

The determination of phenolic compounds as individual molecules in the extracts is, therefore, of great importance for radical scavenging activity [31]. This activity is also dependent on the structure of the compounds, as well as the amount and location of the hydroxyl groups in them [29]. For example, some studies found that caffeic acid, which has two hydroxyl groups, is a compound with greater antiradical activity than coumaric acid, a homolog of caffeic acid, but with only one hydroxyl group [29]. Therefore, the different phenolic combinations of the compounds will have an impact on the antioxidant activity of these [31].

4. Conclusions

Extraction yield, TPC and antioxidant activity from macroalgae extracts obtained by the UAE method using water/ethanol (50:50, *v:v*) as the extraction solvent turned out to be higher than microalgae extracts obtained in the same way, meaning that macro-algae extracts, specially BB extract, are more suitable to be used as possible high-polyphenol antioxidants in products to be used for human consumption. The combined use of the aforementioned extraction method and solvent was inefficient to obtain microalgae extracts with good extraction yields and antioxidant potential. Therefore, these extracts obtained in this way are not interesting for possible industrial applications, presenting drawbacks, such as the cost or the amount that must be added to the product. Taking into account the data obtained, if additional research is carried out, it should be focused on BB algae extract. In addition, it would be interesting to assess the real impact of antioxidants from both macro- and micro-algae at a cellular level in further research.

Acknowledgments: The authors are grateful to the Instituto Nacional de Investigaciones Agrarias y Alimentarias (INIA) for the award of a predoctoral scholarship (CPR2014-0128) to Rubén Agregán.

Author Contributions: Francisco J. Barba conceived of the experiments. Paulo E.S. Munekata designed the experiments. Rubén Agregán performed the experiments, analyzed the data and wrote the paper. Daniel Franco, Javier Carballo and José M. Lorenzo reviewed the paper before submitting.

Conflicts of Interest: The authors declare no conflict of interest.

References

1. Valko, M.; Leibfritz, D.; Moncol, J.; Cronin, M.T.; Mazur, M.; Telser, J. Free radicals and antioxidants in normal physiological functions and human disease. *Int. J. Biochem. Cell Biol.* **2007**, *39*, 44–84. [CrossRef] [PubMed]
2. Kranl, K.; Schlesier, K.; Bitsch, R.; Hermann, H.; Rohe, M.; Böhm, V. Comparing antioxidative food additives and secondary plant products—Use of different assays. *Food Chem.* **2005**, *93*, 171–175. [CrossRef]
3. Ito, N.; Hirose, M.; Fukushima, S.; Tsuda, H.; Shirai, T.; Tatematsu, M. Studies on antioxidants: Their carcinogenic and modifying effects on chemical carcinogenesis. *Food Chem. Toxicol.* **1986**, *24*, 1071–1082. [CrossRef]
4. Safer, A.M.; Al-Nughamish, A.J. Hepatotoxicity induced by the anti-oxidant food additive, butylated hydroxytoluene (BHT), in rats: An electron microscopical study. *Histol. Histopathol.* **1999**, *14*, 391–406. [PubMed]
5. Holdt, S.L.; Kraan, S. Bioactive compounds in seaweed: Functional food applications and legislation. *J. Appl. Phycol.* **2011**, *23*, 543–597. [CrossRef]
6. Fernando, I.S.; Kim, M.; Son, K.T.; Jeong, Y.; Jeon, Y.J. Antioxidant activity of marine algal polyphenolic compounds: A mechanistic approach. *J. Med. Food* **2016**, *19*, 615–628. [CrossRef] [PubMed]
7. Koivikko, R.; Eränen, J.K.; Loponen, J.; Jormalainen, V. Variation of phlorotannins among three populations of *Fucus vesiculosus* as revealed by HPLC and colorimetric quantification. *J. Chem. Ecol.* **2008**, *34*, 57–64. [CrossRef] [PubMed]
8. Li, Y.X.; Wijesekara, I.; Li, Y.; Kim, S.K. Phlorotannins as bioactive agents from brown algae. *Process Biochem.* **2011**, *46*, 2219–2224. [CrossRef]
9. Lopes, G.; Sousa, C.; Silva, L.R.; Pinto, E.; Andrade, P.B.; Bernardo, J.; Mouga, T.; Valentão, P. Can phlorotannins purified extracts constitute a novel pharmacological alternative for microbial infections with associated inflammatory conditions? *PLoS ONE* **2012**, *7*, e31145. [CrossRef] [PubMed]
10. Rodriguez-Garcia, I.; Guil-Guerrero, J.L. Evaluation of the antioxidant activity of three microalgal species for use as dietary supplements and in the preservation of foods. *Food Chem.* **2008**, *108*, 1023–1026. [CrossRef] [PubMed]
11. Srivastava, A.K.; Bhargava, P.; Rai, L.C. Salinity and copper-induced oxidative damage and changes in the antioxidative defence systems of *Anabaena doliolum*. *World J. Microbiol. Biotechnol.* **2005**, *21*, 1291–1298. [CrossRef]
12. Vigani, M.; Parisi, C.; Rodríguez-Cerezo, E.; Barbosa, M.J.; Sijtsma, L.; Ploeg, M.; Enzing, C. Food and feed products from micro-algae: Market opportunities and challenges for the EU. *Trend Food Sci. Technol.* **2015**, *42*, 81–92. [CrossRef]
13. Giorgis, M.; Garella, D.; Cena, C.; Boffa, L.; Cravotto, G.; Marini, E. An evaluation of the antioxidant properties of *Arthrospira maxima* extracts obtained using non-conventional techniques. *Eur. Food Res. Technol.* **2017**, *243*, 227–237. [CrossRef]
14. Azmir, J.; Zaidul, I.S.M.; Rahman, M.M.; Sharif, K.M.; Mohamed, A.; Sahena, F.; Jahurul, M.H.A.; Ghafoor, K.; Norulaini, N.A.N.; Omar, A.K.M. Techniques for extraction of bioactive compounds from plant materials: A review. *J. Food. Eng.* **2013**, *117*, 426–436. [CrossRef]
15. Polshettiwar, V.; Varma, R.S. Aqueous microwave chemistry: A clean and green synthetic tool for rapid drug discovery. *Chem. Soc. Rev.* **2008**, *37*, 1546–1557. [CrossRef] [PubMed]
16. Herrero, M.; Cifuentes, A.; Ibañez, E. Sub-and supercritical fluid extraction of functional ingredients from different natural sources: Plants, food-by-products, algae and microalgae: A review. *Food Chem.* **2006**, *98*, 136–148. [CrossRef]
17. Wang, L.; Weller, C.L. Recent advances in extraction of nutraceuticals from plants. *Trends Food Sci. Technol.* **2006**, *17*, 300–312. [CrossRef]
18. Hahn, T.; Lang, S.; Ulber, R.; Muffler, K. Novel procedures for the extraction of fucoidan from brown algae. *Process Biochem.* **2012**, *47*, 1691–1698. [CrossRef]
19. Roselló-Soto, E.; Galanakis, C.M.; Brnčić, M.; Orlien, V.; Trujillo, F.J.; Mawson, R.; Knoerzer, K.; Tiwari, B.K.; Barba, F.J. Clean recovery of antioxidant compounds from plant foods, by-products and algae assisted by ultrasounds processing. Modeling approaches to optimize processing conditions. *Trends Food Sci. Technol.* **2015**, *42*, 134–149. [CrossRef]

20. Corbin, C.; Fidel, T.; Leclerc, E.A.; Barakzoy, E.; Sagot, N.; Falguiéres, A.; Renouard, S.; Blondeau, J.P.; Ferroud, C.; Doussot, J.; et al. Development and validation of an efficient ultrasound assisted extraction of phenolic compounds from flax (*Linum usitatissimum* L.) seeds. *Ultrason. Sonochem.* **2015**, *26*, 176–185. [CrossRef] [PubMed]
21. Kadam, S.U.; O'Donnell, C.P.; Rai, D.K.; Hossain, M.B.; Burgess, C.M.; Walsh, D.; Tiwari, B.K. Laminarin from Irish brown seaweeds *Ascophyllum nodosum* and *Laminaria hyperborea*: Ultrasound assisted extraction, characterization and bioactivity. *Mar. Drugs* **2015**, *13*, 4270–4280. [CrossRef] [PubMed]
22. Moreira, R.; Chenlo, F.; Sineiro, J.; Arufe, S.; Sexto, S. Drying temperature effect on powder physical properties and aqueous extract characteristics of *Fucus vesiculosus*. *J. Appl. Phycol.* **2016**, *28*, 2485–2494. [CrossRef]
23. Rodrigues, D.; Sousa, S.; Silva, A.; Amorim, M.; Pereira, L.; Rocha-Santos, T.A.; Gomes, A.M.; Duarte, A.C.; Freitas, A.C. Impact of enzyme-and ultrasound-assisted extraction methods on biological properties of red, brown, and green seaweeds from the central west coast of Portugal. *J. Agric. Food Chem.* **2015**, *63*, 3177–3188. [CrossRef] [PubMed]
24. ISO 1442. *International Standards Meat and Meat Products—Determination of Moisture Content*; International Organization for Standardization: Geneva, Switzerland, 1997.
25. Medina-Remón, A.; Barrionuevo-González, A.; Zamora-Ros, R.; Andres-Lacueva, C.; Estruch, R.; Martínez-González, M.Á.; Diez-Espino, J.; Lamuela-Raventos, R.M. Rapid Folin–Ciocalteu method using microtiter 96-well plate cartridges for solid phase extraction to assess urinary total phenolic compounds, as a biomarker of total polyphenols intake. *Anal. Chim. Acta* **2009**, *634*, 54–60. [CrossRef] [PubMed]
26. Ou, B.; Hampsch-Woodill, M.; Prior, R.L. Development and validation of an improved oxygen radical absorbance capacity assay using fluorescein as the fluorescent probe. *J. Agric. Food Chem.* **2001**, *49*, 4619–4626. [CrossRef] [PubMed]
27. Dávalos, A.; Bartolomé, B.; Suberviola, J.; Gómez-Cordovés, C. Orac-fluorescein as a model for evaluating antioxidant activity of wines. *Pol. J. Food Nutr. Sci.* **2003**, *12*, 133–136.
28. Re, R.; Pellegrini, N.; Proteggente, A.; Pannala, A.; Yang, M.; Rice-Evans, C. Antioxidant activity applying an improved ABTS radical cation decolorization assay. *Free Radic. Biol. Med.* **1999**, *26*, 1231–1237. [CrossRef]
29. Brand-Williams, W.; Cuvelier, M.E.; Berset, C.L.W. T. Use of a free radical method to evaluate antioxidant activity. *LWT-Food Sci. Technol.* **1995**, *28*, 25–30. [CrossRef]
30. Benzie, I.F.; Strain, J.J. The ferric reducing ability of plasma (FRAP) as a measure of "antioxidant power": The FRAP assay. *Anal. Biochem.* **1996**, *239*, 70–76. [CrossRef] [PubMed]
31. Farvin, K.S.; Jacobsen, C. Phenolic compounds and antioxidant activities of selected species of seaweeds from Danish coast. *Food Chem.* **2013**, *138*, 1670–1681. [CrossRef] [PubMed]
32. Matanjun, P.; Mohamed, S.; Mustapha, N.M.; Muhammad, K.; Ming, C.H. Antioxidant activities and phenolics content of eight species of seaweeds from north Borneo. *J. Appl. Phycol.* **2008**, *20*, 367. [CrossRef]
33. Agregán, R.; Lorenzo, J.M.; Munekata, P.E.; Dominguez, R.; Carballo, J.; Franco, D. Assessment of the antioxidant activity of *Bifurcaria bifurcata* aqueous extract on canola oil. Effect of extract concentration on the oxidation stability and volatile compound generation during oil storage. *Food Res. Int.* **2016**, *99*, 1095–1102. [CrossRef] [PubMed]
34. Tierney, M.S.; Smyth, T.J.; Hayes, M.; Soler-Vila, A.; Croft, A.K.; Brunton, N. Influence of pressurised liquid extraction and solid–liquid extraction methods on the phenolic content and antioxidant activities of Irish macroalgae. *Int. J. Food Sci. Technol.* **2013**, *48*, 860–869. [CrossRef]
35. Barba, F.J.; Grimi, N.; Vorobiev, E. New approaches for the use of non-conventional cell disruption technologies to extract potential food additives and nutraceuticals from microalgae. *Food Eng. Rev.* **2015**, *7*, 45–62. [CrossRef]
36. Dufossé, L.; Galaup, P.; Yaron, A.; Arad, S.M.; Blanc, P.; Murthy, K.N.C.; Ravishankar, G.A. Microorganisms and microalgae as sources of pigments for food use: A scientific oddity or an industrial reality? *Trends Food Sci. Technol.* **2005**, *16*, 389–406. [CrossRef]
37. Kwang, H.C.; Lee, H.J.; Koo, S.Y.; Song, D.G.; Lee, D.U.; Pan, C.H. Optimization of pressurized liquid extraction of carotenoids and chlorophylls from *Chlorella vulgaris*. *J. Agric. Food Chem.* **2009**, *58*, 793–797.
38. Plaza, M.; Santoyo, S.; Jaime, L.; Avalo, B.; Cifuentes, A.; Reglero, G.; Reina, G.G.B.; Señoráns, F.J.; Ibáñez, E. Comprehensive characterization of the functional activities of pressurized liquid and ultrasound-assisted extracts from *Chlorella vulgaris*. *LWT-Food Sci. Technol.* **2012**, *46*, 245–253. [CrossRef]

39. Ahmed, F.; Fanning, K.; Netzel, M.; Turner, W.; Li, Y.; Schenk, P.M. Profiling of carotenoids and antioxidant capacity of microalgae from subtropical coastal and brackish waters. *Food Chem.* **2014**, *165*, 300–306. [CrossRef] [PubMed]
40. Targett, N.M.; Arnold, T.M. Minireview—Predicting the effects of brown algal phlorotannins on marine herbivores in tropical and temperate oceans. *J. Phycol.* **1998**, *34*, 195–205. [CrossRef]
41. Van Altena, I.A.; Steinberg, P.D. Are differences in the responses between North American and Australasian marine herbivores to phlorotannins due to differences in phlorotannin structure? *Biochem. Syst. Ecol.* **1992**, *20*, 493–499. [CrossRef]
42. Chew, Y.L.; Lim, Y.Y.; Omar, M.; Khoo, K.S. Antioxidant activity of three edible seaweeds from two areas in South East Asia. *LWT-Food Sci. Technol.* **2008**, *41*, 1067–1072. [CrossRef]
43. Connan, S.; Goulard, F.; Stiger, V.; Deslandes, E.; Ar Gall, E. Interspecific and temporal variation in phlorotannin levels in an assemblage of brown algae. *Bot. Mar.* **2004**, *47*, 410–416. [CrossRef]
44. Amsler, C.D.; Fairhead, V.A. Defensive and sensory chemical ecology of brown algae. *Adv. Bot. Res* **2005**, *43*, 1–91.
45. Ragan, M.A.; Jensen, A. Quantitative studies on brown algal phenols. II. Seasonal variation in polyphenol content of *Ascophyllum nodosum* (L.) Le Jol. and *Fucus vesiculosus* (L.). *J. Exp. Mar. Biol. Ecol.* **1978**, *34*, 245–258. [CrossRef]
46. Sampath-Wiley, P.; Neefus, C.D.; Jahnke, L.S. Seasonal effects of sun exposure and emersion on intertidal seaweed physiology: Fluctuations in antioxidant contents, photosynthetic pigments and photosynthetic efficiency in the red alga *Porphyra umbilicalis* Kützing (Rhodophyta, Bangiales). *J. Exp. Mar. Biol. Ecol.* **2008**, *361*, 83–91. [CrossRef]
47. Ahn, G.N.; Kim, K.N.; Cha, S.H.; Song, C.B.; Lee, J.; Heo, M.S.; Yeo, I.K.; Lee, N.H.; Jee, Y.H.; Kim, J.S.; et al. Antioxidant activities of phlorotannins purified from *Ecklonia cava* on free radical scavenging using ESR and H_2O_2-mediated DNA damage. *Eur. Food Res. Technol.* **2007**, *226*, 71–79. [CrossRef]
48. Goiris, K.; Muylaert, K.; Fraeye, I.; Foubert, I.; De Brabanter, J.; De Cooman, L. Antioxidant potential of microalgae in relation to their phenolic and carotenoid content. *J. Appl. Phycol.* **2012**, *24*, 1477–1486. [CrossRef]
49. Maadane, A.; Merghoub, N.; Ainane, T.; El Arroussi, H.; Benhima, R.; Amzazi, S.; Bakri, Y.; Wahby, I. Antioxidant activity of some Moroccan marine microalgae: PUFA profiles, carotenoids and phenolic content. *J. Biotechnol.* **2015**, *215*, 13–19. [CrossRef] [PubMed]

medicines

MDPI

Article

In Vitro Assessment of Total Phenolic and Flavonoid Contents, Antioxidant and Photoprotective Activities of Crude Methanolic Extract of Aerial Parts of *Capnophyllum peregrinum* (L.) Lange (Apiaceae) Growing in Algeria

Mostefa Lefahal [1], Nabila Zaabat [1], Radia Ayad [1], El hani Makhloufi [1], Lakhdar Djarri [1], Merzoug Benahmed [2], Hocine Laouer [3], Gema Nieto [4,*] and Salah Akkal [1,*]

[1] Valorization of Natural Resources, Bioactive Molecules and Biological Analysis Unit, Department of Chemistry, University of Mentouri Constantine, Constantine 25000, Algeria; mlefahal@gmail.com (M.L.); z_nabila2002@yahoo.fr (N.Z.); radia.ayad@yahoo.fr (R.A.); makhloufi_el_hani@yahoo.fr (E.h.M.); djarri62@gmail.com (L.D.)

[2] Department of Chemistry, Faculty of Science, University of Tebessa, Tebessa 12000, Algeria; Riad43200@yahoo.fr

[3] Laboratory of Natural Biological Resources Valorization, Faculty of Sciences, University of Setif, Setif 19000, Algeria; hocine_laouer@yahoo.fr

[4] Department of Food Technology, Nutrition and Food Science, Faculty of Veterinary Sciences, University of Murcia, Campus de Espinardo, Espinardo, 30100 Murcia, Spain

* Correspondence: gnieto@um.es (G.N.); salah4dz@yahoo.fr (S.A.); Tel.: +34-868-889-624 (G.N.); +213-31-811-102 (S.A.)

Received: 17 February 2018; Accepted: 21 March 2018; Published: 22 March 2018

Abstract: Background: *Capnophyllum peregrinum* (L.) Lange (Apiaceae) is the unique taxon of *capnophyllum* genus in Algerian flora. It has never been investigated in regards to its total phenolic and flavonoid contents and antioxidant and photoprotective activities. **Methods:** *C. peregrinum* aerial parts extracted with absolute methanol. The total flavonoid and phenolic contents of the extract were evaluated to determine their correlation with the antioxidant and photoprotective activities of the extract. **Results:** The methanolic extract demonstrated a significant amount of phenolics and flavonoids (74.06 ± 1.23 mg GAE/g, 44.09 ± 2.13 mg QE/g, respectively) and exhibited good antioxidant activity in different systems, especially in 1,1-Diphenyl-2-picrylhydrazyl (DPPH), reducing power and total antioxidant capacity assays. Furthermore the extract showed high photoprotective activity with the sun protection factor (SPF) value = 35.21 ± 0.18. **Conclusions:** The results of the present study show, that the methanolic extract could be used as a natural sunscreen in pharmaceutics or cosmetic formulations and as a valuable source of natural antioxidants.

Keywords: *Capnophyllum peregrinum*; antioxidant activity; photoprotective activity

1. Introduction

Since ancient times, medicinal plants have been used for their medicinal virtues and nutriment values. Presently, the crude extracts from both medicinal and aromatic plants have attracted keen interest in the development and preparation of alternative traditional medicine and food additives [1].

Apiaceae is one of the best-known families of flowering plants, which comprises of about 300–455 genera and 3000–3750 species worldwide [2]. In Algerian flora this family is represented by 55 genera and 130 species [3]. Several Apiaceae members are aromatic plants that are popularly used in medicine and in cooking, such as *Anethum graveolens*, *Angelica archangelica*, *Apium graveolens*,

Carum carvi, *Coriandrum sativum*, and *Foeniculum vulgare* [4]. *Capnophyllum* Gaertner belongs to the Apiaceae family, which is a genus of small annual herbs, and its name is derived from the Greek (Capnos = smoke, phyllon = leaf) [5]. This genus is represented in the Algerian flora by unique taxon known as *Capnophyllum peregrinum* (L.) Lange [3]. Concerning the uses of this species, it has been mentioned that its roots are used as vegetables [6]. Regarding the phytochemical investigations on this taxon, only one data item has been published so far, indicating the presence of phtalides, such as Z-ligustilide, in its roots [6].

Natural products from plant sources have the ability to reduce oxidative stress by acting as antioxidants [7]. Hence, plants still present a large source of natural antioxidants that could be taken into account for searching and developing the novel drugs. In fact, phenolic compounds from natural sources are well known as radical scavengers, metal chelators, reducing agents, and hydrogen donors. Thus, plants with high levels of polyphenols have attracted significant importance to be used as natural antioxidants [8].

The ultraviolet radiation is divided into three categories: UV-A (320–400 nm), UV-B (290–320 nm), and UV-C (200–290 nm). The prolonged exposure to these radiations can generate harmful effects which can cause several skin ailments (in particular, UV-B radiation (290–320 nm)) that can cause erythema, sunburns, DNA damage, and premature aging of skin [9]. They also led to the generation of reactive oxygen species (ROS) [10]. Thus, protecting human skin against UV radiation is evident and the effective protection results in the use of formulations containing solar filters (chemicals that absorb UV radiations) known as sunscreens [11]. Recently, plant extracts with antioxidant properties have been used in phytocosmetic field to be used as sunscreens. In fact, that they comprise ingredients that could inactivate ROS and prevent erythema and premature aging of the skin [12].

To find new natural sources which could be used as natural antioxidants and as sunscreens in pharmaceutical or cosmetic preparations, the main aim of this study was to evaluate the in vitro total phenolic and flavonoid contents, antioxidant, and photoprotective activities of crude methanolic extract of aerial parts of *C. peregrinum* growing in Algeria.

2. Materials and Methods

2.1. Plant Materials

C. peregrinum aerial parts were collected in May 2015 from Elkala (eastern Algerian). The plant was identified by Prof. Dr. H. Laouer from the Department of biology and plant ecology, Ferhat Abbas University (Setif, Algeria) and a voucher specimen were deposited in the Herbarium of our laboratory.

Preparation of Extracts

C. peregrinum aerial parts were dried in a shade at room temperature. A total of 20 g of dried aerial parts were soaked in absolute methanol in ratio (1/10) at room temperature for 72 h. The macerate was filtered using Watman N° 1 filter paper. The obtained filtrate was concentrated to dryness under reduced pressure at 40 °C using a rotary evaporator. The extract is stored at 4 °C until the experiments were performed [13].

2.2. Chemicals

2,2-azinobis-3-ethylbenzothiazoline-6-sulfonic acid (ABTS), 1,1-Diphenyl-2-picrylhydrazyl (DPPH), Potassium ferricyanide [$K_3Fe(CN)_6$], Trichloroacetic acid ($C_2HCl_3O_2$), Ferric chloride ($FeCl_3$), Sodium phosphate (NaH_2PO_4), Ammonium molybdate ($(NH_4)_2MoO_4$), Sulfuric acid, Folin–Ciocalteu, Aluminium chloride ($AlCl_3$), Sodium carbonate (Na_2CO_3), Gallic acid, Quercetin, Ascorbic acid, Butylated hydroxytoluene (BHT), Butylated hydroxyanisole (BHA), α-tocopherol were obtained from Sigma Aldrich (St. Louis, MO, USA). All the chemicals used, including the solvents, were of analytical grade.

2.2.1. Determination of Total Phenolic Content (TPC)

Total phenolic content of crude methanolic extract of *C. peregrinum* was determined by the Folin–Ciocalteu method adopted by Tanguy [14]. A volume of 300 μL of extract solution (1 mg/mL in methanol) was mixed with 1500 μL of Folin–Ciocalteu reagent (diluted 10 fold). After 4 min, 1200 μL of Na_2CO_3 (75 g/L) was added. The mixture was incubated at room temperature in the dark for 2 h. The absorbance of the reaction mixture was measured at 765 nm with UV/VIS spectrophotometer. Gallic acid was used as a standard for calibration curve and results were expressed as Gallic acid equivalents (μg GAE/mg).

2.2.2. Determination of Total Flavonoid Content (TFC)

Total flavonoid content of crude methanolic extract of *C. peregrinum* was performed by aluminium chloride colorimetric method adopted by Djeridane et al. [15]. A volume of 1 mL of 2% $AlCl_3$ ethanol solution was mixed with 1 mL of sample solution (1 mg/mL). After incubation for 10 min at room temperature, the absorbance was measured at 415 nm with UV/VIS spectrophotometer (Thermo, Waltham, MA, USA). Quercetin was used as a standard for calibration curve and the results were expressed as Quercetin equivalents (μg QE/mg).

2.3. In Vitro Antioxidative Activity

2.3.1. DPPH Radical Scavenging Assay

Free radical scavenging activity of crude methanolic extract of *C. peregrinum* was determined spectrophotometrically according to the modified Blois methods [16]. Forty microliters of crude methanolic extract and standards (BHT, BHA) at various concentrations (12.5–800 μg/mL) were added to 160 μL of a methanol solution of DPPH (0.4 M) in a 96 well plate. The mixture was vigorously shaken and then incubated at room temperature for 30 min in the dark. The absorbance of the mixture was measured at 517 nm with UV/VIS spectrophotometer. The scavenging activity on the DPPH radical was expressed as inhibition percentage using the following equation:

$$\%\ \text{Inhibition} = [(A_{control} - A_{sample})/A_{control}] \times 100$$

where $A_{control}$ is the absorbance of the control reaction (containing all reagents except the test extract or standard), and A_{sample} is the absorbance of the test extract or standard.

2.3.2. ABTS Radical Scavenging Assay

The ABTS radical scavenging activity was determined according to the method adopted by Re et al. [17]. The stock solution which was allowed to stand in the dark for 12 h at room temperature contained equal volumes of 7 mM ABTS salt and 2.4 mM potassium persulfate. The resultant $ABTS^+$ solution was diluted with ethanol until an absorbance of 0.708 ± 0.025 at 734 nm was obtained. Forty microliters of varying concentrations (12.5–800 μg/mL) of the crude methanolic extract and standards (BHT, BHA) were allowed to react with 160 μL of the $ABTS^+$ for 10 min. The absorbance of mixture was recorded at 734 nm with UV/VIS spectrophotometer.

The scavenging activity on the $ABTS^+$ radical was expressed as inhibition percentage using the following equation:

$$\%\ \text{Inhibition} = [(A_{control} - A_{sample})/A_{control}] \times 100$$

where $A_{control}$ is the absorbance of the control reaction (containing all reagents except the test extract or standard), and A_{sample} is the absorbance of the extract or standard.

2.3.3. Reducing Power Assay

This assay was performed following the method of Oyaizu [18]. A volume of 1 mL in different concentrations of crude methanolic extract and standards (BHA, α-tocopherol) at various concentrations (3.125–200 μg/mL) and 0.75 mL of distilled water were mixed with 1 mL of 0.2 M sodium phosphate buffer (pH 6.6) and, a volume of 1 mL of potassium ferricyanide (1%) was added to the mixture. Following incubation at 50 °C for 20 min, the reaction mixture was acidified with 1 mL of trichloroacetic acid (10%) and 0.25 mL of $FeCl_3$ (0.1%) was added to this solution. The absorbance was measured at 700 nm with UV/VIS spectrophotometer.

2.3.4. Total Antioxidant Capacity by Phosphomolybdenum Method

Total antioxidant capacity (TAC) of the crude methanolic extract was evaluated by the phosphomolybdenum method according to the procedure described by Prieto et al. [19]. An aliquot 300 μL (2 mg/mL) of crude methanolic extract was added in 3 mL of reagent solution containing (0.6 M sulfuric acid, 28 mM sodium phosphate and 4 mM ammonium molybdate). The mixture solution was subjected to incubation in a water bath at 95 °C for 90 min. The absorbance was measured at 695 nm with UV/VIS spectrophotometer. The total antioxidant capacity was expressed as Ascorbic acid equivalents (μg AAE/mg).

2.4. *Photoprotective Activity*

The photoprotective activity of crude methanolic extract was measured by determination in vitro of sun protection factor (SPF), which is considered to be one of the most frequently used indicators for the classification of protection levels afforded by sunscreen products against sunburn due mainly to harmful UV-B radiation [20]. In order to perform the photoprotective activity of *C. peregrinum* aerial parts, the crude methanolic extract was diluted in absolute methanol to obtain a concentration of 2 mg/mL. Spectrophotometric scanning was performed at wavelengths between 290 and 320 nm, with intervals of 5 nm with UV/VIS spectrophotometer. The readings were performed using 1 cm quartz cell and methanol used as a blank. SPF value was obtained according to the equation developed by Mansur et al. [21]:

$$\mathrm{SPF} = \mathrm{CF} \sum_{290}^{320} \mathrm{EE}\ (\lambda)\ \mathrm{I}\ (\lambda)\ \mathrm{A}\ (\lambda)$$

where EE(λ) is the erythemal effect spectrum; I(λ) is the solar intensity spectrum; Abs(λ) is the absorbance; and CF is the correction factor (=10).

The values of EE(λ) × I(λ) (Table 1) are constants, and they were determined by Sayre et al. [22].

Table 1. The Normalized product function used in the calculation of sun protection factor (SPF).

Wavelength (nm)	EE × I (Nomalized)
290	0.0150
295	0.0817
300	0.2874
305	0.3278
310	0.1864
315	0.0839
320	0.0180

2.5. *Statistical Analysis*

All data were expressed as means ± SD for at least three replications for each prepared sample. Statistical analysis was performed using one-sample *t*-test. The results are considered to be significant when $p < 0.05$.

3. Results

3.1. Total Phenolic and Flavonoid Content Evaluation

The total phenolic content of the crude methanolic extract of *C. peregrinum* was estimated by Folin–Ciocalteu reagent and expressed in gallic acid equivalents (GAE) and it was calculated from the linear regression equation of standard curve (y = 0.0143x + 0.2567, R^2 = 0.9929). The results showed that the crude methanolic extract was found to contain a high amount of phenols (74.06 ± 1.23 µg GAE/mg).

The total flavonoid content of crude methanolic extract was determined via aluminum chloride colorimetric method and it was calculated from the linear regression equation of standard curve of quercetin (y = 0.0225x + 0.0078, R^2 = 0.9965) and expressed as quercetin equivalent per gram of plant extract. The tested extract was found to contain high amounts of flavonoids (44.09 ± 2.13 µg QE/mg).

3.2. Antioxidant Activity

The antioxidant activity is a complex process, usually happening via several mechanisms. Thus evaluation of plant extracts antioxidant activity must be carried out by more than one test [23]. DPPH free radical scavenging, ABTS free radical scavenging, ferric-reducing power and total antioxidant capacity assays were used to evaluate the in vitro antioxidant effect of crude methanolic extract of *C. peregrinum*.

3.2.1. DPPH Radical Scavenging Assay

DPPH free radical scavenging activity of crude methanolic extract is shown in (Table 2). The results reveal that the percentage inhibition of DPPH radical was found to be increased with concentration. The methanolic extract showed maximum activity of 85.21 ± 0.67% at 100 µg/mL; whereas positive standards, BHT and BHA exhibited 94.00 ± 0.31% and 84.18 ± 0.10% inhibition respectively. The IC_{50} value of the extract was determined, and which is defined as the concentration of the extract required to scavenge 50% of DPPH free radical. Low IC_{50} value represents high antioxidant activity. In this study the IC_{50} values of extract and standards (BHT, BHA) were: 48.68 ± 1.71 µg/mL, 12.99 ± 0.41 µg/mL and 6.14 ± 0.41 µg/mL. The results showed that the methanolic extract has a good DPPH radical scavenging effect.

Table 2. Antioxidant activity by the 1,1-Diphenyl-2-picrylhydrazyl (DPPH) assay *C. peregrinum* methanolic extract.

Concentration µg/mL	% Inhibition in DPPH Assay		
	MeOH Extract	BHA	BHT
12.5	16.97 ± 1.06	76.55 ± 0.48	49.09 ± 0.76
25	30.26 ± 2.07	79.89 ± 0.26	72.63 ± 2.06
50	53.90 ± 1.65	81.73 ± 0.10	88.73 ± 0.89
100	85.21 ± 0.67	84.18 ± 0.10	88.73 ± 0.89
200	86.63 ± 0.51	87.13 ± 0.17	94.97 ± 0.08
400	86.92 ± 0.17	89.36 ± 0.19	95.38 ± 0.41
800	86.46 ± 0.19	90.14 ± 0.00	95.02 ± 0.23
IC50 µg/mL	**48.68 ± 1.71**	**6.14 ± 0.41**	**12.99 ± 0.41**

3.2.2. ABTS Radical Scavenging Assay

In case of ABTS assay the experimental data (Table 3) reveal that the crude methanolic extract was found to be effective in scavenging the $ABTS^+$ radical. The percentage inhibition of $ABTS^+$ radical was concentration-dependent. The scavenging effect was 91.91 ± 0.28% at higher concentrations 800 µg/mL; whereas positive standards BHT and BHA exhibited 96.68 ± 0.39%, 95.86 ± 0.10% inhibition respectively. The IC_{50} values of the extract and the standards BHT and BHA were found to be: 63.62 ± 0.66, 1.29 ± 0.30 and 1.81 ± 0.10 μg/mL, respectively, this suggests that the tested extract has a weak $ABTS^{+}$ free radical scavenging activity when compared with standards.

Table 3. Antioxidant activity by the 2,2-azinobis-3-ethylbenzothiazoline-6-sulfonic (ABTS) assay *C. peregrinum* methanolic extract.

Concentration μg/mL	% Inhibition in ABTS Assay		
	MeOH Extract	BHA	BHT
12.5	5.01 ± 0.93	69.21 ± 0.40	92.83 ± 1.42
25	7.22 ± 0.47	78.23 ± 1.34	94.68 ± 0.42
50	13.85 ± 0.09	88.12 ± 1.28	94.95 ± 0.90
100	28.30 ± 0.37	88.76 ± 3.07	95.32 ± 0.25
200	42.75 ± 0.43	90.85 ± 1.74	95.59 ± 0.47
400	68.36 ± 0.09	90.95 ± 0.51	95.83 ± 0.15
800	91.91 ± 0.28	96.68 ± 0.39	95.86 ± 0.10
IC50 μg/mL	**63.62 ± 0.66**	**1.29 ± 0.30**	**1.81 ± 0.10**

3.2.3. Reducing Power Assay

The reducing power of the crude methanolic extract was evaluated using ferric to ferrous reducing activity as determined spectrophotometrically from the formation of Perl's Prussian blue colour complex [24]. In our study, the reducing power of the methanolic extract was compared with α-Tocopherol and BHA. The results are shown in (Table 4). The results showed that the reducing power activity of the crude methanolic extract increases with the increase in concentrations of the extract solutions. The methanolic extract exhibited (0.94 ± 0.02) average absorbance at 700 nm in 200 μg/mL concentration; whereas the positive standards α-Tocopherol and BHA exhibited (1.81 ± 0.09) (1.86 ± 0.46) average absorbance in the same concentrations.

Table 4. Antioxidant activity by the reducing power assay of *C. peregrinum* methanolic extract.

Concentration μg/mL	Absorbance		
	MeOH Extract	BHA	α-Tocopherol
3.125	0.08 ± 0.01	0.28 ± 0.02	0.11 ± 0.00
6.25	0.09 ± 0.01	0.54 ± 0.02	0.16 ± 0.00
12.5	0.13 ± 0.01	0.75 ± 0.07	0.21 ± 0.03
25	0.19 ± 0.02	1.28 ± 0.28	0.35 ± 0.03
50	0.29 ± 0.03	1.49 ± 0.11	0.73 ± 0.03
100	0.58 ± 0.04	1.79 ± 0.16	1.37 ± 0.08
200	0.94 ± 0.02	1.86 ± 0.46	1.81 ± 0.09

3.2.4. Total Antioxidant Capacity by Phosphomolybdenum Method

Total antioxidant capacity of crude methanolic extract of *C. peregrinum* was evaluated by the phosphomolybdenum method and was expressed as ascorbic acid equivalent per mg of plant extract. The results reveal that the crude methanolic extract was found to possess strong total antioxidant capacity (130.91 ± 4.40 μg AAE/mg).

3.3. *Photoprotective Activity*

The photoprotective activity of the crude methanolic extract was evaluated by calculation of SPF; the SPF parameter was determined by the spectrophotometric method developed by Mansur et al. [21], using the UV-B region, considered to be the region of greatest incidence during the day in which people are exposed for longer [10], in this way it has been reported that in SPF ratings, SPF values 2–12, 12–30 and ≥30 are considered as having respectively minimum, moderate and high sun protective activity [25]. As shown in experimental data (Table 5) the extract showed high absorbance values ranged between 3.45 and 3.58 at 290–320 nm, and the SPF value was found to be 35.21 ± 0.18. The results indicate that the methanolic extract have displayed high photoprotective activity.

Table 5. Photoprotective activity of *C. peregrinum* methanolic extract.

Wavelength (nm)	EE × I	Absorbance
290	0.0150	3.583 ± 0.011
295	0.0817	3.561 ± 0.026
300	0.2874	3.53 ± 0.011
305	0.3278	3.52 ± 0.036
310	0.1864	3.484 ± 0.02
315	0.0839	3.478 ± 0.039
320	0.0180	3.453 ± 0.03
$SPF = CF \sum_{290}^{320} EE(\lambda)\, I(\lambda)\, A(\lambda) = 35.21 \pm 0.18$		

4. Discussion

In the present study, phenolic and flavonoid composition as well as antioxidant and photoprotective activities of *Capnophyllum peregrinum* were investigated the first time in an attempt to unravel new possible uses of this plant. Concerning total phenolic and flavonoid contents, the results suggest that phenolics and flavonoids are important components of the crude methanolic extract. These results are in accordance with previous findings reported in other Apiaceae species extracted with methanol such as *Prangos ferulacea* Lindl, *Prangos meliocarpoides* Boiss and *Prangos uechtritzii* Boiss. & Hausskn [26], *Pituranthos chloranthus* Benth and Hook [13]. Because of polyphenols are linked to the cell-wall matrix through a glycosidic/ester linkage, their water solubility may be reduced [27]. Thus several authors displayed that alcohols are suitable solvents for the extraction of phenolic and flavonoids compounds. For example, methanol or ethanol are mostly used for the separation of this class of natural products [28] according to their best solubility in alcohols, particularly in methanol [13]. Also, it has been observed that methanolic extracts of medicinal plants exhibited high phenolic and flavonoids contents as well as antioxidant activities more than water, ethyl acetate, chloroform and acetone extracts [13,29,30]. From literature, it has been well noted that medicinal plants with high amounts of phenols and flavonoids have potent antioxidant actions [31–34]. This may explain the antioxidant activity of *C. peregrinum*. In term of DPPH-scavenging potential of methanolic extract, our results are in accordance with those of previous works, indicating close relationship between DPPH radical scavenging effect and total phenolic and flavonoid contents of Apiaceae species such as *Ammi majus* L. [35], *Ferula gummosa* Boiss [36], *Daucus carota* Linn [37], *Sesili libanotis* (L.) Koch, *Sesili libanotis* (L.) Koch [38], *Coriandrum sativum* [39], *Foeniculum vulgare, Anethum graveolens* [40]. Concerning the reducing power and the total antioxidant capacity, the effectiveness of the methanolic extract may be explained by its high phenol and flavonoid contents. In this context, the results of our investigation are in accordance with those published earlier, which mentioned that containing flavonoids and polyphenols may play an important role in reducing power [7] and they contribute significantly to the total antioxidant activity of many fruits such as red grape [41], Star Apple [42] and medicinal plants [43].

In case of photoprotective activity, it has been well mentioned that flavonoids have significant photoprotective effects because of their UV absorbing capacity and their antioxidants effects [44]. Thus, some flavonoids such as quercetin, kaempferol, galanin and apigenin have been evaluated for their photoprotective activity [9]. Recently, it is well reported that plant extracts rich in flavonoids are capable of absorbing ultraviolet light in the UV-B and UV-A regions [11]. In this context, several authors have associated the photoprotective activity of plant extracts with their flavonoids content [45–47]. Thus the photoprotective potential of the methanolic extract of *C. peregrinum* could be explained by its flavonoids content. Indeed, it has been reported that UV-B rays absorbed by the skin led to the production of aggressive free radicals such as (O_2, $^1O_2$, HO_2, OH, ROO) [48]. Hence, the incorporation of antioxidants is now widely recommended in sunscreens. In this context, it also has been reported that the evaluation of most effective extracts for the antioxidant activity would be important for the development of more effective sunscreens [49]. Since, the methanolic extract exhibited antioxidant effects, is having a possibility to be used as sunscreen in pharmaceutics or cosmetics formulations.

5. Conclusions

In conclusion, our study evaluates, for the first time, total phenolic and flavonoid contents in addition to antioxidant and photoprotective activities of aerial parts of *Capnophyllum peregrinum* (L.) Lange (Apiaceae) growing in Algeria, our findings revealed that the methanolic extract was found to have a high phenolic and flavonoid contents as well as antioxidant and photoprotective activities. Therefore, it appears to be used a sunscreen in pharmaceutical or cosmetic preparations and as a natural source of antioxidant. Also, it can be speculated that the findings of our work could make the background for further investigation of this species, especially research concerning individual phenolic compounds.

Acknowledgments: The authors gratefully acknowledge the Ministry of Higher Education and Scientific Research, Algeria, for financial support.

Author Contributions: Mostefa Lefahal, Nabila Zaabat, Radia Ayad and El hani Makhloufi contributed to the experiments. Lakhdar Djarri and Merzoug Benahmed contributed to the data handling. Hocine Laouer contributed for the botanical identification of the plant. Salah Akkal and Gema Nieto contributed for the writing of the paper.

Conflicts of Interest: The authors report no financial or nonfinancial conflict of interest. The authors alone are responsible for the content and writing of the paper.

References

1. Amzad, H.M.; Al-Rakmi, K.A.S.; Al-Mijizy, Z.H.; Weli, A.M.; Al-Riyami, Q. Study of total phenol, flavonoids contents and phytochemical screening of various leaves crude extracts of locally grown *Thymus vulgar*. *Asian Pac. J. Trop. Biomed.* **2013**, *3*, 705–710.
2. Lamamra, M.; Laouer, H.; Amira, S.; Ilkay, E.O.S.; Sezer, S.F.; Demereci, B.; Akkal, S. Chemical Composition and Cholinesterase Inhibitory Activity of Different Parts of *Daucus aristidis* Coss. Essential Oils from Two Locations in Algeria. *Rec. Nat. Prod.* **2017**, *11*, 147–156.
3. Quezel, P.; Santa, S. New flora of Algeria and southern desert regions. *J. Agric. Trop. Bot. Appl.* **1965**, *12*, 784.
4. El-Kolli, M.; Laouer, H.; El-Kolli, H.; Akkal, S.; Sahli, F. Chemical analysis, antimicrobial and anti-oxidative properties of *Daucus gracilis* essential oil and its mechanism of action. *Asian Pac. J. Trop. Biomed.* **2016**, *6*, 8–15. [CrossRef]
5. Magee, A.R.; Van Wyk, B.E.; Tilney, P.M.; Downie, S.R. A taxonomic revision of *Capnophyllum* (Apiaceae: Apioideae). *S. Afr. J. Bot.* **2009**, *75*, 283–291. [CrossRef]
6. Gijbels, M.J.M.; Fischer, F.C.; Scheffer, J.J.C.; Baerheim Svendsen, A. Phthalides in Roots of *Capnophyllum peregrinum* and *Peucedanum ostruthium*. *Planta Med.* **1984**, *50*, 110. [CrossRef] [PubMed]
7. Ghribia, L.; Ghouilaa, H.; Omrib, A.; Besbesb, M.; Ben Janneta, H. Antioxidant and anti-acetylcholinesterase activities of extracts and secondary metabolites from *Acacia cyanophylla*. *Asian Pac. J. Trop. Biomed.* **2014**, *4* (Suppl. 1), S417–S423. [CrossRef] [PubMed]
8. Senthilkumar, R.; Parimelazhagan, T.; Chaurasia, O.P.; Srivastava, R.B. Free radical scavenging property and antiproliferative activity of *Rhodiola imbricata* Edgew extracts in HT-29 human colon cancer cells. *Asian Pac. J. Trop. Med.* **2013**, *6*, 11–19. [CrossRef]
9. Stevanato, R.; Bertelle, M.; Fabris, S. Photoprotective characteristics of natural antioxidant polyphenols. *Regul. Toxicol. Pharmacol.* **2014**, *69*, 71–77. [CrossRef] [PubMed]
10. De-Oliveira-Junior, R.G.; Ferraz, C.A.A.; Souza, G.R.; Leite Guimaraes, A.; Paula de Oliveira, A.; Gomes de Lima-Saraiva, S.R.; Araújo Rolim, L.; José Rolim-Neto, P.; Guedes da Silva Almeida, J.R. Phytochemical analysis and evaluation of antioxidant and photoprotective activities of extracts from flowers of *Bromelia laciniosa* (Bromeliaceae). *Biotechnol. Biotechnol. Equit.* **2017**, *31*, 600–605. [CrossRef]

11. Costa, S.C.C.; Detoni, C.B.; Branco, C.R.C.; Botura, M.B.; Branco, A. In vitro photoprotective effects of *Marcetia taxifolia* ethanolic extract and its potential for sunscreen formulations. *Rev. Bras. Farmacogn.* **2015**, *25*, 413–418. [CrossRef]
12. Reis Mansura, M.C.P.P.; Leitaoa, S.G.; Cerqueira-Coutinhoa, C.; Vermelhob, A.B.; Silva, R.S.; Presgravec, O.A.F.; Leitaod, A.A.C.; Leitaoe, G.G.; Ricci-Juniora, E.; Santosa, E.P. In vitro and in vivo evaluation of efficacy and safety of photoprotective formulations containing antioxidant extracts. *Rev. Bras. Farmacogn.* **2016**, *26*, 251–258. [CrossRef]
13. Khettaf, A.; Belloula, N.; Dridi, S. Antioxidant activity, phenolic and flavonoid contents of some wild medicinal plants in southeastern Algeria. *Afr. J. Biotechnol.* **2016**, *15*, 524–530.
14. Tanguy, J. Phenol metabolism and the hypersensitive reaction in Nicotiana infected with tobacco mosaic virus. *Physiol. Veg.* **1971**, *9*, 169–187.
15. Djeridane, A.; Yous, M.; Nadjemi, B.; Boutassouna, D.; Stocker, P.; Vidal, N. Antioxidant activity of some Algerian medicinal plants extracts containing phenolic compounds. *Food Chem.* **2006**, *97*, 654–660. [CrossRef]
16. Blois, M.S. Antioxidant determinations by the use of a stable free radical. *Nature* **1958**, *181*, 1199–1200. [CrossRef]
17. Re, R.; Pellegrini, N.; Proteggente, A.; Pannala, A.; Yang, M.; Rice-Evans, C. Antioxidant activity applying an improved ABTS radical cation decolorization assay. *Free Radic. Biol. Med.* **1999**, *26*, 1231–1237. [CrossRef]
18. Oyaizu, M. Studies on products of browning reactions: Antioxidative activities of browning reaction prepared from glucosamine. *Jpn. J. Nutr.* **1986**, *44*, 307–315. [CrossRef]
19. Prieto, P.; Pineda, M.; Aguilar, M. Spectrophotometric Quantitation of Antioxidant Capacity through the Formation of a Phosphomolybdenum Complex: Specific Application to the Determination of Vitamin E1. *Anal. Biochem.* **1999**, *269*, 337–341. [CrossRef] [PubMed]
20. Miksa, S.; Lutz, D.; Guy, C. New approach for a reliable in vitro sun protection factor method Part I: Principle and mathematical aspects. *Int. J. Cosmet. Sci.* **2015**, *37*, 555–566. [CrossRef] [PubMed]
21. Mansur, J.S.; Breder, M.V.R.; Mansur, M.C.A. Determinacao do fator de protecao solar por espectrofotometria. *An. Bras. Dermatol.* **1986**, *61*, 121–124.
22. Sayre, R.M.; Agin, P.P.; Levee, G.J.; Marlowe, E. A comparison of in vivo and in vitro testing of sunscreening formulas. *Photochem. Photobiol.* **1979**, *29*, 559–566. [CrossRef] [PubMed]
23. El Jemli, M.; Kamal, R.; Marmouzi, I.; Doukkali, Z.; Bouidida, E.H.; Touati, D.; Nejjari, R.; El Guessabi, L.; Cherrah, Y.; Alaoui, K. Chemical composition, acute toxicity, antioxidant and anti-inflammatory activities of Moroccan *Tetraclinis articulata* L. *J. Tradit. Complement. Med.* **2017**, *7*, 281–287. [CrossRef] [PubMed]
24. Hossain, M.D.I.; Sharmin, F.A.; Akhter, S.; Bhuiyan, M.A.; Shahriar, M. Investigation of cytotoxicity and *in-vitro* antioxidant activity of *Asparagus racemosus* root extract. *Int. Curr. Pharm. J.* **2012**, *1*, 250–257. [CrossRef]
25. Ratnasooriya, W.D.; Pathirana, R.N.; Dissanayake, A.S.; Samanmali, B.L.C.; Desman, P.K. Evaluation of in vitro sun screen activities of salt marshy plants *Suaeda monoica*, *Suaeda maritima* and *Halosarcia indica*. *Int. J. Pharm. Res. Allied Sci.* **2016**, *5*, 15–20.
26. Ahmed, J.; Guvenec, A.; Kucukboyaci, N.; Baldemir, A.; Coskun, M. Total phenolic contents and antioxidant activities of Prangos Lindl. (Umbelliferae) species growing in Konya province (Turkey). *Turk. J. Biol.* **2011**, *35*, 353–360.
27. Rasouli, H.; Hosein-Farzaei, M.; Khodarahmi, R. Polyphenols and their benefits: A review. *Int. J. Food Prop.* **2017**, *20*, S1700–S1741. [CrossRef]
28. Ignat, I.; Volf, I.; Popa, V.I. A critical review of methods for characterisation of polyphenolic compounds in fruits and vegetables. *Food Chem.* **2011**, *126*, 1821–1835. [CrossRef] [PubMed]
29. Tripathi, Y.C.; Jhumka, Z.; Anjum, N. Evaluation of Total Polyphenol and Antioxidant Activity of Leaves of *Bambusa nutans* and *Bambusa vulgaris*. *J. Pharm. Res.* **2015**, *9*, 271–277.
30. Nino, J.; Anjum, N.; Tripathi, Y.C. Phytochemical screening and evaluation of polyphenols, flavonoids and antioxidant activity of *Prunus cerasoids*. D. Don leaves. *J. Pharm. Res.* **2016**, *10*, 502–508.
31. Dehshiri, M.M.; Aghamollaei, H.; Zarini, M.; Nabavi, S.M.; Mirzaei, M.; Loizzo, M.R.; Nabavi, S.F. Antioxidant activity of different parts of *Tetrataenium lasiopetalum*. *Pharm. Biol.* **2013**, *51*, 1081–1085. [CrossRef] [PubMed]
32. Da Silva, J.F.M.; De Souza, M.C.; Matta, S.R. Correlation analysis between phenolic levels of Brazilian propolis extracts and their antimicrobial and antioxidant activities. *Food Chem.* **2006**, *99*, 431–435. [CrossRef]

33. Ksouri, R.; Falleh, H.; Megdiche, W.; Trabelsi, N.; Mhamdi, B.; Chaieb, K.; Bakrouf, A.; Magné, C.; Abdelly, C. Antioxidant and antimicrobial activities of the edible medicinal halophyte *Tamarix gallica* L. and related polyphenolic constituents. *Food Chem. Toxicol.* **2009**, *47*, 2083–2091. [CrossRef] [PubMed]
34. Falleh, H.; Medini, F.; Ksouri, R.; Guyot, S.; Abdelly, C.; Magné, C. Antioxidant activity and phenolic composition of the medicinal and edible halophyte *Mesembryanthemum edule* L. *Ind. Crops Prod.* **2011**, *34*, 1066–1071. [CrossRef]
35. Al-Hadhrami, R.M.S.; Hossain, M.A. Evaluation of antioxidant, antimicrobial and cytotoxic activities of seed crude extracts of *Ammi majus* grown in Oman. *Egypt. J. Basic Appl. Sci.* **2016**, *3*, 329–334. [CrossRef]
36. Ebrahimzadeh, M.A.; Nabavi, S.M.; Nabavi, S.F.; Dehbour, A.A. Antioxidant activity of hydroalcoholic extract of *Ferula gummosa* Boiss roots. *Eur. Rev. Med. Pharm. Sci.* **2011**, *15*, 658–664.
37. Chatatikun, M.; Chiabchalard, A. Phytochemical screening and free radical scavenging activities of orange baby carrot and carrot (*Daucus carota* Linn.) root crude extracts. *J. Chem. Pharm. Res.* **2013**, *5*, 97–102.
38. Matejić, J.S.; Džamić, A.M.; Mihajilov-Krstev, T.; Ranđelović, V.N.; Krivošej, Z.D.; Marin, P.D. Total phenolic content, flavonoid concentration, antioxidant and antimicrobial activity of methanol extracts from three *Seseli* L. taxa. *Cent. Eur. J. Biol.* **2012**, *7*, 1116–1122.
39. Shah, M.R.; Satardekar, K.V.; Barve, S.S. Screening of phenolic content, antioxidant and in vitro eye irritation activities from Apiaceae family (dry seeds) for potential cosmetic applications. *Int. J. Pharm. Sci. Res.* **2014**, *5*, 4366–4374.
40. Bagdassarian, V.L.C.; Bagdassarian, K.S.; Atanassova, M.S. Phenolic profile, antioxidant and antimicrobial activities from Apiaceae family (dry seeds). *Mintage J. Pharm. Med. Sci.* **2013**, *2*, 26–31.
41. Negro, C.; Tommasi, L.; Miceli, A. Phenolic compounds and antioxidant activity from red grape marc extracts. *Bioresour. Technol.* **2003**, *87*, 41–44. [CrossRef]
42. Luo, X.D.; Basile, M.J.; Kennelly, E.J. Polyphenolic antioxidants from the fruits of *Chrysophyllum cainito* L. (star apple). *J. Agric. Food Chem.* **2002**, *50*, 1379–1382. [CrossRef] [PubMed]
43. Bourgou, S.; Ksouri, R.; Bellila, A.; Skandrani, I.; Falleh, H.; Marzouk, B. Phenolic composition and biological activities of Tunisian *Nigella sativa* L. shoots and roots. *C. R. Biol.* **2008**, *331*, 48–55. [CrossRef] [PubMed]
44. Saewan, N.; Jimtaisong, A. Photoprotection of natural flavonoids. *J. Appl. Pharm. Sci.* **2013**, *3*, 129–141.
45. Souza, M.S.K.; Dos Santos, A.T.; Alves, F.C.A.; Paula, O.A.; Almeida, A.V.; Alves, S.F.J.; Cavalcante da Cruz, A.E.; Guedes da Silva, A.J.R.; Darklei Santos, S.N.; Pereira, N.X. Identification of flavonol glycosides and *in vitro* photoprotective and antioxidant activities of *Triplaris gardneriana* Wedd. *J. Med. Plants Res.* **2015**, *9*, 207–215.
46. Silva, E.E.S.; Alencar-Filho, J.M.T.; Oliviera, A.P.; Guimaraes, A.L.; Iqueira-Filho, J.A.; Almeida, J.R.G.S.; Araujo, E.C.C. Identification of glycosil flavones and determination in vitro of antioxidant and photoprotective activities of *Alternanthera braziliana* L. Kuntze. *Res. J. Phytochem.* **2014**, *8*, 148–154.
47. De-Oliveira-Junior, R.G.; Souza, G.R.; Guimarães, A.L.; Paula de Oliveira, A.; Silva Morais, A.C.; Araújo, E.C.C.; Nunes, X.P.; Almeida, J.R.G.S. Dried extracts of *Encholirium spectabile* (Bromeliaceae) present antioxidant and photoprotective activities in vitro. *J. Young Pharm.* **2013**, *5*, 102–105. [CrossRef] [PubMed]
48. Ratnasooriya, W.D.; Chandra-Jayakody, J.R.A.; Denzil-Rosa, S.R.; Ratnasooriya, C.D.T. In vitro sun screening activity of Sri Lankan orthodox black tea (*Camellia sinensis* linn). *World J. Pharm. Sci.* **2014**, *2*, 144–148.
49. Napagoda, M.T.; Shamila, B.M.A.M.; Abayawardana, S.A.K.; Qader, M.M.; Jayasingh, L. Photoprotective potential in some medicinal plants used to treat skin diseases in Sri Lanka. *BMC Complement. Altern. Med.* **2016**, *16*, 479. [CrossRef] [PubMed]

medicines

MDPI

Communication

Characterisation of Polyphenol-Containing Extracts from *Stachys mucronata* and Evaluation of Their Antiradical Activity

Spyros Grigorakis [1] and Dimitris P. Makris [2,*]

1 Food Quality & Chemistry of Natural Products, Mediterranean Agronomic Institute of Chania (M.A.I.Ch.), International Centre for Advanced Mediterranean Agronomic Studies (CIHEAM), P.O. Box 85, 73100 Chania, Greece; grigorakis@maich.gr

2 Department of Food Technology, Technological Educational Institute (T.E.I.) of Thessaly, N. Temponera Street, 43100 Karditsa, Greece

* Correspondence: dmakris@aegean.gr; Tel.: +30-22540-83114

Received: 9 January 2018; Accepted: 26 January 2018; Published: 27 January 2018

Abstract: Background: The aromatic plant *Stachys mucronata* (Lamiaceae) is endemic to the island of Crete (southern Greece), but as opposed to other native Greek members of this family, this species has never been investigated in the past with regard to its polyphenolic composition and antioxidant potency. **Methods**: Aerial parts of *S. mucronata* were exhaustively extracted and partly fractionated through partition, using *n*-butanol and dichloromethane. **Results**: Following an initial examination, which consisted of estimating the total polyphenol content and the antiradical activity, the *n*-butanol extract was found to be by far the richest in polyphenols, exhibiting much stronger antiradical activity compared with the dichloromethane counterpart. On this basis, the *n*-butanol extract was analysed by liquid chromatography-diode array-mass spectrometry, to tentatively characterise the principal polyphenolic components, which were shown to be flavonol but mainly flavone derivatives. **Conclusions**: The most potent radical-scavenging compounds were detected in the *n*-butanol fraction of the extracts, suggesting that the most active antioxidants in *S. mucronate* are relatively polar. The analyses suggested the major constituents to be derivatives of the flavone luteolin, accompanied by apigenin analogues, as well as flavonol glycosides and chlorogenate conjugates.

Keywords: antioxidants; Lamiaceae; polyphenols; *Stachys mucronata*

---

1. Introduction

Numerous secondary plant metabolites have been proven to possess pharmaceutical properties, and various multidisciplinary approaches have been attempted to open novel opportunities for the production of innovative plant-derived pharmaceuticals. In this direction, several strategies have been developed to integrate the knowledge of medicinal plants into drug design [1]. Out of the enormous diversity of bioactive substances occurring in botanicals, the class of polyphenols appears as a prominent phytochemical family, embracing an outstanding range of compounds with a wide spectrum of biological effects [2]. Thus, over the past few years polyphenols and/or polyphenol-containing botanical extracts have been a subject of intensive examination, pertaining to their isolation, identification, and their health- and medical-related properties [3].

The Mediterranean flora exhibits a broad biodiversity including a notably high number of native medicinal and aromatic plants, many of which may have several pharmacological potencies. The island of Crete (southern Greece) in particular is unique among the Mediterranean regions, embracing more than 1700 plant species [4], the polyphenolic composition of which is largely uncharacterised. The Lamiaceae family is a distinct botanical group, which includes several well-studied species, such as

Salvia and *Origanum*, with powerful antioxidant properties [5]. However, species belonging to *Stachys* are rather scarcely studied. In the framework of recent studies on the polyphenolic composition and antioxidant activity of native Cretan Lamiaceae species [4,6], this investigation was carried out with the aim of partly fractionating extracts from the aerial parts of *Stachys mucronata*, a relatively uncommon member of the Lamiaceae family, and characterising their polyphenolic profile and antiradical activity.

2. Materials and Methods

2.1. Chemicals and Reagents

Solvents used for liquid chromatography were of HPLC grade. Hexane, methanol, dichloromethane, *n*-butanol, Folin-Ciocalteu reagent, trolox®, 2,2-diphenyl-picrylhydrazyl (DPPH•) stable radical, anhydrous magnesium sulphate, and gallic acid were from Sigma-Aldrich (Darmstadt, Germany). Sodium carbonate was from Penta (Prague, Czechia).

2.2. Plant Material

The aerial parts of *Stachys mucronata* (Lamiaceae) were collected and provided by the Mediterranean Plant Conservation Centre (Chania, Greece). The plant material was left to dry in a dark and dry chamber for seven days and then ground in a domestic blender and stored in sealed plastic vessels at room temperature, in the dark.

2.3. Sample Preparation and Extraction

An amount of 10.1 g of ground plant material was defatted using the Soxhlet technique with hexane for 6 h. The defatted material was freed from residual hexane at room temperature (23 ± 1 °C) and then extracted overnight with methanol, under continuous stirring at 300 rpm. The mixture was filtered through a paper filter (grade 1, pore size 11 μm) and the clear extract was dried in a rotary evaporator (T = 40 °C). The solid residue was dissolved by adding hot water (approximately 90 °C) and then left to cool down to ambient temperature. The aqueous solution was then filtered to remove undissolved material.

2.4. Solvent Partition

The aqueous solution (approximately 100 mL) was first partitioned with an equal volume of dichloromethane, and this was repeated three times (3 × 100 mL). The dichloromethane extracts were combined, dried over magnesium sulphate, filtered, and the solvent was removed in vacuo. The solid residue (280 mg) was dissolved in a minimum volume of methanol (usually 2–3 mL) and stored at −20 °C until further analysis. The same procedure was followed with the dichloromethane partition using *n*-butanol, and afforded 580 mg of solid material (Figure 1).

2.5. Total Polyphenol and Antiradical Activity Determination

For total polyphenol determination, a previously reported methodology was used [7]. Results were expressed as milligrams of gallic acid equivalents (GAE) per gram of extract. Antiradical activity was measured using DPPH as the chromophore probe, using a well-established protocol [8]. Results were expressed as mM trolox equivalents (TRE).

2.6. Qualitative Liquid Chromatography-Diode Array-Mass Spectrometry (LC-DAD-MS)

A Finnigan MAT Spectra System P4000 pump was used coupled with a UV6000LP diode array detector and a Finnigan AQA mass spectrometer. Analyses were carried out on an end-capped Superspher RP-18, 125 × 2 mm, 4 μm, column (Merck, Darmstadt, Germany), protected by a guard column packed with the same material, and maintained at 40 °C. Analyses were carried out employing electrospray ionisation (ESI) at the positive ion mode, with acquisition set at 5 and 50 eV, capillary voltage 4 kV, source voltage 25 V, detector voltage 650 V, and probe temperature 400 °C. Eluent (A) and eluent (B) were 2% acetic acid and methanol, respectively. The flow rate was 0.33 mL min^{-1}, and the elution programme used was as follows: 0–2 min, 0% B; 2–52 min, 100% B; 60 min, 100% B.

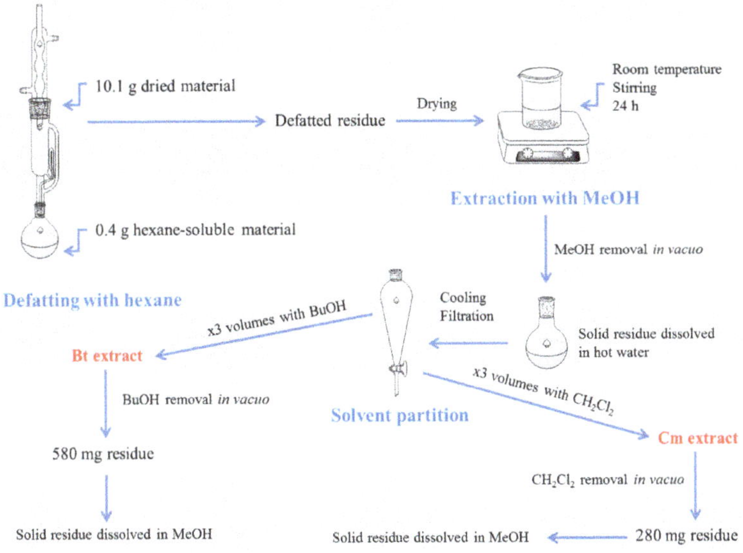

Figure 1. Overview of the analytical procedure followed to generate dichloromethane (Dcm) and *n*-butanol (Bt) fractions of *S. mucronata*.

2.7. Statistics

All determinations were repeated at least three times and the results were averaged and given with standard deviation. For all analyses, Microsoft Excel® 2010 and SigmaPlot® 12.0 (Systat Software Inc., San Jose, CA, USA) were used.

3. Results and Discussion

3.1. Polyphenolic Content and Antiradical Activity

Extracts were first partly fractionated through partition with dichloromethane and *n*-butanol, to obtain evidence regarding the polarity of the major polyphenols occurring in the aerial parts of *S. mucronate*. As can be seen in Figure 2, the fraction obtained with *n*-butanol (Bt) had a total polyphenol content of 632.0 ± 50.0 mg GAE g^{-1}, whereas the dichloromethane (Dcm) fraction displayed a total polyphenol content of 40.0 ± 3.7 mg GAE g^{-1}. This finding strongly suggested that the tissue extracted contained relatively polar polyphenols.

As a further step, the extracts were assayed using a representative radical scavenging test (DPPH) to ascertain the presence of antioxidant compounds. Indeed, the results demonstrated that the Bt fraction contained by far more potent antiradical substances compared with the Dcm counterpart (Figure 3). Moreover, the antiradical activity exhibited by both fractions was dose-dependent, showing linear response as a function of total polyphenol concentration ($R^2 > 0.98$). Based on this outcome, it was concluded that the Bt fraction was particularly enriched in antioxidant polyphenols, and it was chosen for the characterisation of its polyphenolic composition.

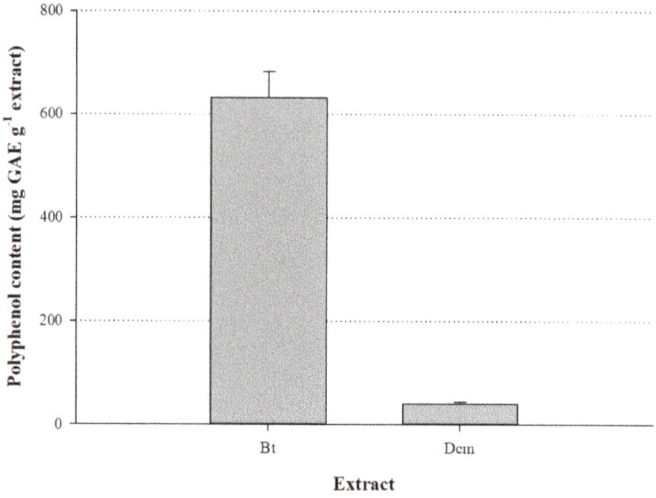

Figure 2. Total polyphenol content of the dichloromethane (Dcm) and *n*-butanol (Bt) fractions of *S. mucronata*. Bars indicate standard deviation.

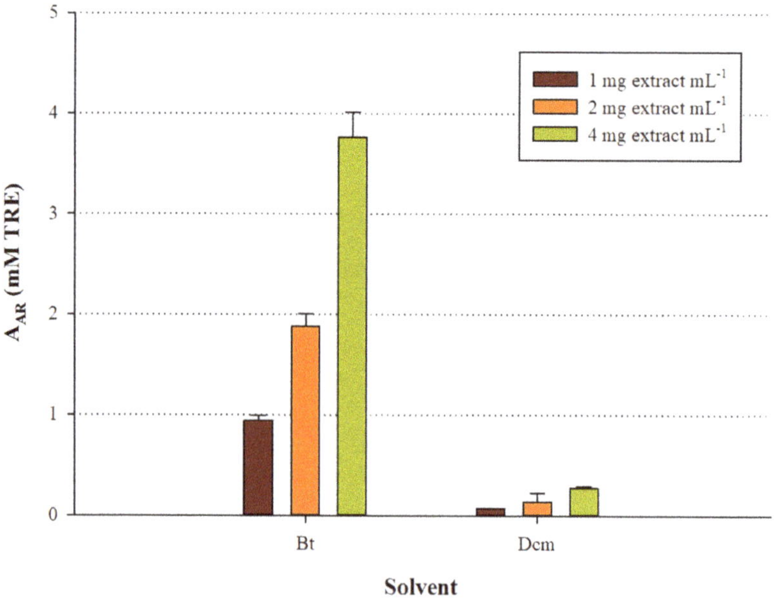

Figure 3. Graph illustrating the A_{AR} of the *S. mucronata* fractions as a function of extract quantity. Bars indicate standard deviation.

3.2. Polyphenolic Composition

The Bt fraction was subjected to LC-DAD-MS analysis to tentatively identify the principal polyphenolic constituents. By obtaining the polyphenolic profile through the total ion current (Figure 4) and the UV-vis spectral characteristics, it was made possible to assign putative structures to 13 compounds (Table 1). Peak #1 displayed a typical hydroxycinnamate UV-vis spectrum, and the diagnostic fragments at m/z = 355 and 163 (caffeoyl unit) pointed to a chlorogenate derivative [9]. The UV-vis spectrum of peak #2 was consistent with a flavonol structure and the ion at m/z = 303 suggested a quercetin derivative. Considering the ion at m/z = 465, this compound might correspond to a substance with a quercetin glucoside or galactoside backbone [9]. Likewise, peak #5 gave a molecular ion at m/z = 669 and a diagnostic fragment at m/z = 303, evidencing a hydroxyquercetin acetylallosylglucoside [10].

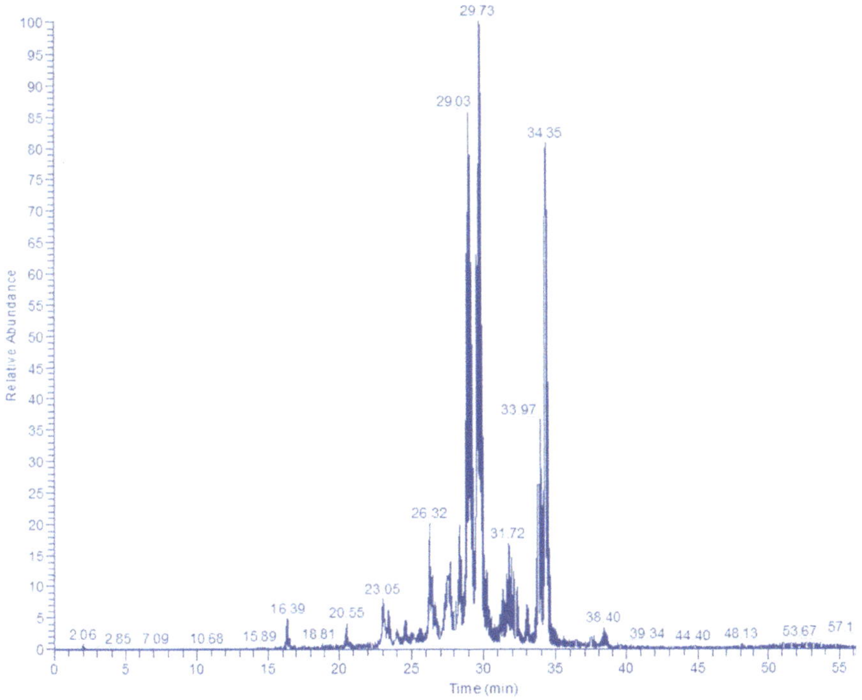

Figure 4. Total ion current (TIC) showing the major polyphenolic phytochemicals detected in *n*-butanol fraction of *S. mucronata*.

Peak #3 yielded a molecular ion at m/z = 449 and a diagnostic fragment at m/z = 287, suggesting a luteolin glucoside [10]. Peak #6 also gave the ion at m/z = 449, but the molecular ion at m/z = 653 along with the UV-vis characteristics indicated the presence of isoscutellarein acetylallosylglucoside [10]. However, peaks #4 and 8 with molecular ions at m/z = 653 afforded characteristic fragments at m/z = 287, a finding pointing to luteolin derivatives. In the same line, peak #9 showed a molecular ion at m/z = 695 and fragments at m/z = 653 and 287, indicating common structural features. On the other hand, peaks #11 and 12 also gave molecular ions at m/z = 695, confirmed by their Na^+ adducts, but yielded fragment ions only at m/z = 287.

Finally, peaks #7, 10, and 13 had a common diagnostic fragment at m/z = 271, evidence of apigenin derivatives. For peak #7, the molecular ion at m/z = 433 and the UV-vis pattern were in accordance with those reported for apigenin *C*-glucoside [11]. Peak #10 might correspond to apigenin rutinoside [12], but the UV-vis spectral characteristics of peak #13 might indicate a *p*-coumaric acid derivative of apigenin glucoside [10].

Table 1. UV-vis and mass spectral characteristics of the main polyphenolic phytochemicals detected in the Bt extracts of *S. mucronata*.

Peak	Rt (min)	λ_{max} (nm)	$[M + H]^+$ (*m*/*z*)	Other Ions (*m*/*z*)	Tentative Identity
1	16.39	298 (s), 322	779	765, 751, 731, 503, 489, 457, 355, 163	Chlorogenate derivative
2	24.68	242, 292 (s), 344	763	627, 465, 441, 393, 371, 303	Quercetin derivative
3	25.11	250, 348	449	287	Luteolin glucoside
4	26.32	278, 300 (s), 344	653	611, 287	Luteolin derivative
5	26.52	242, 374 (s), 392	669	653, 517, 303	Quercetin derivative
6	26.72	272, 300, 330	653	449	Isoscutellarein acetylallosylglucoside
7	26.88	265, 340	433	271	Apigenin *C*-glucoside
8	29.03	270, 304 (s), 358	653	287	Luteolin derivative
9	29.73	252, 280, 344	695	653, 287	Luteolin derivative
10	32.74	234, 336	579	447, 271	Apigenin derivative
11	33.73	264, 302 (s), 364	695	717 $[M + Na]^+$, 287	Luteolin derivative
12	33.97	232, 276, 306, 332	695	717 $[M + Na]^+$, 287	Luteolin derivative
13	34.35	234, 268, 316, 344	579	601 $[M + Na]^+$, 271	Apigenin derivative

4. Conclusions

In this study, a partial fractionation of *S. mucronata* extracts was carried out in an effort to obtain a polyphenol-enriched fraction. Out of the two fractions generated, the *n*-butanol one showed particularly high polyphenolic content and powerful, dose-dependent antiradical activity. The characterisation of this extract by means of liquid chromatography-diode array-mass spectrometry enabled the tentative identification of 13 polyphenols, which were mainly flavone glycosides, accompanied by flavonol glycosides and a chlorogenic acid derivative. Similar compounds have been detected in several other Lamiaceae species, which possess a variety of beneficial bioactivities. To the best of the authors' knowledge, this is the first report on the polyphenolic composition of the native Cretan *S. mucronata*, and may provide valuable data for future studies that will aim at investigating the possible biological effects of this particular botanical species, which remain unexamined to date. Since the results from the in vitro examination of the antioxidant activity are only indicative of the antioxidant effects of the extracts, future studies should include both in vitro (e.g., cell lines) and in vivo assays to clearly demonstrate the possible pharmacological potency of *S. mucronata*.

Acknowledgments: The authors acknowledge the kind donation of certified plant material from the Mediterranean Plant Conservation Centre (Chania, Greece).

Author Contributions: Spyros Grigorakis and Dimitris P. Makris commonly contributed to the analyses, data handling, and the writing of the paper.

Conflicts of Interest: The authors declare no conflict of interest.

References

1. Wang, Y. Needs for new plant-derived pharmaceuticals in the post-genome era: An industrial view in drug research and development. *Phytochem. Rev.* **2008**, *7*, 395–406. [CrossRef]
2. Li, A.-N.; Li, S.; Zhang, Y.-J.; Xu, X.-R.; Chen, Y.-M.; Li, H.-B. Resources and biological activities of natural polyphenols. *Nutrients* **2014**, *6*, 6020–6047. [CrossRef] [PubMed]
3. Dai, J.; Mumper, R.J. Plant phenolics: Extraction, analysis and their antioxidant and anticancer properties. *Molecules* **2010**, *15*, 7313–7352. [CrossRef] [PubMed]

4. Tair, A.; Weiss, E.-K.; Palade, L.M.; Loupassaki, S.; Makris, D.P.; Ioannou, E.; Roussis, V.; Kefalas, P. *Origanum* species native to the island of Crete: In vitro antioxidant characteristics and liquid chromatography–mass spectrometry identification of major polyphenolic components. *Nat. Prod. Res.* **2014**, *28*, 1284–1287. [CrossRef] [PubMed]
5. Krishnaiah, D.; Sarbatly, R.; Nithyanandam, R. A review of the antioxidant potential of medicinal plant species. *Food Bioprod. Process.* **2011**, *89*, 217–233. [CrossRef]
6. Atwi, M.; Weiss, E.-K.; Loupassaki, S.; Makris, D.P.; Ioannou, E.; Roussis, V.; Kefalas, P. Major antioxidant polyphenolic phytochemicals of three *Salvia* species endemic to the island of Crete. *J. Herbs Spices Med. Plants* **2016**, *22*, 27–34. [CrossRef]
7. Karakashov, B.; Grigorakis, S.; Loupassaki, S.; Mourtzinos, I.; Makris, D.P. Optimisation of organic solvent-free polyphenol extraction from *Hypericum triquetrifolium* Turra using Box–Behnken experimental design and kinetics. *Int. J. Ind. Chem.* **2015**, *6*, 85–92. [CrossRef]
8. Dourtoglou, V.G.; Mamalos, A.; Makris, D.P. Storage of olives (*Olea europaea*) under CO_2 atmosphere: Effect on anthocyanins, phenolics, sensory attributes and in vitro antioxidant properties. *Food Chem.* **2006**, *99*, 342–349. [CrossRef]
9. Karakashov, B.; Grigorakis, S.; Loupassaki, S.; Makris, D.P. Optimisation of polyphenol extraction from *Hypericum perforatum* (St. John's Wort) using aqueous glycerol and response surface methodology. *J. Appl. Res. Med. Aromat. Plants* **2015**, *2*, 1–8. [CrossRef]
10. Marin, P.D.; Grayer, R.J.; Grujic-Jovanovic, S.; Kite, G.C.; Veitch, N.C. Glycosides of tricetin methyl ethers as chemosystematic markers in *Stachys* subgenus Betonica. *Phytochemistry* **2004**, *65*, 1247–1253. [CrossRef] [PubMed]
11. Karageorgou, I.; Grigorakis, S.; Lalas, S.; Makris, D.P. Enhanced extraction of antioxidant polyphenols from *Moringa oleifera* Lam. leaves using a biomolecule-based low-transition temperature mixture. *Eur. Food Res. Technol.* **2017**, *243*, 1839–1848. [CrossRef]
12. Dedousi, M.; Mamoudaki, V.; Grigorakis, S.; Makris, D.P. Ultrasound-assisted extraction of polyphenolic antioxidants from olive (*Olea europaea*) leaves using a novel glycerol/sodium-potassium tartrate low-transition temperature mixture (LTTM). *Environments* **2017**, *4*, 31. [CrossRef]

medicines

MDPI

Article

Dose-Dependent Effects of Green Tea or Maté Extracts on Lipid and Protein Oxidation in Brine-Injected Retail-Packed Pork Chops

Sisse Jongberg [1,*], Mari Ann Tørngren [2] and Leif H. Skibsted [1]

[1] Department of Food Science, University of Copenhagen, Rolighedsvej 30, DK-1958 Frederiksberg, Denmark; ls@food.ku.dk

[2] Danish Meat Research Institute, Danish Technological Institute, Gregersensvej 9, DK-2630 Taastrup, Denmark; matn@teknologisk.dk

* Correspondence: jongberg@food.ku.dk; Tel.: +45-3533-2181; Fax: +45-3533-3344

Received: 11 December 2017; Accepted: 16 January 2018; Published: 22 January 2018

Abstract: Background: Phenolic plant extracts are added as antioxidants in meat to prevent lipid oxidation, but depending on the concentration applied, may affect proteins either through covalent interactions or by serving as a prooxidant. **Methods:** Brine-injected pork chops prepared with green tea extract (25–160 ppm gallic acid equivalents (GAE)), or maté extract (25–160 ppm GAE) and stored (5 °C, 7 days) in high-oxygen atmosphere packaging (MAP: 80% O2 and 20% CO2) were analyzed for color changes, lipid oxidation by thiobarbituric acid reactive substances (TBARS), and protein oxidation evaluated by thiol loss and protein radical formation by electron spin resonance (ESR) spectroscopy, and compared to a control without antioxidant. **Results:** Extract of maté and green tea showed significant and comparable antioxidative effects against formation of TBARS in brine-injected pork chops for all concentrations applied compared to the control. Protein radical formation decreased significantly by addition of 25 ppm maté extract, but increased significantly by addition of 80–160 ppm green tea extract, when monitored as formation of protein radicals. Meanwhile, protein thiol groups disappeared when applying the extracts by reactions assigned to addition reactions of oxidized phenols from the extracts to protein thiols. **Conclusion:** Maté is accordingly a good source of antioxidants for protection of both lipids and proteins in brine-injected pork chops chill-stored in high-oxygen atmosphere, though the dose must be carefully selected.

Keywords: brine injection; pork; green tea extract; maté extract; lipid oxidation; protein oxidation; modified atmosphere packaging

1. Introduction

Modified atmosphere packaging and storage of meat has been attracting attention of producers, consumers, and scientists, as packaging in high oxygen concentration combined with carbon dioxide is a valuable tool for extending the microbiological shelf-life of meat. However, high-oxygen modified atmosphere packaging (MAP) may impair meat quality due to both lipid and protein oxidation [1], and these hazardous effects of MAP have been thoroughly explored in meat sold for retail, whereas meat produced and distributed for food service (canteens, nursing homes, and schools) has been given little consideration in regard to the effects of high-oxygen MAP. The food service sector is an expanding marked with a turnover of more than 5.6 billion euro per year in Denmark. Meat produced for food service must benefit from increased robustness, as the meat often is cooked and eaten in different places often undergoing reheating and longer distribution times. Especially, the tenderness and juiciness are often compromised because the meat is commonly heat-treatment to minimum 75 °C once or twice before consumption. Such robust meat products can be produced by brine-injection, which are found to stabilize the tenderness and juiciness [2]. In 2007, 28% pork and 16% beef in the US were enhanced by adding moisture through brine injection [3]. Salt and sugar added to the brine, bind water in the meat, and the meat products become more robust, gain weight, and show improved tenderness and increased juiciness after cooking [4].

Meat cuts sold for food service are distributed both in MAP and in vacuum, and both chilled and/or frozen. As recently reviewed by Suman et al. [5], high oxygen MAP improves meat color, but impairs the eating quality by accelerating oxidation of lipids and proteins, resulting in off-flavor formation, and less tender and juicy meat. Phenolic antioxidants extracted from herbs and spices and other botanicals, have been shown to stabilize meat color and to be efficient protectors against lipid oxidation when added to animal feed [6,7], when mixed into minced meat products [8,9], or when used in marinades for entire meat cuts [10,11]. The phenols in the plant extracts act as radical scavengers and metal chelators, inhibiting reactive oxygen species from initiating oxidation of lipids. With regards to protein oxidation, phenols have also been shown to be able to hamper oxidative protein modifications, such as in frankfurters prepared from Iberian pigs and added rosemary essential oil (150–600 ppm), where the protein carbonyl content was reduced during storage (4 °C/60 days) [12]. However, the same group found a prooxidative effect on protein carbonyls for the same experimental set-up using white pigs [13], indicating unexpected effects of phenolic antioxidants on protein oxidation, which highly depends on unknown parameters. Furthermore, studies have shown that the phenols are likely to react with the thiols or other nucleophiles in meat protein, generating protein-phenol adducts [14,15]. Any effects of formation of such adducts in fresh whole meat cuts are so far unidentified, but it has been suggested that the adduct formation may increase the protein cross-linking and polymerization, and hence increase meat toughness [14]. Most studies considering the effects of natural antioxidants applied to meat, explore the effects in minced meat of various animal origins. However, the effects of phenolic antioxidants injected into roast or chops, are less explored, even though injection-enhancement is a commonly used technology in meat production worldwide. Investigations focusing on this technology seem accordingly relevant, since phenolic antioxidants may preserve meat tenderness, a sensory quality of far more importance to whole meat cuts than for minced meats.

The aim of the present study was to investigate the dose-dependent effects of phenolic extracts from green tea and maté on the oxidative stability of MAP pork chops. Green tea (*Camellia sinensis*) is commonly used as antioxidant in various food products [16], whereas maté (*Ilex paraguariensis*) is a less utilized source of phenols. Maté consists of leaves from a South American bush and is rich in caffeic acid derivatives [17], and has successfully been used as an antioxidant added to meat or as a feed supplement for chicken and cattle protecting against lipid oxidation [7,18,19]. In the present study, the oxidative stability with regards to color, lipid, and protein was explored in MAP retail-packed pork chops cut from injection-enhanced loins containing three different levels of green tea or maté extract to compare the two sources of antioxidants including their dose-dependence on the oxidative stability of pork.

2. Materials and Methods

2.1. Plant Extracts and Chemicals

Green tea (*Camellia sinensis*) extract "Guardian Green Tea 20 M", a commercial product with Product description PD 215033-6.0EN) was obtained from DuPont Nutrition and Biosciences ApS, Brabrand, Denmark. Maté (*Ilex paraguariensis*) extract from Centroflora, Botucatu, Sao Paulo, Brazil, was kindly provided by Daniel Cardoso at University of Sao Paulo in Sao Carlos. Details regarding extract composition and extraction method are previously published [19]. All other reagents were of analytical grade. Double-deionized water (Milipore, Bedford, MA, USA) was used throughout.

2.2. Total Phenolic Content in Extracts

In order to control the amount of phenols injected into the pork, the total phenolic content was determined in the maté extract by Folin Ciocalteu's method as described by Singleton and Rossi [20]. The total phenolic content in the green tea extract was previously determined to be 23.8% [21], and this concentration was applied throughout this investigation. In brief, 100 μL 1 mg/mL maté extract dissolved to a total volume of 1500 μL double-deionized water, was left to react with 125 μL Folin–Ciocalteu phenol reagent (Sigma-Aldrich, St. Louis, MO, USA) for 8 min. Subsequently, 375 μL 20% sodium carbonate was added and the reaction mixture was left to incubate at 20 °C for 2 h. The phenol concentration was determined spectrophotometrically at 765 nm against a standard curve prepared from gallic acid. The concentrations are given in gallic acid equivalents (g/100 g dry extract; % *w*/*w*).

2.3. Preparation and Storage of Injected Pork Loins

Twelve pork loins (*logissimus dorsi*) from 6 female pigs slaughtered on the same day and with similar and normal pH (~5.6) were collected from a Danish slaughterhouse and transported to the Danish Meat Research Institute (Roskilde, Denmark). The loins were divided in half to obtain 24 half loins, and four loins from the same pig were injected with either salt brine or salt brine added three different concentrations of extract. The neutral salt brine was based on water and contained 6.6% NaCl and 5.5% dextrose, which is the common composition used by the industry. The brines with extract were based on the results from the Folin Ciocalteu analysis of total phenolic content, and the neutral salt brine was added 0.10, 0.31, or 0.63% green tea extract, or 0.11, 0.34, or 0.69% maté extract, to obtain 100, 350 or 700 ppm extract, or 25, 80, or 160 ppm phenolic compounds (gallic acid equivalents, GAE) in the injected loins with an expected gain of 12% (*w*/*w*). Both left and right loins from three pigs were used for the treatment with green tea extract ($n = 3$, A, B, C), and left and right loins from three other pigs were used for the treatment with maté extract ($n = 3$, A, B, C). The loins were divided in halves, and three half loins were added the low concentration of phenolics (25 ppm), another added the medium concentration (80 ppm), and a third the high concentration (160 ppm). Additionally, one half loin from each pig were injected with salt brine, resulting in six replicates of the control without antioxidant (A–F). Samples treated with 25, 80 or 160 ppm GAE green tea extract are named GT1, GT2, GT3, respectively, and samples treated with 25, 80 or 160 ppm GAE maté extract are named M1, M2, M3, respectively. The half loins were weighted prior to injection for the determination of weight-gain. The weight-gain was further used to calculate the exact amount of phenolic compounds present in the meat:

Calculation example:

(1) Phenol content in brine: 0.10% extract in brine correspond to 0.1 g/100 mL 23.8% = 0.238 mg/mL phenol in brine
(2) Phenol in loin (2.02 kg) for a weight-gain of 229 g (mL): 229 mL 0.238 mg/mL phenol = 54.5 mg phenol
(3) Phenol (ppm) in loin: 54.5 mg phenol/2.02 kg meat = 27.0 mg phenol/kg meat = 27 ppm.

The injections were performed using a multichannel brine injector (FMG 26/52, Fomaco A/S, Køge, Denmark) with 66 punch/minute, 1.0 bar pressure, and 3.0 bar up-pressure. The injected half loins were covered in plastic bags to avoid evaporation from the surface and left to equalize overnight in the dark at 2–5 °C. Next day, the loins were dabbed with tissue and weighted for calculation of total weight-gain. The final concentration of phenolic compounds in ppm was calculated based on the total weight-gain for each loin. Every half loin was subsequently sliced in 8 pork chops of 2.0 cm and the whole loin numbered 1–16, having number 1–8 starting from the hip-end and 9–16 ending in the neck-end. The pork chops were then randomized for the various analyses, and the pork chops to be analyzed on day 1 were vacuum packed and stored cold until analysis the next day. The pork chops to be stored for day 7 were packed in modified atmosphere packaging (MAP, 80% O_2/20% CO_2) using a traysealer (T200, Multivac, Wolfertschwenden, Germany). Tray (K2190-53H clear/MAPET) and film

(Toplex HB PET EP40 code 2600/040, oxygen permeability: 2.5 cc/m^2/24 h) for MAP were obtained from Færch Plast (Holstebro, Denmark). No soaker pads were applied. Trays were transported to University of Copenhagen (Frederiksberg, Denmark) and stored for 7 days at 5 °C in a display cabinet with light exposure (~950 lux as measured on product surface) for 10 h daily. At the end of storage, the surface color was measured for all samples before mincing. The mince was afterwards carefully mixed, divided in smaller portions, vacuum packed and stored at −80 °C until analysis.

2.4. Color Analysis

Color was measured on all samples through the packaging film using a Konica Minolta Spectrophotometer CM-600d (illuminant D65, 10° standard observer, 8 mm aperture) and the corresponding Color Data Software CM-S100w SpectraMagic™ NX (Konica Minolta Sensing Inc., Osaka, Japan). CIE (Commission International de l'Éclairage) 1976 L* (lightness), a* (redness), b* (yellowness), C* (chroma), and h (hue angle) values were determined. Reflectance spectra within the visual spectrum (400–700 nm in 10 nm intervals) were measured simultaneously. Each value of the color parameters and reflectance represents an average of five measurements per sample. From L*, a*, and b* the total color difference (ΔE) was calculated [22]:

$$\Delta E = \sqrt{(\Delta L^2 + \Delta a^2 + \Delta b^2)} \tag{1}$$

2.5. Lipid Oxidation by TBARS

Lipid oxidation in the pork loins was determined by TBARS analysis according to Vyncke [23] and Sørensen & Jørgensen [24] as described in Jongberg et al. [25]. TBARS were determined in the meat spectrophotometrically after reaction with 2-thiobarbituric acid at 532 nm using 600 nm as baseline. Results are expressed as 2-thiobarbituric reactive substances (TBARS) in mg MDA (malondialdehyde equivalents)/kg dry matter using a standard curve and are presented as mean ± sd (n = 3, but for control sample, n = 6).

2.6. Myofibrillar Protein Isolates (MPI)

Myofibrillar proteins were isolated from the pork chops according to the method described by Park et al. [26] with slight modifications as described by Koutina et al. [27]. Three replicates were prepared per sample type (n = 3). The myofibrillar protein isolates (MPI) were lyophilized and stored at −20 °C until analysis.

2.7. Protein Thiol Concentration

Protein thiol groups were determined in the MPI after derivatization with DTNB (5,5 dithiobis(2-nitrobenzoic acid, Sigma-Aldrich, St. Louis, MO, USA) [28] as previously described [29].

2.8. Protein Radical Detection

MPI was transferred to clear fused quartz ESR tubes (inner diameter 4 mm, wall 0.5 mm, Wilmad, Buena, NJ, USA) to reach approximately 5 cm filling of the tube. The tubes were placed in the cavity of a JEOL JES-FR30X ESR spectrometer (JEOL Ltd., Tokyo, Japan) and measured according to Gravador et al. [6]. The radical signal intensity relative to a Mn(II) standard was calculated based on the density of the sample measured as g/cm in the ESR tube [Radical intensity (Spin) = (signal area sample/signal area Mn(II))/density sample (g/cm)].

2.9. Statistical Data Analysis

Statistical analysis was performed using R© version 3.4.2., The R Foundation for Statistical Computing (ISBN: 3-900051-07-0). Data were analyzed by analysis of variance using a linear model with mixed effects with the variables "Treatment" and "Phenol concentration" as fixed effects, and "End" as random effect. Where "Phenol concentration" was found insignificant for the statistical model, it was excluded as a variable. The significance level used was $p < 0.05$. A partial least square regression (PLSR) plot without standardization on individual observations (three per treatment) was conducted using Unscrambler (version 9.8) by applying a design matrix of injection brine, phenolic concentration and day as X-matrix, and color and oxidation parameters as Y-matrix.

3. Results

A PLSR plot gave an overview of the parameters investigated in the present study (Figure 1). The correlation loadings plot shows that the variation in PC1 was primarily explained by differences between day 1 and day 7 resulting in a gradient of time going from right (day 1) to left (day 7). Day 1 associated with redness (a*) and the concentration of thiol groups, whereas day 7 associated with hue and lightness. The variation in PC2 was explained by the difference in brine with the control (salt brine) and green tea extract or the phenol concentration extending the axis in each direction. The control sample were associated with chroma, yellowness (b*) and TBARS, and green tea extract and the phenol concentration were associated with radical intensity. Maté extract was found in the middle, and closest to the control.

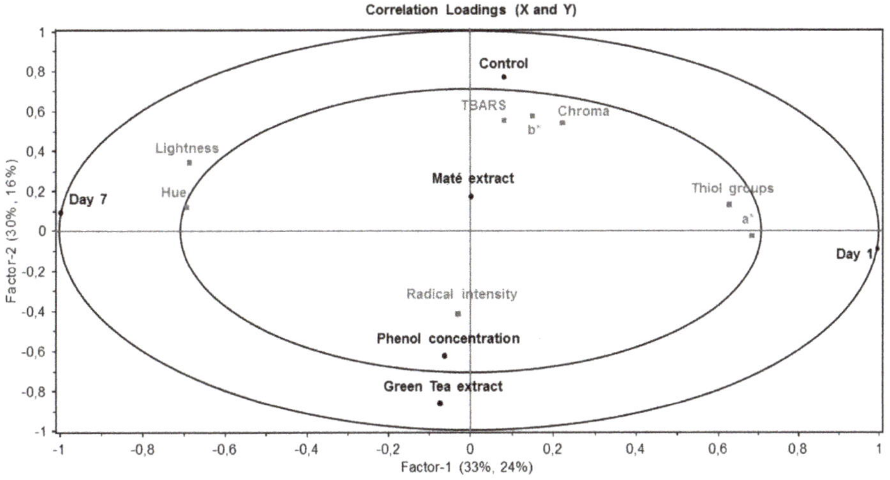

Figure 1. Oxidation parameters presented as a PLSR correlation loadings plot for PC1 versus PC2 of pork chops injected with three different concentrations of green tea or maté extract (25–180 ppm gallic acid equivalents), and chill stored in high-oxygen modified atmosphere packaging (MAP) for 1 or 7 days. The model was derived from treatment variables (injection brine [Control, Green tea, or maté extract], phenol concentration, and day) in the X-matrix, and color parameters and oxidation parameters in the Y-matrix. Ellipses represent $r^2 = 0.5$ and 1.0.

3.1. *Weight-Gain and Phenolic Content*

The concentration of extract in the brine injected half loins was based on the total phenolic content determined in gallic acid equivalents by the Folin-Ciocalteu method. The phenolic content in the green tea extract was 23.8 g/100 g [21] and for the maté extract 21.7 g/100 g. The final phenol content in the brine-injected pork loins was calculated with respect to the actual weight gain in each half loin after injection and equalization (Table 1).

The calculated phenol content was found to vary more for the phenol concentration levels at 80 and 160 ppm. The variation was assigned to the variation in weight-gain between the hip- and neck-end of the loins. The gain for the hip-end was in average 8.8 ± 2.3%, which is significantly lower than for the neck-end, which was in average 13.8 ± 2.0%. From a technological point of view, this means that when injecting pork loins, the injection procedure must be adjusted according to whether it is the hip or neck part that is being subject to injection. This will ensure minimum variation in weight-gain, and hence, low variation in the extract concentration applied to each half loin. For the discussion of the results in the present study, the actual phenol concentration in each half loin is accordingly taken into consideration when evaluating the results.

Table 1. Concentration of extract (aimed) and phenols (aimed and calculated, mean ± sd) in brine injected-pork chops.

Treatment	$[Extract]_{Aimed}$ (~ppm)	$[Phenols]_{Aimed}$ (~ppm GAE *)	$[Phenols]_{Calculated}$ ** (ppm GAE)
Control	-	-	-
GT1	100	25	29 ± 0 ^{d}
GT2	350	80	68 ± 13 ^{c}
GT3	700	160	105 ± 36 ^{b}
M1	100	25	28 ± 4 ^{d}
M2	350	80	83 ± 11 ^{b,c}
M3	700	160	150 ± 33 ^{a}

* GAE = gallic acid equivalents. ** Calculated from the weight-gain of brine-injected pork loins. $^{a-d}$ Different letters (a–d) denotes significant ($p < 0.05$) difference between calculated concentrations of phenols.

3.2. *Color Changes*

The color of the injected pork loins was evaluated after 7 days of storage in MAP. Data showed that the lightness, the b-value, and chroma value were significantly different depending on the injection brines (Table 2). In the CIELAB color space, the b axis extends from blue (−b) to yellow (+b) and chroma is perceived as the strength of surface color, also defined as the brightness or colorfulness of the object.

Table 2. Color parameters (mean ± sd) and the total color difference (ΔE) in brine-injected pork chops.

Treatment *	Color Parameter			ΔE
	Lightness	*b*-Value	Chroma	
Control	58.78 ± 1.65 ^{a}	7.34 ± 0.18 ^{a,b}	7.37 ± 0.18 ^{a,b}	0.0
GT1	56.45 ± 0.49 ^{b,c}	4.70 ± 0.01 ^{b,c}	4.71 ± 0.01 ^{c}	3.1
GT2	55.96 ± 1.30 ^{c}	6.06 ± 0.95 ^{b}	6.13 ± 0.96 ^{b,c}	3.1
GT3	56.60 ± 0.51 ^{b,c}	4.83 ± 0.62 ^{c}	4.86 ± 0.65 ^{c}	3.3
M1	57.98 ± 1.41 ^{a,b,c}	6.34 ± 0.90 ^{a,b}	6.43 ± 0.97 ^{a,b}	1.3
M2	58.64 ± 1.36 ^{a,b}	7.20 ± 0.28 ^{a}	7.26 ± 0.29 ^{a}	0.2
M3	56.21 ± 0.62 ^{b,c}	6.46 ± 0.76 ^{a,b}	6.48 ± 0.77 ^{a,b}	2.7

* Stored in high-oxygen modified atmosphere packaging (MAP) for 7 days (5 °C). $^{a-c}$ Different letters (a–c) denotes significant ($p < 0.05$) values within the same column.

Results indicated that application of green tea or maté extract to the brine reduced the lightness, b* and chroma, resulting in less yellow and less bright colored pork loins. No effect of the extract concentration or interaction between injection brine and concentration on any of the color parameters were observed. Calculation of total color difference (ΔE), which is a metric for understanding how the human eye perceives color difference, resulted in ΔE > 3 for the pork chops added green tea extract. Typically, values ~2.3 corresponds to JND *(just noticeable difference)* [22]. The pork chops added the low and intermediate concentration of maté extract were <2.3 and hence, not noticeable by the human eye, whereas the high concentration of maté with ΔE = 2.7 also were within the category of JND.

3.3. Lipid Oxidation

The secondary lipid oxidation products measured as TBARS were quantified after 1 and 7 days of storage. At day 1, no significant difference in TBARS was observed between any of the treatments (data not shown), and the average concentration was found to be 8.6 ± 1.8 µmol MDA/kg DM (mean ± sd). On the other hand, at day 7 the level of TBARS differed between treatments ($p = 0.0018$) as TBARS were found to be lower in the pork loins injected with green tea extract or with maté extract. As seen from Figure 2A, the decrease tended to be dependent on the concentration level of phenolic compounds, but no significant difference was observed between the two extracts, or between concentration levels.

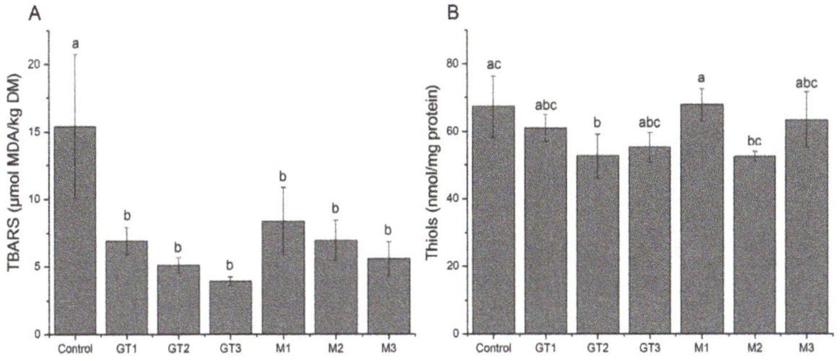

Figure 2. (**A**) Secondary lipid oxidation products as determined by TBARS (µmol MDA equivalents per kg dry matter) and (**B**) protein thiol concentration (nmol/mg protein) in pork chops injected with three different concentrations (denoted 1, 2, or 3 corresponding to 25, 80, and 160 ppm phenolic compounds, respectively) of green tea (GT) or maté extract (M) and chill stored in high-oxygen modified atmosphere packaging (MAP) for 7 days. Different letters (a–c) denotes significant ($p < 0.05$) difference between samples.

Even though the brine contained equal concentrations of phenolics, based on gallic acid equivalents determined by the Folin-Ciocalteu method, the actual phenol concentrations varied between samples as shown in Table 1. For the high dose, the concentration of green tea was found to be significantly lower than the concentration of maté, which makes it difficult to compare across treatment for the high concentration level. The phenolic composition of green tea is different from the composition of maté extract, and this may also affect their antioxidative effect, as the different phenolics may have different mode of action. So, even though the reducing capacity against the Folin-Ciocalteu reagent is the same, it does not a priori provide any information about the actual mechanism by which the extracts serve as an antioxidant protecting the lipids.

The phenolic composition of green tea extract has been widely characterized and consists primarily of flavonoids, such as catechin, epicatechin, epicatechin gallate, epigallocatechin gallate, and quercetin, with lower levels of hydrocinnamic acids, caffeic, coumaric, and ferulic acid [16]. In contrast, maté extract consists primarily of caffeoyl derivatives including caffeic acid, chlorogenic acid, as well as various dicaffeoylquinic acids [17]. The maté extract used in the present study contains 58.2% chlorogenic acid and 28.4% 1,5-dicaffeoylquinic acid [19]. In meat, one of the primary oxidation initiators is the hydrogen peroxide-activated hypervalent myoglobin species, and a recent study demonstrated, that extracts from green tea and maté were equally effective in reducing the perferrylmyoglobin radical, and that the total phenolic content had more impact on the reducing capacity rather than the specific phenolic composition [30]. However, when it comes to protecting against lipid oxidation as determined by the formation of secondary lipid oxidation products, TBARS, the present study shows that green tea extract is more effective as an antioxidant as compared to maté. Figure 3 shows that both extracts protected against TBARS in a dose-dependent manner, and that the increment in effect was similar (comparable slopes) for both extracts by increasing concentrations. However, green tea is 3-fold more effective in lowering TBARS (50 ppm phenolics from green tea extract resulted in the same TBARS concentration as 160 ppm phenolics from maté extract). The correlation coefficients for the linear regressions presented in Figure 3 indicate a large variation in the pork chops added extracts. This was especially distinguished for the pork chops that had added maté extract, which makes it difficult to predict antioxidative effects in large-scale productions. This aspect has already been further investigated in our laboratory.

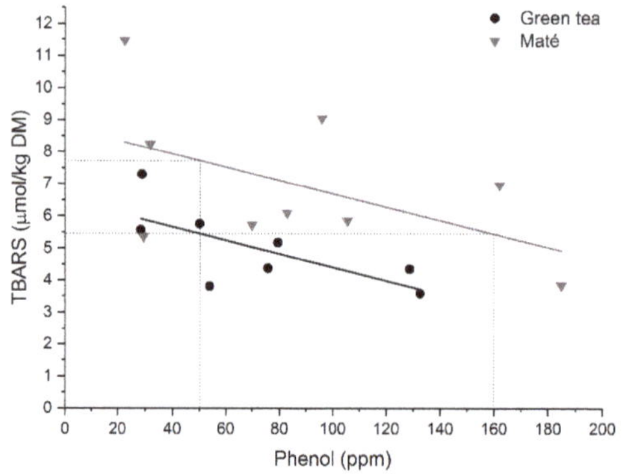

Figure 3. TBARS plotted as a function of phenolic content for all samples containing green tea or maté extract. Linear fit for samples added green tea extract (●): y = −0.0210x · 6.50, R^2 = 0.488, and for samples added maté extract (▼): y = −0.0208x · 8.77, R^2 = 0.272. Dashed lines indicate the concentration of phenol needed to obtain comparable TBARS levels.

3.4. Protein Oxidation

Protein oxidation as evaluated by the loss of thiol groups were quantified in the myofibrillar fraction of the meat proteins, the MPI. No significant differences between samples were observed at day 1 (data not shown) and the average concentration was found to be 75.9 ± 10.1 nmol/mg protein (mean ± sd). At day 7, a significant loss in thiols were observed for GT2 (p = 0.0439), and M2 was also close to significantly reducing the thiol concentration (p = 0.0549), as compared to the control without antioxidant (Figure 2B). None of the other concentration levels affected the protein thiols. This suggests that green tea extract, and possibly maté extract, may decrease the thiol concentration when added to pork loins stored in high-oxygen MAP, indicating that these extracts not solely serves as antioxidants protecting against oxidation. Similar results have previously been reported [9,14,25,31], and has been explained by the reaction between the quinones, which are the oxidation products of the phenols, and the protein thiol groups [15,31]. The quinones are strong electrophilic compounds and reacts rapidly with nucleophiles, such as thiol and amino groups forming covalent protein-phenol adducts [32,33]. Addition of green tea extract (as seen for the 25–375 ppm concentration interval of phenolic compounds) to meat emulsions showed that heat treatment (70 ° for 15 min) depleted thiols in a dose-dependent manner, and it was suggested, that the excessive loss of thiols predominantly was caused by thiol-quinone adduct formation [14]. Likewise, recent studies by other groups have demonstrated that addition of chlorogenic acid [34], catechin [35], or (-)-epigallocatechin-3-gallate (EGCG) [36] to myofibrillar proteins change the physicochemical properties of the proteins, especially the gelling properties. The changes are found to be either advantageous or detrimental depending on the concentration applied, and all mentioned studies assign the changes to be caused by the formation of quinone-protein covalent interactions. Application of phenolic rich extracts has a multifaceted role in meat by being both anti- or prooxidative and playing a part in the structural development of proteins especially during heat treatment.

The concentration of protein radicals was quantified using electron spin resonance (ESR) spectrometry on a relative scale expressed as radical intensity. The radical intensity did not develop significantly during the storage time of 7 days in any of the samples, therefore only day 7 results are presented in Figure 4. As seen from the figure, GT2 and GT3 were found to have significantly higher protein radical intensity, whereas M1 was found to have significantly lower protein radical intensity as compared to the control sample without extract (Figure 4B). It appeared that the green tea extract increased the protein radical intensity in a dose-dependent manner, whereas maté had no such effect, but in contrast protected against protein radical formation for the lower concentrations applied. This became evident by comparing the shape of the ESR spectra, where especially GT3 resulted in a distinctly increased signal (Figure 4B).

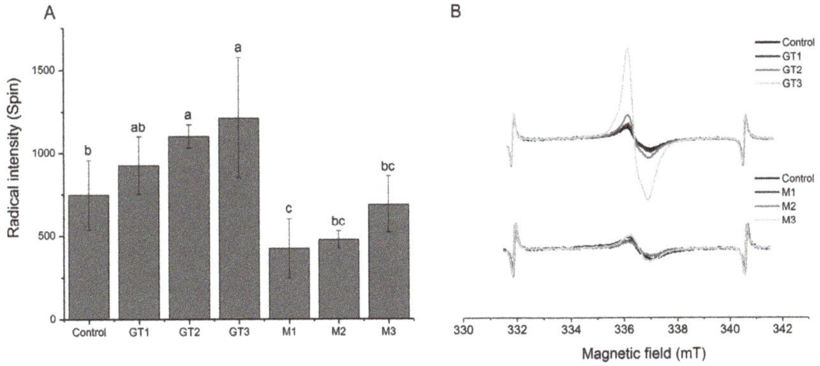

Figure 4. (**A**) Protein radical intensity (Spin) and (**B**) representative ESR spectra of MPI isolated from pork chops injected with three different concentrations (denoted 1, 2, or 3 corresponding to 25, 80, and 160 ppm phenolic compounds, respectively) of green tea (GT) or maté extract (M) and chill stored in high-oxygen modified atmosphere packaging (MAP) for 7 days. Different letters (a–c) denotes significant ($p < 0.05$) difference between samples.

An increased protein radical intensity may be caused by prooxidant effects of phenols added as plant extracts. Especially tea-polyphenols have been found to generate hydrogen peroxide upon oxidation carrying the risk of compromising the oxidative stability of food components in the presence of metal catalysts such as iron through generation of hydroxyl radicals. It has, however, also been demonstrated that food proteins may play an important role in retarding this prooxidant effects of phenolic compounds [37]. In meat, this latter property of the proteins may be essential, due to the high concentration of protein, which then may act as an endogenous antioxidative system. It seems likely, that meat proteins will scavenge radicals generated by oxidation of phenolic compounds catalyzed by transition metals. Meat proteins have high molecular weight and radicals may stabilize within the protein structure, reduce their reactivity, and accumulate in the meat as stable protein radicals. In this way, the increased protein radical intensity observed in the present study may be the result of a prooxidant effect of the green tea extract generating stable protein radicals.

Other explanations for the elevated radical intensity should also be considered. A previous study on Bologna-type sausages added green tea extract as antioxidant showed a similar increase in radical intensity [25]. However, in that study the ESR spectra of the MPI from the control sausage versus the sausage added green tea extract were different, indicating that the radical species formed in the samples were different. It was suggested that the covalent protein-phenol adducts generated through thiol-quinone interactions, could scavenge and stabilize radicals, generating phenoxyl radicals attached to the protein, in effect increasing the radical signal intensity observed. In the present study, when comparing the shape of the ESR signal from the control sample with a sample containing green tea, no apparent difference was observed (data not shown). This indicates that different phenomena take place in the two systems, and that heat treatment might be a crucial factor for the generation of sufficient thiol-quinone adducts to act as protein-bound radical scavengers. The modest reduction in the concentration of protein thiol groups observed in the present study (Figure 4) verifies that phenols from green tea only to a lesser extent had reacted with the protein thiols.

In contrast to the green tea extract, the maté extract decreased the radical intensity of the meat protein, and the lowest concentration of maté extract tested had the highest effect (Figure 4). A decreased radical intensity indicate that protein radicals have not been generated due to low prooxidant activity, or simply that the protein radicals have already reacted and caused damage in other targets of oxidation present in the meat.

3.5. Dose-Dependent Effects of Green Tea or Maté Extracts

For lipid oxidation, though not significantly, a dose-dependent effect of green tea was observed, where higher concentration of green tea extract caused lower TBARS levels. The same tendency was observed by addition of maté extract, still, without a significant decrease. For protein thiols, the level tended to decrease by at the intermediate phenol concentration, however, the dependency was only significant for green tea. For neither the TBARS nor thiol groups any significant differences were observed between green tea and maté extract added with similar phenol concentration. This was on the other hand observed for the protein radical intensity, with a significant difference between addition of the green tea or maté extract. In this case, green tea extract also showed a clear dose-dependence, elevating radical intensity when increasing extract addition. In contrast, addition of maté resulted in reduced or similar radical intensities as compared to the control samples without extract.

The difference in antioxidant mechanisms protecting against protein oxidation between the two extracts may be explained by differences in the structure of phenolic compounds. Green tea extract consists of catechins, which contains catechol structures that when oxidized are likely to form adducts with protein, even acting as prooxidants under oxidative conditions. Maté extract on the other hand, consists of caffeic acid derivatives, which may due to a higher molecular size and rigid structure will only react with nucleophiles in protein structures to a lesser degree. More studies on their individual behavior in meat and interaction with meat proteins are necessary to fully explore the potential of maté as antioxidant agents in injected meat.

4. Conclusions

Green tea and maté extracts reduced the formation of TBARS in brine-injected pork chops after 7 days storage in high oxygen MAP. No difference in the antioxidative protection of lipid oxidation was found between the two extracts, or between the different concentrations applied (25–160 ppm GAE). Furthermore, 25 ppm GAE maté extract reduced the formation of protein radicals as compared to the control, which indicated an antioxidative effect of maté against protein oxidation. In contrast, green tea extract was found to increase protein radical intensity especially for the higher concentrations (80–160 ppm GAE). Meanwhile, both green tea and maté extract tended to reduce protein thiol groups, and 80 ppm GAE green tea extract showed a significant loss of thiols, which may either be caused by prooxidative activity or covalent quinone-protein interactions. Maté is accordingly a good source of antioxidants for protection of both lipids and proteins in brine-injected pork, though the dose must be carefully selected.

Acknowledgments: The authors are grateful for the technical assistance of Daniel Gjerløv Rasmussen from Department of Food Science, University of Copenhagen for conducting the oxidation analyses. The authors thank Ann-Britt Frøstrup and Lars Blaabjerg at the Danish Meat Research Institute (DMRI), Danish Technological Institute and Margit Aaslyng at DMRI for assisting in the multivariate data analysis. The authors also thank The Danish Council for Independent Research Technology and Production within The Danish Agency for Science Technology and Innovation for granting the project entitled: "Antioxidant mechanisms of natural phenolic compounds against protein cross-link formation in meat and meat systems" (11-117033), and the Danish Pig

Levy Fund for funding experimental work performed at DMRI. The funding source had no involvement in the preparation of this article.

Author Contributions: Sisse Jongberg and Mari Ann Tørngren conceived and designed the experiments; Sisse Jongberg performed the experiments and analyzed the data; Mari Ann Tørngren and Leif H. Skibsted contributed with raw material, pilot plant facilities, reagents, and analysis tools; Sisse Jongberg, Mari Ann Tørngren, and Leif H. Skibsted wrote the paper.

Conflicts of Interest: The authors declare no conflict of interest.

References

1. McMillin, K.W. Where is MAP Going? A review and future potential of modified atmosphere packaging for meat. *Meat Sci.* **2008**, *80*, 43–65. [CrossRef] [PubMed]
2. Sheard, P.R.; Tali, A. Injection of salt, tripolyphosphate and bicarbonate marinade solutions to improve the yield and tenderness of cooked pork loin. *Meat Sci.* **2004**, *68*, 305–311. [CrossRef] [PubMed]
3. Crews, J. The 2007 national meat case study sheds new light on retail protein offerings. *Meat Poult.* **2007**, *53*, 42–52.
4. Grobbel, J.P.; Dikeman, M.E.; Hunt, M.C.; Milliken, G.A. Effects of different packaging atmospheres and injection-enhancement on beef tenderness, sensory attributes, desmin degradation, and display color. *J. Anim. Sci.* **2008**, *86*, 2697–2710. [CrossRef] [PubMed]
5. Suman, S.P.; Hunt, M.C.; Nair, M.N.; Rentfrow, G. Improving beef color stability: Practical strategies and underlying mechanisms. *Meat Sci.* **2014**, *98*, 490–504. [CrossRef] [PubMed]
6. Gravador, R.S.; Jongberg, S.; Andersen, M.L.; Luciano, G.; Priolo, A.; Lund, M.N. Dietary citrus pulp improves protein stability in lamb meat stored under aerobic conditions. *Meat Sci.* **2014**, *97*, 231–236. [CrossRef] [PubMed]
7. Racanicci, A.M.C.; Menten, J.F.M.; Alencar, S.M.; Buissa, R.S.; Skibsted, L.H. Mate (*Ilex paraguariensis*) as dietary additive for broilers: Performance and oxidative stability of meat. *Eur. Food Res. Technol.* **2011**, *232*, 655–661. [CrossRef]
8. Mitsumoto, M.; O'Grad, M.N.; Kerry, J.P.; Buckley, D.J. Addition of tea catechins and vitamin C on sensory evaluation, colour and lipid stability during chilled storage in cooked or raw beef and chicken patties. *Meat Sci.* **2005**, *69*, 773–779. [CrossRef] [PubMed]
9. Jongberg, S.; Skov, S.H.; Tørngren, M.A.; Skibsted, L.H.; Lund, M.N. Effect of white grape extract and modified atmosphere packaging on lipid and protein oxidation in chill stored beef patties. *Food Chem.* **2011**, *128*, 276–283. [CrossRef] [PubMed]
10. Kim, Y.J.; Jin, S.K.; Park, W.Y.; Kim, B.W.; Joo, S.T.; Yang, H.S. The effect of garlic or onion marinade on the lipid oxidation and meat quality of pork during cold storage. *J. Food Qual.* **2010**, *33*, 171–185. [CrossRef]
11. Mielnik, M.B.; Sem, S.; Egelandsdal, B.; Skrede, G. By-products from herbs essential oil production as ingredient in marinade for turkey thighs. *LWT Food Sci. Technol.* **2008**, *41*, 93–100. [CrossRef]
12. Estévez, M.; Ventanas, S.; Cava, R. Protein oxidation in frankfurters with increasing levels of added rosemary essential oil: Effect on color and texture deterioration. *J. Food Sci.* **2005**, *70*, C427–C432. [CrossRef]
13. Estévez, M.; Cava, R.N. Effectiveness of rosemary essential oil as an inhibitor of lipid and protein oxidation: Contradictory effects in different types of frankfurters. *Meat Sci.* **2006**, *72*, 348–355. [CrossRef] [PubMed]
14. Jongberg, S.; Terkelsen, L.D.; Miklos, R.; Lund, M.N. Green tea extract impairs meat emulsion properties by disturbing protein disulfide cross-linking. *Meat Sci.* **2015**, *100*, 2–9. [CrossRef] [PubMed]
15. Jongberg, S.; Gislason, N.E.; Lund, M.N.; Skibsted, L.H.; Waterhouse, A.L. Thiol-quinone adduct formation in myofibrillar proteins detected by LC-MS. *J. Agric. Food Chem.* **2011**, *59*, 6900–6905. [CrossRef] [PubMed]
16. Brewer, M.S. Natural Antioxidants: Sources, Compounds, Mechanisms of Action, and Potential Applications. *Compr. Rev. Food Sci. F* **2011**, *10*, 221–247. [CrossRef]
17. Heck, C.I.; De Mejia, E.G. Yerba Mate tea (*Ilex paraguariensis*): A comprehensive review on chemistry, health implications, and technological considerations. *J. Food Sci.* **2007**, *72*, R138–R151. [CrossRef] [PubMed]
18. Racanicci, A.M.C.; Allesen-Holm, B.H.; Skibsted, L.H. Sensory evaluation of precooked chicken meat with mate (*Ilex paraguariensis*) added as antioxidant. *Eur. Food Res. Technol.* **2009**, *229*, 277–280. [CrossRef]

19. De Zawadzki, A.; Arrivetti, L.O.R.; Vidal, M.P.; Catai, J.R.; Nassu, R.T.; Tullio, R.R.; Berndt, A.; Oliveira, C.R.; Ferreira, A.G.; Neves-Junior, L.F.; et al. Mate extract as feed additive for improvement of beef quality. *Food Res. Int.* **2017**, *99*, 336–347. [CrossRef] [PubMed]
20. Singleton, V.L.; Rossi, J.A. Colorimetry of total phenolics with phosphomolybdic-phosphotungstic acid reagents. *Am. J. Enol. Vitic.* **1965**, *16*, 144–158.
21. Jongberg, S.; Lund, M.N.; Østdal, H.; Skibsted, L.H. Phenolic Antioxidant Scavenging of Myosin Radicals Generated by Hypervalent Myoglobin. *J. Agric. Food Chem.* **2012**, *60*, 12020–12028. [CrossRef] [PubMed]
22. Sharma, G.; Bala, R. *Digital Color Imagine Handbook*, 1st ed.; CRC Press: Boca Raton, FL, USA, 2002.
23. Vyncke, W. Direct determination of the thio barbituric-acid value in trichloro acetic-acid extracts of fish as a measure of oxidative rancidity. *Fett Wiss Technol.* **1970**, *72*, 1084–1091.
24. Sørensen, G.; Jørgensen, S.S. A critical examination of some experimental variables in the 2-thiobarbituric acid (TBA) test for lipid oxidation in meat products. *Zeitschrift Für Lebensmittel-Untersuchung Und-Forschung* **1996**, *202*, 205–210. [CrossRef]
25. Jongberg, S.; Tørngren, M.A.; Gunvig, A.; Skibsted, L.H.; Lund, M.N. Effect of green tea or rosemary extract on protein oxidation in Bologna type sausages prepared from oxidatively stressed pork. *Meat Sci.* **2013**, *93*, 538–546. [CrossRef] [PubMed]
26. Park, D.; Xiong, Y.L.L.; Alderton, A.L. Concentration effects of hydroxyl radical oxidizing systems on biochemical properties of porcine muscle myofibrillar protein. *Food Chem.* **2007**, *101*, 1239–1246. [CrossRef]
27. Koutina, G.; Jongberg, S.; Skibsted, L.H. Protein and lipid oxidation in Parma ham during production. *J. Agric. Food Chem.* **2012**, *60*, 9737–9745. [CrossRef] [PubMed]
28. Ellman, G.L. Tissue sulfhydryl groups. *Arch. Biochem. Biophys.* **1959**, *82*, 70–77. [CrossRef]
29. Jongberg, S.; Wen, J.; Tørngren, M.A.; Lund, M.N. Effect of high-oxygen atmosphere packaging on oxidative stability and sensory quality of two chicken muscles during chill storage. *Food Pack. Shelf Life* **2014**, *1*, 38–48. [CrossRef]
30. Jongberg, S.; Lund, M.N.; Skibsted, L.H.; Davies, M.J. Competitive Reduction of Perferrylmyoglobin Radicals by Protein Thiols and Plant Phenols. *J. Agric. Food Chem.* **2014**, *62*, 11279–11288. [CrossRef] [PubMed]
31. Jongberg, S.; Lund, M.N.; Waterhouse, A.L.; Skibsted, L.H. 4-Methyl catechol inhibits protein oxidation in meat but not disulfide formation. *J. Agric. Food Chem.* **2011**, *59*, 10329–10335. [CrossRef] [PubMed]
32. Kroll, N.G.; Rawel, H.M.; Rohn, S. Reactions of plant phenolics with food proteins and enzymes under special consideration of covalent bonds. *Food Sci. Technol. Int.* **2003**, *9*, 205–218. [CrossRef]
33. Li, Y.; Jongberg, S.; Andersen, M.L.; Davies, M.J.; Lund, M.N. Quinone-induced protein modifications: Kinetic preference for reaction of 1,2-benzoquinones with thiol groups in proteins. *Free Radic. Biol. Med.* **2016**, *97*, 148–157. [CrossRef] [PubMed]
34. Cao, Y.; Xiong, Y.L. Chlorogenic acid-mediated gel formation of oxidatively stressed myofibrillar protein. *Food Chem.* **2015**, *180*, 235–243. [CrossRef] [PubMed]
35. Jia, N.; Wang, L.; Shao, J.; Liu, D.; Kong, B. Changes in the structural and gel properties of pork myofibrillar protein induced by catechin modification. *Meat Sci.* **2017**, *127*, 45–50. [CrossRef] [PubMed]
36. Feng, X.; Chen, L.; Lei, N.; Wang, S.; Xu, X.; Zhou, G.; Li, Z. Emulsifying Properties of Oxidatively Stressed Myofibrillar Protein Emulsion Gels Prepared with (−)-Epigallocatechin-3-gallate and NaCl. *J. Agric. Food Chem.* **2017**, *65*, 2816–2826. [CrossRef] [PubMed]
37. Zhou, L.; Elias, R.J. Investigating the hydrogen peroxide quenching capacity of proteins in polyphenol-rich foods. *J. Agric. Food Chem.* **2011**, *59*, 8915–8922. [CrossRef] [PubMed]

medicines

MDPI

Article

Protein Oxidation and Sensory Quality of Brine-Injected Pork Loins Added Ascorbate or Extracts of Green Tea or Maté during Chill-Storage in High-Oxygen Modified Atmosphere

Sisse Jongberg [1,*], Mari Ann Tørngren [2] and Leif H. Skibsted [1]

[1] Department of Food Science, University of Copenhagen, Rolighedsvej 30, DK-1958 Frederiksberg, Denmark; ls@food.ku.dk

[2] Danish Meat Research Institute, Danish Technological Institute, Gregersensvej 9, DK-2630 Taastrup, Denmark; matn@teknologisk.dk

* Correspondence: jongberg@food.ku.dk; Tel.:+45-35-33-21-81; Fax: +45-35-33-33-44

Received: 11 December 2017; Accepted: 10 January 2018; Published: 15 January 2018

Abstract: Background: Ascorbate is often applied to enhance stability and robustness of brine-injected pork chops sold for retail, but may affect protein oxidation, while plant extracts are potential substitutes. **Methods:** Brine-injected pork chops (weight-gain ~12%, NaCl ~0.9%) prepared with ascorbate (225 ppm), green tea extract (25 ppm gallic acid equivalents (GAE)), or maté extract (25 ppm GAE) stored (5 °C, seven days) in high-oxygen atmosphere packaging (MAP: 80% O_2 and 20% CO_2) were analyzed for color changes, sensory quality, and protein oxidation compared to a control without antioxidant. **Results:** No significant differences were observed for green tea and maté extracts as compared to ascorbate when evaluated based on lipid oxidation derived off-flavors, except for stale flavor, which maté significantly reduced. All treatments increased the level of the protein oxidation product, α-aminoadipic semialdehyde as compared to the control, and ascorbate was further found to increase thiol loss and protein cross-linking, with a concomitant decrease in the sensory perceived tenderness. **Conclusions:** Green tea and maté were found to equally protect against lipid oxidation derived off-flavors, and maté showed less prooxidative activity towards proteins as compared to ascorbate, resulting in more tender meat. Maté is a valuable substitute for ascorbate in brine-injected pork chops.

Keywords: brine-injected pork; green tea extract; maté extract; ascorbate; protein oxidation; sensory quality; high-oxygen modified atmosphere packaging

1. Introduction

Meat produced and distributed for the food service sector, canteens, nursing homes, and schools needs more robustness to withstand common practice, which includes several cycles of heating often to high temperatures (usual above 75 °C) and subsequent chilling [1,2]. Addition of salt binds water in the meat, and results in a weight-gain and improved tenderness and juiciness, which collectively gives a more robust meat product that better tolerates several heating/chilling cycles [3]. Meat cuts sold for the food service sector are distributed both in modified atmosphere packaging (MAP) and in vacuum, and are stored chilled or frozen (Nassu, Juarez, Uttaro, & Aalhus, 2010). As reviewed by Suman et al. [4], high-oxygen MAP improves meat color, but impairs the eating quality by accelerating oxidation of lipids and proteins, resulting in off-flavor formation, and decreased tenderness and reduced juiciness. High-oxygen MAP has, moreover, been found to reduce the otherwise positive effects of injection-enhancement on shear force, tenderness, and juiciness of beef steaks and concomitantly increase off-flavor associated with lipid oxidation [3].

Ascorbate is commonly added to injection brines as an antioxidant for protecting color and lipids of fresh and frozen meat products, as it ensures a stable and robust meat product [5]. However, there is a risk that ascorbate may act as a prooxidant at some concentration levels depending on the system [6]. Tea catechins have previously shown superior antioxidant activity when compared to ascorbate during cold storage of cooked or raw beef or chicken patties [7]. Hence, plant extracts may be potential "natural" substitutes for ascorbate to extend the shelf life of brine-injected meat. Such natural antioxidants extracted from plant material rich in phenolic compounds often protect efficiently against lipid oxidation in meat when added to the animal feed [8,9], when mixed into minced meat products [7,10], or when added to brine for whole meat cuts [11,12]. However, most studies considering the effects of natural antioxidants in meat have explored the effects in minced meat or in surface-marinated meat products. Brine-injection is commonly applied to improve tenderness and juiciness; however, the effects of phenolic antioxidants in brine-injected meat products have not been widely researched. Protein oxidation is known to decrease meat tenderness and juiciness in fresh meat [13], and the effects of phenolic antioxidants in the brine on protein oxidation and meat tenderness need accordingly to be considered. Green tea (*Camellia sinensis*) is commonly used as an antioxidant in various food products [14], whereas maté (*Ilex paraguariensis*) from a South American bush rich in caffeic acid derivatives [15] is a new and less utilized source of phenolic antioxidants for foods. Recently, it was shown that maté extract added to cattle feed resulted in more tender meat with higher consumer acceptance [16]. Furthermore, studies show that extracts from green tea and maté injected into pork loins protected against lipid oxidation during chilled storage in a dose-dependent manner, but found that the meat protein radical intensity increased when added increasing doses of green tea extract [17]. This indicated a prooxidative effect of green tea extract on the meat proteins, which needs to be investigated further.

The aim of the present study was to investigate the effect of substituting ascorbate as an antioxidant agent in brine-injected pork loins with phenolic-rich extracts from green tea or maté. Effects on meat protein oxidation as evaluated by thiol loss and formation of protein disulfide cross-link during storage in high-oxygen atmosphere were related to product color and sensory quality including tenderness and juiciness.

2. Materials and Methods

2.1. Plant Extracts and Chemicals

Green tea (*Camellia sinensis*) extract (Guardian Green Tea 20 M), a commercial product with Product description PD 215033-6.0EN) was obtained from DuPont Nutrition and Biosciences ApS, Brabrand, Denmark. Maté (*Ilex paraguariensis*) extract from Centroflora, Botucatu, Sao Paulo, Brazil, was kindly provided by Daniel Cardoso at University of Sao Paulo in Sao Carlos. Details regarding extract composition and extraction method are previously published by de Zawadzki et al. [16]. All other reagents were of analytical grade. Double-deionized water (Milipore, Bedford, MA, USA) was used throughout.

2.2. Total Phenolic Content in Extracts

In order to control the amount of phenols injected into the pork, the total phenolic content was determined in the maté extract by Folin–Ciocalteu's method as described by Singleton and Rossi [18]. The total phenolic content in the green tea extract was previously determined to be 23.8% [19], and this concentration was applied throughout this investigation. In brief, 100 μL 1 mg/mL maté extract dissolved into a total volume of 1500 μL double-deionized water, was left to react with 125 μL Folin–Ciocalteu phenol reagent (Sigma-Aldrich, St. Louis, MO, USA) for 8 min. Subsequently, 375 μL 20% sodium carbonate was added and the reaction mixture was left to incubate at 20 °C for 2 h. The phenol concentration was determined spectrophotometrically at 765 nm against a standard curve prepared from gallic acid. The concentrations are given in gallic acid equivalents (g GAE/100 g dry extract; % *w*/*w*).

2.3. Preparation and Storage of Injected Pork Loins

Thirty-six pork loins (*logissimus dorsi*) from 18 female pigs slaughtered on the same day and with similar and normal pH (5.61 ± 0.06) were collected from a Danish slaughterhouse and transported to the Danish Meat Research Institute at Technological Institute (Taastrup, Denmark). Pigs 1–6 were used for day 0 samples, pigs 7–12 were used for day 3 samples, and pigs 13–18 were used for day 7 samples under the assumption that six replicates would compensate for any animal variation between the 18 pigs. The loins were divided in half, and hip-ends and neck-ends from the same pig were randomized and injected with either a salt brine, or salt brine with ascorbate, green tea or maté extract, resulting in six replicates (A–F) for each treatment at each day of sampling. The salt brine contained 6.6% NaCl and 5.5% dextrose. The brine containing ascorbate was added 0.21% sodium ascorbate, corresponding to ~225 ppm in the injected loins. The brine containing green tea was added 0.10% green tea extract, and the brine containing maté was added 0.11% maté extract, resulting in a similar level of ~25 ppm phenolic compound in the injected loins with an expected weight gain of 12% (*w*/*w*). The half-loins were weighted prior to injection to determine the exact gain after injection, which were performed using a multichannel brine injector (FMG 26/52, Fomaco A/S, Køge, Denmark) with 66 punch/min, 1.0 bar pressure, and 3.0 bar up-pressure for the hip ends and 66 punch/min, 0.8 bar pressure, and 3.0 bar up-pressure for the neck end. The injected half-loins were covered in plastic bags to avoid evaporation from the surface and left to equalize overnight in the dark at 2–5 °C. The day after brine-injection, the loins were blotted from drip-loss and weighed for calculation of weight-gain. The weight-gain was further used to calculate the exact amount of ascorbate and phenolic compounds present in the meat:

Calculation example:

(1) Phenol content in brine: 0.10% extract in brine gives 0.1 g/100 mL·23.8% = 0.238 mg/mL phenol in brine;
(2) Phenol in loin (2.02 kg) when weight-gain was 193 g (mL): 193 mL·0.238 mg/mL phenol = 44.4 mg phenol;
(3) Phenol (ppm) in loin: 44.4 mg phenol/2.02 kg meat = 22.3 mg phenol/kg meat = 22.3 ppm.

The half-loins were subsequently sliced into 8 chops of 2 cm and numbered 1–16, having numbers 1–8 starting from the hip-end and 9–16 ending in the neck-end. The pork chops were randomized from the various analyses, and the pork chops to be analyzed on day 0 were vacuum packed and frozen (−80 °C) until analysis. The pork chops to be stored for day 3 and day 7 were packed (two in each tray) in modified atmosphere packaging (MAP, 80% O_2/20% CO_2) using a Multivac T200 tray sealer (Multivac, Wolfertschwenden, Germany). Tray (MAPET K 2190-53H, clear) and film (Toplex HB PET EP 40 code 2600/040) with oxygen permeability: 2.5 cc/m^2/24 h were obtained from Færch Plast (Holstebro, Denmark). The MAP pork chops were stored for 3 or 7 days at 5 °C in a display cabinet with light exposure (~1200 lux as measured on product surface) for 12 h daily. After sampling, the surface color was measured before mincing and mixing. The meat was divided into smaller portions, vacuum packed, and stored at −80 °C until analysis.

2.4. Salt Analysis

The concentration of salt was determined according to Nordisk Metodikkomite for Levnedsmidler [20]. In brief, sodium chloride was extracted in hot water, and chloride was subsequently precipitated using silver nitrate. The concentration of salt was determined in 72 samples (from 18 pigs injected with four different brines) and was calculated as an average of a pork chop from the middle of the loin and from the end. Results are presented in g/100 g as mean ± sd (n = 6).

2.5. Color Analysis

The surface color of the pork chops was measured by a videometer (VideometerLab, Videometer A/S—Visionteknologi, Hørsholm, Denmark). Spectra consisting of 1.2 mil pixel were obtained from which lightness (L*), and color (a* and b*) were calculated from the ratio between specific reflection values in correspondence with the original CIE definitions. On each day of take-out (day 0, 3 and 7), 24 samples (4 brines × 6 replicates) were measured. From L*, a* and b* the total color difference (ΔE) was calculated [21]:

$$\Delta E = \sqrt{(\Delta L^2 + \Delta a^2 + \Delta b^2)}.$$

2.6. Isolation of Myofibrillar Proteins (MPI)

Myofibrillar proteins (MPI) were isolated from the pork loins according to the method by Park, Xiong, and Alderton [22] with slight modifications [23]. From each combination of injection brine and day, six replicates were prepared ($n = 6$). The MPI were lyophilized and stored at −20 °C until analysis.

2.7. Protein Thiol Concentration

Protein thiol groups were determined in the MPI after derivatization with DTNB (5,5 dithiobis(2-nitrobenzoic acid, Sigma-Aldrich, St. Louis, MO, USA)) according to Ellman [24] as previously described in detail [25].

2.8. SDS-PAGE

MPI were analyzed by gel-electrophoresis using NuPAGE Novex 3–8% TRIS-acetate gels according to the manufacturer's instructions (Invitrogen, Carlsbad, CA, USA) and as described by Jongberg et al. [25]. Precision Plus Protein Standard All Blue marker was used as protein marker and loading control on the gels. The gels were photographed by a charge-coupled device (CCD) camera (Raytest, Camilla II, Straubenhardt, Germany) and the protein bands were quantified using GelAnalyzer 2010© developed by Dr. Istvan Lazar.

2.9. Determination of α-Aminoadipic Semialdehyde (AAS)

A standard of *N*α-acetyl-α-aminoadipic semialdehyde (AAS) was synthesized from *N*α-acetyl-L-lysine using lysyl oxidase activity from egg shell membrane following the procedure described by Akagawa et al. [26] with slight modifications. Briefly, 10 mM *N*α-acetyl-L-lysine was incubated with constant stirring with 3 g egg shell membrane in 50 mL of 20 mM sodium phosphate buffer, pH 9.0 at 37 °C for 24 h. The egg shell membrane was then removed by centrifugation and the pH of the solution adjusted to 6.0 using 1 M HCl. The resulting aldehyde were reductively aminated with 3 mmol p-amino-benzoic acid (ABA) in the presence of 4.5 mmol sodium cyanoborohydride NaBH3CN at 37 °C for 2 h with constant stirring. Then, the AAS-ABA derivative was hydrolyzed by 50 mL of 12 M HCl at 110 °C for 18 h. The hydrolysates were adjusted to neutral pH 7 using 2.0 M and 0.5 M NaOH and dried in vacuo (40 °C) over night. The purity of the resulting solution and authenticity of the standard compounds obtained following the aforementioned procedures have been checked by using MS and ^{1}H NMR [27,28].

MPI was derivatized with ABA according to the procedure by Utrera et al. [29] with slight modifications. An aliquot of 5.0 mg MPI was treated with 0.5 mL 1% sodium dodecyl sulfate (SDS) and 1 mM diethylenetriaminepentaacetic acid (DTPA), 0.5 mL of 50 mM ABA, and 0.25 mL of 100 mM NaBH3CN. All solutions prepared in 250 mM 2-(*N*-morpholino) ethanesulfonic acid (MES) buffer pH 6.0 and were freshly made at the day of analysis. The derivatization was completed by allowing the mixture to react for 90 min while tubes were immersed in a water bath at 37 °C and stirred every 30 min. The derivatization reaction was stopped by adding 0.25 mL of cold 50% tricholoacetic acid (TCA) followed by a centrifugation at 5000 rpm (4 °C) for 5 min, and subsequently the supernatant was discarded. The proteins were further purified by precipitation with 1.5 mL ice cold 5% TCA followed by a centrifugation at 5000 rpm (4 °C) for 5 min, and subsequently the supernatant was discarded. Protein hydrolysis was performed at 110 °C for 18 h after addition of 1.0 mL 6 M HCl. The hydrolysates were adjusted to neutral pH 7 using 2.0 M and 0.5 M NaOH and dried in vacuo (40 °C) over night. Hydrolysates were finally reconstituted with 1.0 mL Milli-Q water and filtered through hydrophilic polypropylene syringe filters (0.22 μm pore size) for HPLC analysis.

AAS in the ABA-derivatized MPI was quantified using ultrahigh-pressure liquid chromatography (UHPLC, Dionex Ultimate 3000, Thermo Fischer Scientific, Hvidovre, Denmark) equipped with an Accucore-150-C18 column (10 cm × 2.1 mm × 2.6 μm) with guard (Def pk4) (Thermo Fischer Scientific, Hâgersten, Sweden) coupled to a fluoresecnece detector (FLD, Dionex Ultimate 3000, Thermo Fischer Scientific, Hvidovre, Denmark) with excitation wavelength of 283 nm and emissions wavelength of 350 nm. The mobile phase was a mixture of eluent A: 50 mM sodium acetate buffer (pH 5.4) and eluent B: 100% acetonitrile. The injection volume was 1.0 μL, column temperature 30 °C, and the flow rate was 0.5 mL/min. For separation of AAS, a gradient was applied: Eluent B increased from 0 to 8% between 0 and 4.5 min followed by a cleaning procedure consisting of a rapid (10 s) increase to 80% eluent B, which were hold for 2 min, followed by a slow decline to 0% eluent B, which were hold for 1 min resulting in total run time of 12 min per sample. The concentration of AAS-ABA in the standard preparation was determined against a standard curve of ABA (0.05–1 μM). Assuming that the fluorescence emitted by 1 mol of ABA is equivalent to that emitted by 1 mol of derivatized protein carbonyl, a standard curve of AAS-ABA was prepared ranging from 0.1 to 1 μM. Regression coefficients greater than 0.999 were obtained for both the ABA and AAS-ABA standard curves. Identification and quantification of AAS in the MPI was carried out by comparing the retention times (Rt) in the FLD chromatograms with those from the standard AAS-ABA. The peak corresponding to AAS-ABA was manually integrated and the concentration of AAS in the MPI determined in pmol of carbonyl compound per mg MPI (n = 3).

2.10. Sensory Analysis

The brine-injected pork chops were evaluated in double sessions by a trained sensory panel consisting of 8 assessors, one male and 7 female, ranging between 4 to 21 years seniority. All the assessors had participated in two training session in accordance with ISO 4121, ASTM-MNL 13, DIN 13299 and were familiar with sensory assessment of meat. At the training sessions, the 14 descriptors were selected: pre-mature browning (PMB), hardness, tenderness, juiciness, off-flavor, stale flavor, warmed-over flavor, pig flavor, rancid, salt taste, sweet taste, sour flavor, acidic taste, meaty flavor. The descriptors were divided into two categories: *Appearance and texture*, and *Flavor*. All pork chops were analyzed on the day of sampling. Before cooking, the pork chops were tempered to 10–15 °C at room temperature and cooked on a pre-heated pan (170 °C) to a core temperature of 65–68 °C. Four pork chops were used per servings for the eight assessors, who evaluated the chops on a 15-point unstructured scale anchored at the extremes (0 = low intensity and 15 = high intensity). Twenty-four samples were evaluated per double session (4 brines × 6 replicates).

2.11. Statistical Data Analysis

Statistical analysis of salt content, ascorbate and phenol content, color, protein thiols, AAS, and protein cross-linking was performed using R© version 3.4.2., The R Foundation for Statistical Computing, Vienna University of Economics and Business, Institute for Statistics and Mathematics, Vienna, Austria, ISBN: 3-900051-07-0. Analysis of variance were performed using a linear model with mixed effects with Brine, Time and Brine*Time as fixed effects, and Replicates as random effect, where brine, time and/or their interaction were found to be insignificant for the statistical model, and it was excluded as a variable. The level of significance was $p < 0.05$. Sensory data were analyzed using mixed models (SAS, 9.4). The proc mixed model included Brine, Time and Brine*Time as fixed effect and loin end, assessor, and assessor interactions as random effects. Least squares (LSmeans) were calculated and separated using probability of difference.

3. Results

3.1. Product Analyses

The salt content was analyzed in the pork chops prior to storage. In average, the salt concentration was 0.89 ± 0.15 g/100 g brine-injected meat with no significant difference between the different treatments (Table 1). In contrast, significant difference was found between samples prepared for the various storage days (Time, $p = 0.0307$), but this difference originated solely from a significant difference ($p = 0.0155$) between the control pork chops prepared for day 0 and day 7, containing 0.77 ± 0.06 g/100 g and 0.92 ± 0.11 g/100 g, respectively. The ascorbate and phenol concentrations in the brine-injected pork chops were calculated based on the weight gain after injection. The green tea extract had a total phenolic content of 23.8 g GAE/100 g extract [19], and the maté extract was found to contain 21.7 g GAE/100 g extract. The average concentration of salt, ascorbate and phenols, as well as the p-values for Time and Treatment are presented in Table 1.

Table 1. Concentration of NaCl and calculated levels of ascorbate and phenols compounds in brine-injected pork chops.

Treatment [a]	n	NaCl (g/100 g)	Ascorbate [b] (ppm)	Phenols [b] (ppm)	p_{Time}
Control	6	0.85 ± 0.11	-	-	0.0307 (*)
Ascorbate (~225 ppm)	18	0.90 ± 0.18	225.6 ± 40.0	-	0.9878
Green Tea extract (~25 ppm GAE [c])	18	0.86 ± 0.12	-	24.0 ± 2.2	0.1260
Maté extract (~25 ppm GAE [c])	18	0.93 ± 0.15	-	24.5 ± 3.4	0.4670
$p_{\text{Treatment}}$		0.3909	-	0.6141	

[a] Stored in high-oxygen modified atmosphere packaging (MAP) for up to 7 days (5 °C); [b] Calculated from the weight-gain of brine-injected pork loins; [c] GAE = gallic acid equivalents; * Significant difference ($p < 0.05$).

No significant difference was found for ascorbate content between the three storage days, and for the phenolic content, no significant difference was found between the concentrations of green tea or maté extract, or between storage days (Table 1). This indicates a consistent production of brine-injected pork chops, where differentiation of the injection settings according to the hip- or neck-end of the loin, provided a homogenous application of ingredients.

3.2. Color Changes

The color of the brine-injected pork chops stored in high-oxygen MAP was found to differentiate significantly depending on storage time for the three-color parameters lightness (L*), redness (a*), and yellowness (b*) (Table 2).

Table 2. Color parameters and the total color difference (ΔE) in brine-injected pork chops.

Treatment [x]	Storage Time (days)	Lightness (L*)	Redness (a*)	Yellowness (b*)	ΔE
Control (n = 6)	0	60.9 ± 1.5 [b]	17.6 ± 0.6 [a]	15.3 ± 0.2 [a]	0.0
	3	63.2 ± 1.2 [a]	18.0 ± 1.1 [a]	14.9 ± 0.6 [a]	2.4
	7	63.8 ± 1.5 [a]	15.4 ± 1.1 [b]	14.3 ± 0.6 [b]	3.8
Ascorbate (~225 ppm, n = 6)	0	61.1 ± 2.0 [b]	17.0 ± 0.6 [b]	14.9 ± 0.3 [a]	0.0
	3	63.4 ± 0.6 [a]	18.2 ± 0.7 [a]	15.3 ± 0.5 [a]	2.6
	7	64.1 ± 1.3 [a]	16.4 ± 1.0 [b]	14.3 ± 0.5 [b]	3.1
Green Tea extract (~25 ppm GAE [y], n = 6)	0	60.3 ± 1.4 [c]	16.5 ± 0.8 [b]	14.7 ± 0.7 [a,b]	0.0
	3	62.8 ± 1.6 [b]	17.8 ± 1.1 [a]	15.2 ± 0.5 [a]	2.8
	7	64.0 ± 1.0 [a]	15.4 ± 0.9 [c]	14.3 ± 0.5 [b]	3.8
Maté extract (~25 ppm GAE [y], n = 6)	0	60.5 ± 1.2 [b]	16.7 ± 0.5 [b]	14.6 ± 0.2 [a,b]	0.0
	3	62.9 ± 1.1 [a]	17.9 ± 0.9 [a]	14.9 ± 0.6 [a]	3.0
	7	62.9 ± 1.3 [a]	15.8 ± 0.8 [b]	14.1 ± 0.4 [b]	2.7

[x] Stored in high-oxygen modified atmosphere packaging (MAP) for up to 7 days (5 °C); [y] GAE = gallic acid equivalents; [a–c] Different letters (a–c) denotes significant ($p < 0.05$) different values within the same treatment and color parameter.

The brine had no significant influence on the color parameters, and no significant interaction was found between brine and storage time. For all types of brines, the lightness was found to increase over time, leading to significant differences between day 0 and 3, but not between days 3 and 7, indicating that the main increase in lightness occurred during the first days of storage in high-oxygen MAP. Only pork chops added to green tea showed significant increase in lightness between days 3 and 7. Redness (a*) was found to be highest for all samples at day 3 followed by a significant decrease until day 7 for all samples because of discoloration, which may be assigned to oxidation of oxymyoglobin to metmyoglobin. In the pork loins added ascorbate, green tea or maté extracts significantly lower redness was observed at day 0 compared to day 3, which may be explained to increased blooming caused by high oxygen atmosphere (80%) at day 3 compared to atmospheric oxygen level (20%) at day 0. Yellowness (b*) was found to decrease significantly between day 0 and day 7 for the control pork loins. In contrast, for the pork loins added ascorbate or extracts, the highest value for yellowness were found at day 3 with a significant loss at day 7. The total color difference (ΔE) is a metric for understanding how the human eye perceives color difference, and values ~2.3 corresponds to JND (*just noticeable difference*) and values < 2.3 means that differences are not noticeable [21]. For the control and the pork chops injected with ascorbate or green tea ΔE increased over time, showing that storage in high-oxygen MAP affects perception of color in brine-injected pork. After three days of storage, all treatments resulted in JND, with the highest ΔE found for pork added mate ($\Delta E = 3.0$). After 7 seven days of storage, the ΔE increased again for all treatments, except for maté, which dropped to 2.7.

3.3. Sensory Quality

The sensory quality of the brine-injected pork chops was evaluated by descriptors that can be divided into two categories: *Appearance and Texture*, and *Flavor*. The first category describes primarily quality parameters related to protein modifications (pigment and structural proteins), while the latter is related to the formation of secondary lipid oxidation products.

Within the category, *Appearance and Texture*, the descriptor tenderness was significantly affected by the interaction between storage time and brine, where the pork chops injected with ascorbate or maté extract showed opposite effects. The tenderness in the pork chops injected with ascorbate became significantly reduced between days 3 and 7, whereas the tenderness in the pork chops injected with maté extract increased significantly between days 3 and 7. This resulted in significant differences between samples at day 7, where pork chops injected with maté extract were more tender than the pork chops added ascorbate or green tea, and the pork chops added ascorbate was less tender than the control (Figure 1A).

The descriptor juiciness was also significantly affected by the interaction between storage time and brine. The pork chops injected with green tea extract was found to lose juiciness between days 3 and 7, whereas the pork chops injected with maté extract showed a peak in juiciness at day 3, followed by a drop at day 7 (Figure 1B). This resulted in significantly higher juiciness in the pork chops injected with maté extract as compared to the pork chops injected with green tea extract at day 3. Overall, the effects on tenderness and juiciness indicate that ascorbate, green tea and maté extracts all affect the texture and water holding capacity of the meat by interacting with the structural proteins, altering their functional properties, and, in the end, affects the eating quality of the meat. In particular, maté extract had a positive influence on meat tenderness and juiciness, whereas ascorbate had a negative influence on tenderness.

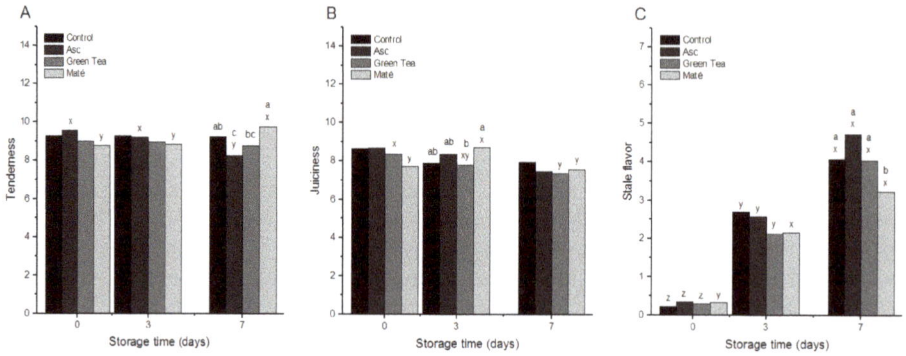

Figure 1. Tenderness (**A**); juiciness (**B**); and stale flavor (**C**) of pork chops injected with salt brine (Control), or brine added 225 ppm ascorbate (Asc), green tea (~25 ppm gallic acid equivalents (GAE)), or maté extract (~25 ppm GAE) and chill stored in high-oxygen modified atmosphere packaging (MAP) for 0, 3 or 7 as evaluated by a trained sensory panel. LSMeans with different letters (a–c) differ significantly ($p < 0.05$) between injection brines within the same day of storage, and LSMeans with different letters (x–z) differ significantly ($p < 0.05$) between days of storage within the same injection brine.

Concerning appearance of the meat, the descriptor pre-mature browning (PMB) was found to increase significantly during the seven days of storage in high-oxygen MAP (data not shown), as previously described by Soerheim and Hoey [30]. Furthermore, PMB was significantly higher for the pork injected with maté extract at day 0, indicating that the natural color of the maté extract (green), or some pro-oxidative interaction between maté extract and the pigments myoglobin, may have affected the appearance of the meat after cooking. Otherwise, no significant differences were observed between storage days or injection-brine, nor their interaction.

Within the category, *Flavor*, the descriptor stale flavor was also affected by the interaction between the injection-brine and storage time, and increased for the control pork chops and the pork chops injected with ascorbate or green tea extract during the seven days of storage (Figure 1). The pork chops injected with maté extract showed no significant increase from day 3 to 7, resulting in a significant reduced stale flavor at day 7 as compared to the three other treatments (Figure 1C). This indicated that the maté extract was able to retard the formation of stale flavor, which is considered a lipid oxidation derived off-flavor. Regarding the remaining descriptors within the category *Flavor*, they were all solely affected by storage time. Warmed-over-flavor, rancidity, and sour taste increased significantly during the seven days of storage in high-oxygen MAP, whereas acidity and meaty flavor decreased significantly (data not shown). Previous studies also show accelerated deterioration related to formation of lipid oxidation products caused by storage in the high-oxygen atmosphere [31,32]. In the present study, neither ascorbate, green tea, nor maté extracts protected against any of the lipid oxidation related descriptors besides stale flavor, which was significantly reduced by the maté extract. The only attribute found to be directly affected by injection brine was the attribute off-flavor, which was found to be significantly higher in the pork chops injected with green tea extract due to the flavor naturally found the green tea extract (data not shown).

From the sensory analysis, it is seen that descriptors such as acidity and meaty flavor are reduced already between day 0 and 3, where also warmed-over-flavor increases. Between days 3 and 7, changes are observed for sour taste and rancidity, which increases significantly, and the meat tenderness, which is either negatively affected by ascorbate or positively affected by maté extract.

3.4. Oxidative Protein Modifications

The protein thiol concentration in the myofibrillar protein isolate from the brine-injected pork chops was found to be similar for all treatments at day 0 (Table 3). No significant loss in thiols was observed after seven days of storage for the pork chops injected with green tea or maté extract. In contrast, ascorbate was found to significantly reduce the thiol concentration at days 3 and 7 as compared to day 0, indicating that ascorbate is unable to preserve protein thiols during storage. The semialdehyde AAS, which is a protein oxidation product of lysine, were also quantified in the brine-injected pork chops, and it was found that at day 0 the pork chops that added maté had a significantly higher concentration of AAS as compared to the other treatments, which showed similar concentrations (Table 3). No clear explanation was found for this difference at day 0 for the pork chops with added maté extract, and the level dropped again at day 3, where no significant differences were found between any of the treatments. After seven days of storage, the pork chops with added ascorbate, green tea and maté extract had all reached AAS concentrations significantly higher than the control, indicating prooxidative effects of both ascorbate and the extracts as compared to the control.

Table 3. Protein thiols and α-amino-adipic semialdehyde (AAS) in myofibrillar protein isolate (MPI) from brine-injected pork.

Marker of Protein Oxidation	Storage Time * (days)	Control	Ascorbate (~225 ppm)	Green Tea Extract (~25 ppm GAE **)	Maté Extract (~25 ppm GAE **)
Protein thiols (nmol/mg protein, $n = 6$)	0	62.2 ± 2.2	61.2 ± 1.8^{x}	$61.5 \pm 1.6^{x,y}$	63.9 ± 2.1^{x}
	3	59.4 ± 3.6^{a}	$56.6 \pm 3.4^{b,y}$	$59.0 \pm 2.6^{a,y}$	$58.1 \pm 2.8^{a,b,y}$
	7	60.6 ± 1.7^{a}	$57.8 \pm 1.7^{b,y}$	$61.7 \pm 1.7^{a,x}$	$61.0 \pm 0.7^{a,y,x}$
AAS (pmol/mg MPI, $n = 3$)	0	62.5 ± 0.0^{b}	$61.1 \pm 7.3^{b,x}$	$55.4 \pm 12.4^{b,y}$	$112.5 \pm 10.2^{a,x}$
	3	82.2 ± 15.3	108.9 ± 17.5^{x}	104.5 ± 3.1^{x}	80.5 ± 3.0^{y}
	7	64.2 ± 4.6^{b}	$114.2 \pm 27.5^{a,x}$	$110.9 \pm 20.6^{a,x}$	$129.2 \pm 9.4^{a,x}$

* Stored in high-oxygen modified atmosphere packaging (MAP) for up to 7 days (5 °C); ** GAE = gallic acid equivalents. $^{a-b}$ Mean ± sd within the same row without a common letter differ significantly ($p < 0.05$). $^{x-y}$ Mean ± sd within the same analysis and within the same column without a common letter differ significantly ($p < 0.05$).

The myofibrillar protein isolates from the brine-injected pork chops were also subjected to gel electrophoresis (SDS-PAGE) to evaluate the formation of protein cross-linking. Lund et al. [13] found that under oxidative conditions, myosin heavy chain (MHC) forms disulfide bonds, which cross-link the myosin heavy chains. The occurrence of cross-linked MHC (CL-MHC) was found to correlate with reduced tenderness and juiciness, and increased hardness in high-oxygen MAP pork *longissimus dorsi* [13]. Running the gel electrophoresis with samples in both their reduced and non-reduced state enabled the detection of disulfide-derived CL-MHC, as disulfides bonds will be reduced by the reducing agent thereby removing the protein cross-links and regenerating MHC. In the present study, control samples from day 0 and day 7 together with samples containing ascorbate, green tea, or maté extract from day 7 were analyzed by SDS-PAGE (Figure 2). For the non-reduced samples, a band assigned as the CL-MHC based on previous LC-MS analysis by Lund et al. [13] was detected for the pork loins added ascorbate, and to a lesser extent for the pork loins added green tea and maté extract at day 7. In contrast, almost no CL-MHC was visible in the reduced samples, indicating that the main part of the protein cross-links was generated through reducible bonds.

Gel chromatography is not a quantitative method, and it is hence difficult to evaluate the exact difference between samples. This uncertainty is also due to the large variation between gels. In order to compare samples, the band intensities were quantified to obtain a semi-quantitative determination of MHC and CL-MHC. Addition of green tea extract to the brine-injected pork loins was found to significantly increase the MHC in the non-reduced samples at day 7 as compared to all the other samples (Figure 3). The same amount of protein was added to each well of the gel, so no clear explanation to this increment was found. Moreover, the green tea extract tended to increase the formation of CL-MHC, although the increase was not significantly different from the control (Figure 3). In contrast, ascorbate was found to significantly increase CL-MHC at day 7 as compared to the control sample at day 0, and the maté sample at day 7 (Figure 3). No significant differences in the CL-MHC levels were found between any samples after reduction (data not shown), indicating that the variations observed for CL-MHC between samples were caused by reducible bonds.

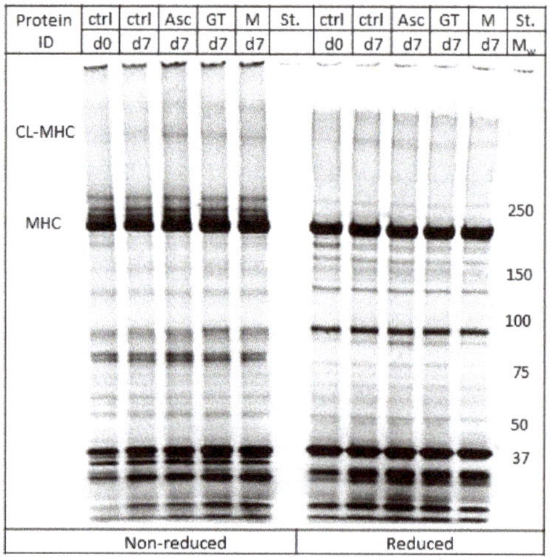

Figure 2. Representative SDS-PAGE of pork loins injected with neutral brine (ctrl) and chill stored in high-oxygen modified atmosphere packaging (MAP) for 0 (d0) or 7 days (d7), and pork loins injected with brine added 225 ppm ascorbate (Asc), green tea extract (GT; ~25 ppm gallic acid equivalents (GAE)), or maté extract (M; ~25 ppm GAE), and chill stored in high-oxygen (MAP) for seven days (d7). Samples were run both in their non-reduced state and reduced state. CL-MHC, cross-linked myosin heavy chain; MHC, myosin heavy chain.

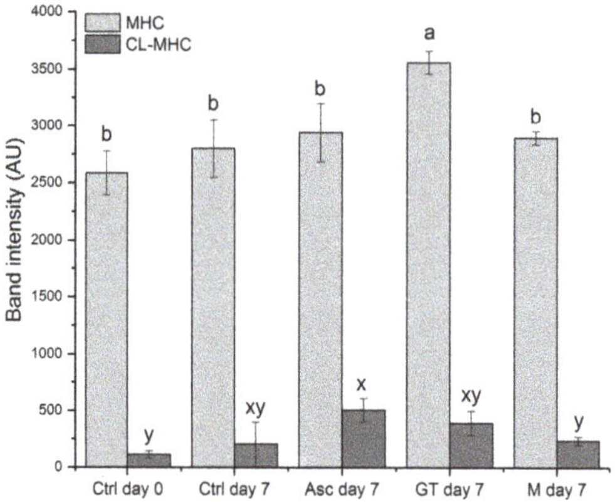

Figure 3. Band intensity of myosin heavy chain (MHC) and cross-linked MHC (CL-MHC) separated by SDS-PAGE in pork chops injected with neutral brine (Ctrl) and chill stored in high-oxygen modified atmosphere packaging (MAP) for 0 or 7 days, and pork loins injected with brine added 225 ppm ascorbate (Asc), green tea (GT, ~25 ppm gallic acid equivalents (GAE)), or maté extract (M, ~25 ppm GAE), and chill stored in high-oxygen (MAP) for seven days. Band intensity expressed as mean ± sd of three independent replicates. Means with different letters (a–b for MHC, and x–y for CL-MHC) differ significantly ($p < 0.05$).

Overall, the results indicated that especially ascorbate, and to some extent green tea extract, increased the protein cross-links in the brine-injected pork chops during storage. However, as the gel chromatography results are merely semi-quantitative, they are less conclusive. Though, in this case, the results correlated well with the protein thiol concentrations determined and the tenderness evaluated by the sensory panel. Significantly lower thiol concentration was found at day 7 in the pork chops added ascorbate as compared to the other three pork chops on the same day (Table 3), confirming that thiols were involved in the protein cross-linking observed for the pork loins injected with ascorbate. Neither green tea nor maté extract were found to affect thiol loss or protein cross-linking significantly over seven days of storage, indicating no such prooxidative effect at the concentration level applied. It is known that oxidation of the phenolic moiety, *o*-catechols, results in the formation of electrophilic *o*-quinones that react rapidly with nucleophiles, such as protein thiol groups in meat proteins and generate protein-phenol adducts [33,34], and a similar reaction is also known for ascorbate with proteins generating a protein-DHA* adduct. After oxidation of ascorbate, dehydroascorbate (DHA) may readily decompose to a reactive 5-carbon compound DHA* that can modify reduced cysteinyl residues in proteins [35].

The reaction of quinones with meat proteins seems to be dose-dependent, as the loss of thiols depends on the concentration of phenolic compounds [36–39]. Preliminary studies in our groups found that the concentration level of 25 ppm phenols, which was used in the present study, minimized protein–quinone interactions as evident by no loss in protein thiols [17]. The low phenol concentration applied in the present study resulted in low to insignificant protection against lipid oxidation off-flavors as evaluated by the sensory panel. Only maté extract was able to protect significantly against stale flavor as compared to the control.

Green tea extract contains mainly catechin and catechin derivatives, while maté extracts contains chlorogenic acid and caffeic acid derivatives [14–16]. All compounds contain catechol moieties, which are excellent for protecting especially lipid against oxidation [14]. However, the catechol moeities may, under certain conditions, serve as prooxidants [40], as was seen for the generation of AAS in the present study by the addition of both extracts. Phenols from plant extracts are otherwise efficient radical scavengers, which protect lipids against oxidation in the water–lipid interfaces [41], but the results of the present study shows that only maté extract at the applied concentration served as potential antioxidant in brine-injected pork. However, it must be taken into consideration that components in the plant extracts may mask lipid oxidation derived flavors and therefore create a false antioxidant protection. In the present study, addition of green tea resulted in significant off-flavor formation related to the natural taste of the extract.

3.5. Ascorbate in Brine-Injected Pork

The results of the present study emphasized the link between MHC cross-linking in pork and product tenderness, as previously demonstrated for pork, beef, and lamb [13,42,43]. However, to our knowledge, this is the first demonstration of a clear correlation between protein cross-linking and tenderness in brine-injected pork chops. Addition of ascorbate to the injection brine promoted protein oxidation by increasing both AAS and thiol oxidation (Table 3), which led to increased protein cross-linking (Figure 3). Overall, these protein modifications resulted in reduced tenderness (Figure 1) directly by the formation of disulfide bonds due to thiol oxidation, and possibly also due to altered structural properties of the meat caused by other protein modifications, such as AAS [44]. In light of these results, ascorbate plays in this sense a double role in the brine-injected pork loins, on one hand added as an antioxidant to protect color and lipids, and on the other hand promoting protein oxidation as shown in the present study, and previously described for beef patties [45], and emulsion-type sausages [46]. This is a well-known phenomenon previously described on a cellular level [47]. In the aqueous phase, ascorbate may as an electron donor together with ascorbate oxidase activate oxygen to generate reactive oxygen species (ROS) and dehydroascorbate (DHA), which in proximity to proteins may oxidize thiols to generate disulfides or form protein-DHA* adducts [35]. Meanwhile, ascorbate is also known to reduce tocopheryl radicals to generate tocopherol and thereby act as an antioxidant protecting lipids from oxidation [47]. In the present study, the exact mechanism by which ascorbate results in thiol loss is unclear; however, the increased protein cross-linking observed indicates that ascorbate served as a prooxidant leading to protein cross-links rather than forming protein-DHA* adducts.

4. Conclusions

Substituting ascorbate in the production of brine-injected pork chops with phenolic-rich green tea or maté extracts showed equal efficiency against most lipid oxidation derived off-flavors. With regards to reduction of stale flavor, the maté extracts showed to be even more effective than green tea extract and ascorbate. Furthermore, ascorbate was found to increase protein thiols and protein cross-linking, with a concomitant reduction in meat tenderness at day 7 as compared to the control. Based on the present results, maté extract is a potential substitution for ascorbate in the production of brine-injected pork over green tea extract, as maté extract did not affect protein cross-linking, tenderness, or juiciness negatively throughout storage. Compared to green tea, maté extract generated no off-flavor, and, hence, based on the findings, is a valuable alternative as an antioxidant in brine-injected meat.

Acknowledgments: The authors thank Ann-Britt Frøstrup and Lars Blaabjerg at the Danish Meat Research Institute (DMRI), Technological Institute, as well as Ramus Harly Nielsen and Daniel Gjerløv Rasmussen from the Faculty of Science, University of Copenhagen for technical assistance. Sisse Jongberg also thanks the Danish Council for Independent Research, Technology and Production within the Danish Agency for Science Technology and Innovation for granting the project entitled: "Antioxidant mechanisms of natural phenolic compounds against protein cross-link formation in meat and meat systems" (11-117033), and the Danish Pig Levy Fund for funding experimental work at DMRI.

Author Contributions: Sisse Jongberg and Mari Ann Tørngren conceived and designed the experiments; Sisse Jongberg performed the experiments and analyzed the data; Mari Ann Tørngren and Leif H. Skibsted contributed with raw material, pilot plant facilities, reagents, and analysis tools; Sisse Jongberg, Mari Ann Tørngren, and Leif H. Skibsted wrote the paper.

Conflicts of Interest: The authors declare no conflict of interest.

References

1. Sheard, P.R.; Tali, A. Injection of salt, tripolyphosphate and bicarbonate marinade solutions to improve the yield and tenderness of cooked pork loin. *Meat Sci.* **2004**, *68*, 305–311. [CrossRef] [PubMed]
2. Walsh, H.; Martins, S.; O'Neill, E.E.; Kerry, J.P.; Kenny, T.; Ward, P. The effects of different cooking regimes on the cook yield and tenderness of non-injected and injection enhanced forequarter beef muscles. *Meat Sci.* **2010**, *84*, 444–448. [CrossRef] [PubMed]
3. Grobbel, J.P.; Dikeman, M.E.; Hunt, M.C.; Milliken, G.A. Effects of different packaging atmospheres and injection-enhancement on beef tenderness, sensory attributes, desmin degradation, and display color. *J. Anim. Sci.* **2008**, *86*, 2697–2710. [CrossRef] [PubMed]
4. Suman, S.P.; Hunt, M.C.; Nair, M.N.; Rentfrow, G. Improving beef color stability: Practical strategies and underlying mechanisms. *Meat Sci.* **2014**, *98*, 490–504. [CrossRef] [PubMed]
5. Cheng, E.H.; Ockerman, H.W. Effect of ascorbic acid with tumbling on lipid oxidation of precooked roast beef 1. *J. Muscle Food* **2004**, *15*, 83–93. [CrossRef]
6. Sato, K.; Hegarty, G.R. Warmed-over flavor in cooked meats. *J. Food Sci.* **1971**, *36*, 1098–1102. [CrossRef]
7. Mitsumoto, M.; O'Grad, M.N.; Kerry, J.P.; Buckley, D.J. Addition of tea catechins and vitamin C on sensory evaluation, colour and lipid stability during chilled storage in cooked or raw beef and chicken patties. *Meat Sci.* **2005**, *69*, 773–779. [CrossRef] [PubMed]
8. Racanicci, A.M.C.; Menten, J.F.M.; Alencar, S.M.; Buissa, R.S.; Skibsted, L.H. Mate (*Ilex paraguariensis*) as dietary additive for broilers: Performance and oxidative stability of meat. *Eur. Food Res. Technol.* **2011**, *232*, 655–661. [CrossRef]
9. Gravador, R.S.; Jongberg, S.; Andersen, M.L.; Luciano, G.; Priolo, A.; Lund, M.N. Dietary citrus pulp improves protein stability in lamb meat stored under aerobic conditions. *Meat Sci.* **2014**, *97*, 231–236. [CrossRef] [PubMed]

10. Jongberg, S.; Skov, S.H.; Tørngren, M.A.; Skibsted, L.H.; Lund, M.N. Effect of white grape extract and modified atmosphere packaging on lipid and protein oxidation in chill stored beef patties. *Food Chem.* **2011**, *128*, 276–283. [CrossRef] [PubMed]
11. Mielnik, M.B.; Sem, S.; Egelandsdal, B.; Skrede, G. By-products from herbs essential oil production as ingredient in marinade for turkey thighs. *LWT Food Sci. Technol.* **2008**, *41*, 93–100. [CrossRef]
12. Kim, Y.J.; Jin, S.K.; Park, W.Y.; Kim, B.W.; Joo, S.T.; Yang, H.S. The effect of garlic or onion marinade on the lipid oxidation and meat quality of pork during cold storage. *J. Food Qual.* **2010**, *33*, 171–185. [CrossRef]
13. Lund, M.N.; Lametsch, R.; Hviid, M.S.; Jensen, O.N.; Skibsted, L.H. High-oxygen packaging atmosphere influences protein oxidation and tenderness of porcine *longissimus dorsi* during chill storage. *Meat Sci.* **2007**, *77*, 295–303. [CrossRef] [PubMed]
14. Brewer, M.S. Natural Antioxidants: Sources, Compounds, Mechanisms of Action, and Potential Applications. *Compr. Rev. Food Sci. Food Saf.* **2011**, *10*, 221–247. [CrossRef]
15. Heck, C.I.; De Mejia, E.G. Yerba Mate tea (*Ilex paraguariensis*): A comprehensive review on chemistry, health implications, and technological considerations. *J. Food Sci.* **2007**, *72*, R138–R151. [CrossRef] [PubMed]
16. De Zawadzki, A.; Arrivetti, L.O.R.; Vidal, M.P.; Catai, J.R.; Nassu, R.T.; Tullio, R.R.; Berndt, A.; Oliveira, C.R.; Ferreira, A.G.; Neves-Junior, L.F.; et al. Mate extract as feed additive for improvement of beef quality. *Food Res. Int.* **2017**, *99*, 336–347. [CrossRef] [PubMed]
17. Jongberg, S.; Mari Ann, T.; Skibsted, L.H. Dose-Dependent Effects of Green Tea or Maté Extracts on Lipid and Protein Oxidation in Brine-Injected Retail-Packed Pork Chops. *Medicines* **2018**. submitted for publication.
18. Singleton, V.L.; Rossi, J.A. Colorimetry of total phenolics with phosphomolybdic-phosphotungstic acid reagents. *Am. J. Enol. Vitic.* **1965**, *16*, 144–158.
19. Jongberg, S.; Lund, M.N.; Østdal, H.; Skibsted, L.H. Phenolic Antioxidant Scavenging of Myosin Radicals Generated by Hypervalent Myoglobin. *J. Agric. Food Chem.* **2012**, *60*, 12020–12028. [CrossRef] [PubMed]
20. Nordisk Metodikkomite for Levnedsmidler Chloride (Salt). *Determination in Foods by Potentiometric Titration*; Nordisk Metodikkomite for Levnedsmidler Chloride: Copenhagen, Denmark, 2004.
21. Sharma, G.; Bala, R. *Digital Color Imagine Handbook*, 1st ed.; CRC Press: Boca Raton, FL, USA, 2002.
22. Park, D.; Xiong, Y.L.L.; Alderton, A.L. Concentration effects of hydroxyl radical oxidizing systems on biochemical properties of porcine muscle myofibrillar protein. *Food Chem.* **2007**, *101*, 1239–1246. [CrossRef]
23. Koutina, G.; Jongberg, S.; Skibsted, L.H. Protein and lipid oxidation in Parma ham during production. *J. Agric. Food Chem.* **2012**, *60*, 9737–9745. [CrossRef] [PubMed]
24. Ellman, G.L. Tissue sulfhydryl groups. *Arch. Biochem. Biophys.* **1959**, *82*, 70–77. [CrossRef]
25. Jongberg, S.; Wen, J.; Tørngren, M.A.; Lund, M.N. Effect of high-oxygen atmosphere packaging on oxidative stability and sensory quality of two chicken muscles during chill storage. *Food Packag. Shelf Life* **2014**, *1*, 38–48. [CrossRef]
26. Akagawa, M.; Sasaki, D.; Ishii, Y.; Kurota, Y.; Yotsu-Yamashita, M.; Uchida, K.; Suyama, K. New method for the quantitative determination of major protein carbonyls, alpha-aminoadipic and gamma-glutamic semialdehydes: Investigation of the formation mechanism and chemical nature in vitro and in vivo. *Chem. Res. Toxicol.* **2006**, *19*, 1059–1065. [CrossRef] [PubMed]
27. Akagawa, M.; Suyama, K.; Uchida, K. Fluorescent detection of a-aminoadipic and g-glutamic semialdehydes in oxidized proteins. *Free Radic. Biol. Med.* **2009**, *46*, 701–706. [CrossRef] [PubMed]
28. Estévez, M.; Morcuende, D.; Ventanas, S. Determination of oxidation. In *Handbook of Processed Meats and Poultry Analysis*; CRC Press: New York, NY, USA, 2009.
29. Utrera, M.; Morcuende, D.; Rodríguez-Carpena, J.G.; Estévez, M. Fluorescent HPLC for the detection of specific protein oxidation carbonyls-α-aminoadipic and γ-glutamic semialdehydes—In meat systems. *Meat Sci.* **2011**, *89*, 500–506. [CrossRef] [PubMed]
30. Soerheim, O.; Hoey, M. Effects of food ingredients and oxygen exposure on premature browning in cooked beef. *Meat Sci.* **2013**, *93*, 105–110. [CrossRef] [PubMed]
31. Clausen, I.; Jakobsen, M.; Ertbjerg, P.; Madsen, N.T. Modified atmosphere packaging affects lipid oxidation, myofibrillar fragmentation index and eating quality of beef. *Packag. Technol. Sci.* **2009**, *22*, 85–96. [CrossRef]
32. Zakrys, P.I.; Hogan, S.A.; O'Sullivan, M.G.; Allen, P.; Kerry, J.P. Effects of oxygen concentration on the sensory evaluation and quality indicators of beef muscle packed under modified atmosphere. *Meat Sci.* **2008**, *79*, 648–655. [CrossRef] [PubMed]

33. Rawel, H.M.; Kroll, J.; Hohl, U.C. Model studies on reactions of plant phenols with whey proteins. *Mol. Nutr. Food Res.* **2001**, *45*, 72–81. [CrossRef]
34. Jongberg, S.; Lund, M.N.; Waterhouse, A.L.; Skibsted, L.H. 4-Methyl catechol inhibits protein oxidation in meat but not disulfide formation. *J. Agric. Food Chem.* **2011**, *59*, 10329–10335. [CrossRef] [PubMed]
35. Kay, P.; Wagner, J.R.; Gagnon, H.; Day, R.; Klarskov, K. Modification of Peptide and Protein Cysteine Thiol Groups by Conjugation with a Degradation Product of Ascorbate. *Chem. Res. Toxicol.* **2013**, *26*, 1333–1339. [CrossRef] [PubMed]
36. Cao, Y.; Xiong, Y.L. Chlorogenic acid-mediated gel formation of oxidatively stressed myofibrillar protein. *Food Chem.* **2015**, *180*, 235–243. [CrossRef] [PubMed]
37. Feng, X.; Chen, L.; Lei, N.; Wang, S.; Xu, X.; Zhou, G.; Li, Z. Emulsifying Properties of Oxidatively Stressed Myofibrillar Protein Emulsion Gels Prepared with (−)-Epigallocatechin-3-gallate and NaCl. *J. Agric. Food Chem.* **2017**, *65*, 2816–2826. [CrossRef] [PubMed]
38. Jia, N.; Wang, L.; Shao, J.; Liu, D.; Kong, B. Changes in the structural and gel properties of pork myofibrillar protein induced by catechin modification. *Meat Sci.* **2017**, *127*, 45–50. [CrossRef] [PubMed]
39. Jongberg, S.; Terkelsen, L.D.; Miklos, R.; Lund, M.N. Green tea extract impairs meat emulsion properties by disturbing protein disulfide cross-linking. *Meat Sci.* **2015**, *100*, 2–9. [CrossRef] [PubMed]
40. Zhou, L.; Elias, R.J. Investigating the hydrogen peroxide quenching capacity of proteins in polyphenol-rich foods. *J. Agric. Food Chem.* **2011**, *59*, 8915–8922. [CrossRef] [PubMed]
41. Shah, M.A.; Bosco, S.J.D.; Mir, S.A. Plant extracts as natural antioxidants in meat and meat products. *Meat Sci* **2014**, *98*, 21–33. [CrossRef] [PubMed]
42. Zakrys-Waliwander, P.I.; O'Sullivan, M.G.; O'Neill, E.E.; Kerry, J.P. The effects of high oxygen modified atmosphere packaging on protein oxidation of bovine, *M. longissimus dorsi* muscle during chilled storage. *Food Chem.* **2012**, *131*, 527–532. [CrossRef]
43. Kim, Y.H.; Huff-Lonergan, E.; Sebranek, J.G.; Lonergan, S.M. High-oxygen modified atmosphere packaging system induces lipid and myoglobin oxidation and protein polymerization. *Meat Sci.* **2010**, *85*, 759–767. [CrossRef] [PubMed]
44. Estévez, M. Protein carbonyls in meat systems: A review. *Meat Sci.* **2011**, *89*, 259–279. [CrossRef] [PubMed]
45. Lund, M.N.; Hviid, M.S.; Skibsted, L.H. The combined effect of antioxidants and modified atmosphere packaging on protein and lipid oxidation in beef patties during chill storage. *Meat Sci.* **2007**, *76*, 226–233. [CrossRef] [PubMed]
46. Rysman, T.; Van Hecke, T.; De Smet, S.; Van Royen, G. Ascorbate and Apple Phenolics Affect Protein Oxidation in Emulsion-Type Sausages during Storage and in Vitro Digestion. *J. Agric. Food Chem.* **2016**, *64*, 4131–4138. [CrossRef] [PubMed]
47. Bánhegyi, G.; Csala, M.; Szarka, A.; Varsányi, M. Role of ascorbate in oxidative folding. *Biofactors* **2003**, *17*, 37–46. [CrossRef] [PubMed]

medicines

MDPI

Article

The Determination of Blood Glucose Lowering and Metabolic Effects of *Mespilus germanica* L. Hydroacetonic Extract on Streptozocin-Induced Diabetic Balb/c Mice

Fatemeh Shafiee [1], Elnaz Khoshvishkaie [1], Ali Davoodi [2,3], Ayat Dashti Kalantar [4], Hossein Bakhshi Jouybari [2] and Ramin Ataee [4,5,*]

1 Student Research Committee, Pharmaceutical Sciences Research Center, Mazandaran University of Medical Sciences, Sari 4847193698, Iran; fatemehshafiee0@gmail.com (F.S.); Elnaz.K@yahoo.com (E.K.)
2 Department of Pharmacognosy, Faculty of Pharmacy, Mazandaran University of Medical Sciences, Sari 4847193698, Iran; adavoodi.pharm@gmail.com (A.D.); ma_2253@yahoo.com (H.B.J.)
3 Medicinal Plants Research Center, Ayatollah Amoli Branch, Islamic Azad University, Amol 4635143358, Iran
4 Pharmaceutical Sciences Research Center, Hemoglobinopathy Institute, Mazandaran University of Medical Sciences, Sari 4847193698, Iran; dashti68612@gmail.com
5 Thalassamia Research Center, Hemoglobinopathy Institute, Mazandaran University of Medical Sciences, Sari 4847193698, Iran
* Correspondence: raminataee1349@gmail.com; Tel.: +98-113-354-3083; Fax: +98-113-354-3084

Received: 20 October 2017; Accepted: 29 December 2017; Published: 1 January 2018

Abstract: Background: The serum glucose lowering, normalization animal body weight, and antioxidative stress effects of *Mespilus germanica* L. leaf extract were investigated in normal and streptozotocin-induced Balb/C mice. **Methods:** The phenol and flavonoid of the leaves of *M. germanica* were extracted by percolation and concentrated using a rotary evaporator. Its total phenol and flavonoid content was determined using folin and aluminum chloride methods, respectively. The study was conducted on 48 matured male Balb/C mice (20–30 g) divided into 6 groups ($n = 8$). Diabetes mellitus was induced by single intraperitoneal injection of 35 mg/kg of streptozotocin (STZ). Extracts of *Mespilus germanica* were used orally at the dose of 50, 100, and 200 mg/kg body weight per day for 21 days. **Results:** Oral administrations of the *M. germanica* L. leaf extract significantly decreased serum glucose, oxidative stress, and lipid peroxidation and maintained animal body weight during treatment period ($p < 0.05$) compared to metformin (200 mg/kg) in over 100 mg/kg, 200 mg/kg, and 50 mg/kg dosages, respectively. **Conclusions:** The present study indicated that the *Mespilus germanica* leaf extract significantly decreased serum glucose and maintained normal body weight in Balb/C diabetic mice.

Keywords: flavonoids; diabetes; Rosaceae; *Mespilus germanica*; mice

1. Introduction

Diabetes mellitus (DM) is a metabolism disorder and exocrine system dysfunction that represent an insulin deficiency or resistance of cells for insulin hormone. DM can be classified in two basic types, Type I and Type II, Type I DM resulting from the pancreatic cell's failure to produce endogen insulin. Type II DM illustrates a condition of quickly hyperglycemia due to cell insulin receptors resistance [1,2]. The present number (as of 2014) of diabetic humans in worldwide is about 300 million, and this is likely to be increased to about 600 million or more by the year 2030. Reasons for this include a decrease in lifestyle levels, the consumption of high energetic diets, and obesity. [3].

Many medicinal plants have been recommended for the treatment of diabetes mellitus. Drugs of plant sources are frequently considered to be less toxic and almost free from adverse effects in conventional uses [4–6]. *Mespilus germanica* is a large shrub or small tree common in northern forest regions of Iran that grows to a height of 2–6 m. It is a member of the Rosaceae family and has very nutritive and therapeutic usages in Iran. The fresh and dried fruits and leaves of the plant are usually used in treating wounds, oral abscess, diabetes mellitus, microbial infections, etc. [7–9]. *M. germanica* fruits are rich in phytochemicals, nutrition, and therapeutic ingredients. It contains proteins, carbohydrates, lipids, and phenolic compounds such as flavonoids and tannins. These phytochemicals induce the therapeutic effects of the plant [10].

Despite the absence of studies on the anti-diabetic effect of this plant, except for those proposed for the measurement of its phenol and flavanoid components and the anti-oxidative stress properties of the related compounds, this research was designed to experimentally determine the serum glucose lowering, normalization animal body weight, and antioxidative stress effects of *Mespilus germanica* leaf hydro acetonic extract used in normal and streptozotocin-induced Balb/c mice.

2. Materials and Methods

2.1. Plant

Mespilus germanica leaves were collected from Jouybar city of Mazandaran province in Iran (latitude: 36.644272; longitude: 54.963289) in the spring of 2015. The plant was identified by Department of Pharmacognosy, and Faculty of Pharmacy of Mazandaran University of Medical Sciences in Sari, Iran. The voucher number of this plant is defined as E_1-223202. The voucher specimen is stored in the Department of Pharmacognosy Herbarium.

2.2. Extract Preparation

Fresh *M. germanica* leaves were dried and placed in a percolator to extract with 70% acetone via percolation. Briefly, 100 g of powdered leaves were macerated in 1000 mL solvents for 24 h. Then, the same amount of solvent was used for continuous extraction. After extraction, the solvent was evaporated in 40 °C with a rotavap, and extracts were freeze-dried. The obtained acetonic extract was stored at −10 °C until being used [11].

2.3. Phenols and Flavonoids Assay

Total phenolic contents of *M. germanica* leaf extract were determined by Folin–Ciocalteu's method. The Folin reagent was diluted 2-fold with distilled water. One milliliter of extracts (1 mg/mL) was added to 1.5 mL of reagent and allowed to stand at room temperature for 5 min. Sodium carbonate solution (1.25 mL, 20%) was added to the mixture and stored at room temperature for an additional 60 min, and absorptions at 725 nm were recorded. Calibration curve was created by a standard concentration of tannic acid and total phenolic compounds of extract were obtained by calibration curve [12,13].

The total flavonoid content of the extract was determined by aluminum chloride ($ALCl_3$). The sample solution (1 mL) was mixed with 1 mL of aluminum trichloride (2%) in methanol. Moreover, a blank solution was prepared by adding an extract solution (1 mL) to 1 mL of methanol without $AlCl_3$. The extract and blank absorbance were recorded at 415 nm after 10 min of incubation at 25 °C. The total flavonoid content was expressed as equivalents of quercetin. Furthermore, calibration curve was prepared by a standard solution of quercetin [12,14].

2.4. Animal Studies

2.4.1. Animal Conditions

Male Balb/C mice weighing 20–30 g were housed in clean cages at room temperature (22–25 °C), 12-h light/12-h dark cycle and relative air humidity 40–60%. Mice had continuous access to food and tap water. All procedures involving animals were approved by the ethical committee of Mazandaran University of Medical Sciences. With ethical code 294 , 25 August 2016.

2.4.2. Preparation of Diabetic Mice

The animals were injected with streptozocin (35 mg/kg, IP). Five days after injection, the mice with fasting blood glucose higher than 250 mg/dL were used for the experiments. Eight mice were used in each experiment. In addition, each animal was used once only in all of experiments. The dietary food and water were removed from cages 12 h before testing [5].

2.4.3. Drug Administration

The extract was suspended in distilled water and administered orally through oro-gastric tube at doses of 50, 100, and 200 mg/kg body weight. The volume of administrated extract was calculated 1 unit of insulin syringe per gram of weight for each animal [5].

2.4.4. Experimental Design

In the present study, 48 Balb/C mice (40 diabetics, 8 normal mice) were used. The mice were divided into six groups. In addition, eight mice were used in each group.

Group 1: Normal control mice were administrated 1 unit of insulin syringe per gram of weight of distilled water daily for 21 days.

Groups 2: Diabetic mice were administrated 1 unit of insulin syringe per gram of weight of distilled water daily for 21 days.

Group 3: Diabetic mice were administrated metformin (200 mg/kg body weight) daily for 21 days.

Groups 4–6: Diabetic mice were administrated *M. germanica* extract (50, 100, and 200 mg/kg body weight) daily using a gavage tube for 21 days [5].

2.4.5. Serum Glucose Assay

After 21 days of treatments, blood samples were drawn from the hearts of the mice, and serum glucose was determined. Serum glucose was estimated with a digital blood glucose analyzer [13].

2.4.6. Glutathione and Lipid Peroxidation Assay

Tissue Preparation and Subcellular Fractionation

The animal groups were killed after 21 days, and livers were taken out and kept on a low temperature condition. The livers were homogenized separately in a phosphate buffer (10 mM phosphate buffer, pH 7.0) and centrifuged at 1000× *g* for 10 min at 4 °C to separate the nuclear debris. The aliquot obtained was used for the lipid peroxidation [15].

Lipid Peroxidation Assay

The procedure was used for the estimation of the rate of lipid peroxidation. Homogenate tissue (0.5 mL) was pipetted in a 15 × 100 mm glass tube and incubated at 37 ± 1 °C in a shaker (100 cycles per min) for 60 min. Another 0.5 mL of the same homogenate was pipetted in a centrifuge tube and placed at 0 °C. After 1 h of incubation, 0.5 mL of 5% chilled TCA followed by 1 mL of 0.67% TBA was added to each glass tube and centrifuge tube and mixed after each addition. The aliquot amounts of each tube were centrifuged at 2000× *g* for 20 min. Then, the supernatant was placed in a boiling water bath. After 10 min, the test tubes were taken out and cooled, and the absorbance of the color was read at 535 nm [15].

Glutathione Assay

Reduced glutathione was assayed using a spectroscopic method. Post-mitochondrial supernatant (0.5 mL) was precipitated with 0.5 mL of sulfosalicylic acid (2%). The samples were kept at 4 °C for 2 h and then subjected to centrifugation at 1500× *g* for 10 min at 4 °C. The assay mixture contained 0.5 mL of filtered residue, 2.3 mL of phosphate buffer (0.2 M, pH 7.4), and 0.2 mL of DTNB (0.5% in phosphate buffer 0.2 M, pH 7.4) and was calculated immediately at 412 nm [15,16].

2.4.7. Statistical Analysis

Statistical analyses were performed using one-way analysis of variance and a Student's *t*-test by SPSS 16. The differences between the means were considered significant at the probability level $p < 0.05$ [17].

3. Results

The dried hydroacetonic extracts yielded 18.6% (*w*/*w*). The total phenol and flavonoid content of the extract were 720 and 500 (mg/100 g), respectively. The blood sugar levels and animal weights measured in normal and experimental Balb/C mice before and after 21 days of treatment are shown in Figures 1 and 2.

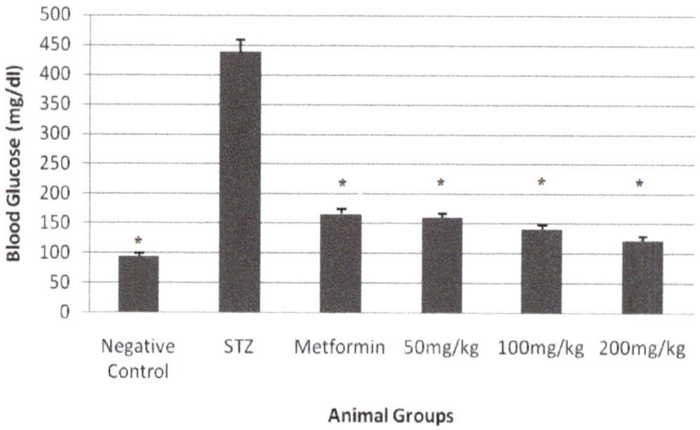

Figure 1. Effect of extract on blood glucose (mg/dL) in mice. * $p < 0.05$ compared with Streptozocin (STZ).

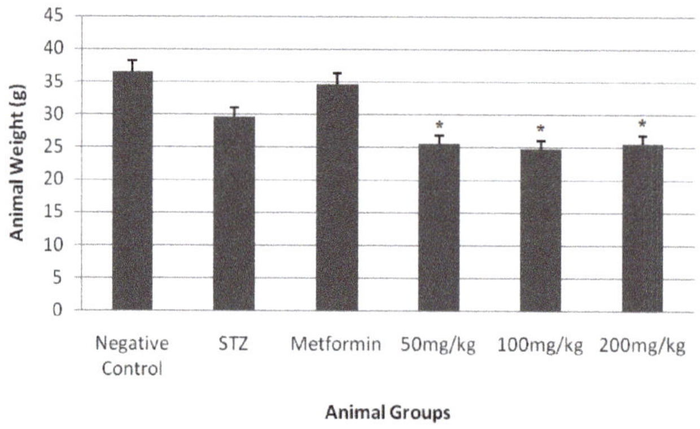

Figure 2. Effect of extract on body weight in mice (g). * $p < 0.05$ compared with negative control.

Additionally, the preventive effects of *M. germanica* leaf extract on stress oxidative and lipid peroxidation in Balb/C mice shown in Figure 3.

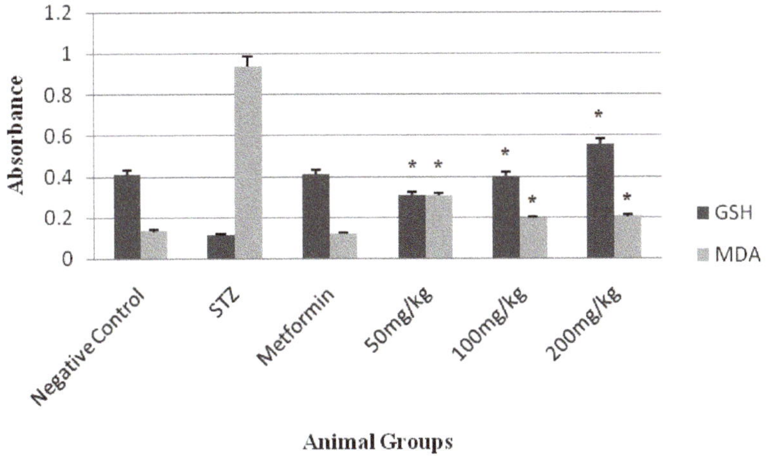

Figure 3. Effects of extract on stress oxidative and lipid peroxidation in mice. GSH: glutathione as an indicator of oxidative stress; MDA: malonyl dealdehyde as an indicator for lipid peroxidation; * $p < 0.05$ compared with STZ.

According to the results shown in Figure 1, the extract reduced the blood sugar almost in a dose-dependent manner, more evenly than metformin at doses of 100 and 200 mg/kg; however, as shown in Figure 2, the extract reduced the weight unexpectedly but was maintained in a constant range.

As in Figure 3, STZ had reduced glutathione (GSH) as an indicator for oxidative stress and increased malonyl dealdehyde as an indicator for lipid peroxidation. Metformin prevented MDA reducing and GSH increasing and the extract reduced MDA and increased GSH in a dose-dependent manner.

4. Discussion

According to the obtained data, *M. germanica* leaf hydroacetonic extract is effective in reducing blood glucose. This extract also significantly increased glutathione and decreased lipid peroxidation in a dose-dependent manner. Although the extract could not improve the weight of animal and evenly decreased the weights, this reduction was maintained, was not dose-dependent, and may be due to toxicities of the extract. As the extract had anti-oxidative stress properties, its sugar-reducing effect was most likely due to its protection effect on mitochondrias of the liver and not because of its toxicities. Additionally, the high total phenol and flavonoid contents of the extract can emphasize its anti-oxidant effects and the decreasing intestinal absorption of dietary sugars, which can also explain its weight reductions.

In diabetic conditions, auto-oxidation of excessive glucose leads to an accumulation of reactive oxygen species (ROS), the overproduction of which is said to be related to complications associated with diabetes. This has been supported by studies reporting improvement in diabetic complications through antioxidant treatment, including antioxidant chemicals or plant extracts [18]. Indeed, the underlying DM induction mechanism of STZ is based on the formation of superoxide radicals in pancreatic beta cells in consequence of several reactions [18]. GSH is considered a non-enzymatic antioxidant and has free radical scavenging potential in the cellular defense system [18]. MDA is an end product of lipid peroxidation and is a marker of oxidative stress related to membrane damage [18]. *M. germanica* extracts are comprised of polyphenolic compounds that are known to have antioxidant properties. One of these compounds, quercetin, is a flavonoid and is also able to inhibit glucose absorption in the intestines [18–21].

In our study, elevated MDA levels and decreased GSH activities in diabetic rats proved the key role of oxidative stress in the pathophysiology of liver damage in DM, and the extract could improve them.

Different studies have shown antidiabetic effects for some plants due to the presence of phytochemicals in their herbal organs [19,20]. Flavonoids and other phenolic compounds are potentially antidiabetic effects by glucose absorption inhibition in gastro-intestinal tract [21] and the antidiabetic effect of *M. germanica* is most likely due to flavanoid content such as quercetin.

Our study was also in parallel with other studies, such as those by Panjeshahin MR et al. on the antidiabetic activity of different extracts of *Myrtus communis* in streptozotocin-induced diabetic rats [5], those by Sokri G et al. on the anti-diabetic effects of the hydroalcoholic extract of green tea and cinnamon on diabetic rats [13], and those by Hatice B et al. on the anti-diabetic effects of aqueous extract of *Myrtus communis* L. leaves in diabetic rats [18]. In all of these studies, the herbal extract role of phenol and flavanoids such as quercetin as anti-oxidative stress compounds have been considered. Since we found a high percentage of phenols and flavanaoids in *M. germanica*, we can suggest that the compounds of this plant have an anti-diabetic effect, but more studies are needed for purifications of these components and for more precise toxicology and pharmacologic assay.

5. Conclusions

The present study indicated that the *Mespilus germanica* leaf extract significantly decreased serum glucose and maintained normal body weight in Balb/C diabetic mice as compared with control groups. In addition, this extract decreased oxidative stress and lipid peroxidation. In conclusion, this species and other citable plants are very valuable and should be evaluated in experimental and clinical trials for their pharmacological efficacy and the discovery of new approved drugs for diabetes mellitus.

Acknowledgments: This study was supported by Student Research Committee of Mazandaran University of Medical Sciences in Sari, Iran. We would like to thank laboratory personnel of department of Pharmacognosy and Department of Toxicology and Pharmacology in faculty of pharmacy of Mazandaran University of Medical Sciences. We also thank Mohammad Azadbakht from the Department of Pharmacognosy, Faculty of Pharmacy, Mazandaran University of Medical Sciences in Sari, Iran, for approving the authenticity of the plant used in the research. The analysis was supported by Mazandaran University of Medical Sciences with a project number of 294 from the student research committee.

Author Contributions: Fatemeh Shafiee was a study investigator and contributed to the analysis of the data. Elnaz Khoshvishkaie was a study investigator and contributed to the analysis of the data. Ali Davoodi participated in data interpretation and critically revised the manuscript. Ayat Dashti Kalantar participated in the practical processes. Hossein Bakhshi Jouybari participated in the practical processes. Ramin Ataee was a study investigator, contributed to the analysis of the data, and critically revised the manuscript.

Conflicts of Interest: The authors declare no conflict of interest.

References

1. Unnikrishnan, A. Diabetes secondary to endocrine and pancreatic disorders. *Ind. J. Med. Res.* **2016**, *143*, 670. [CrossRef]
2. Goldstein, B.J.; Müller-Wieland, D. *Type 2 Diabetes: Principles and Practice*; CRC Press: Boca Raton, FL, USA, 2016; Available online: https://scholar.google.com/scholar?q=Goldstein+BJ (accessed on 31 December 2017).
3. Guariguata, L.; Whiting, D.; Hambleton, I.; Beagley, J.; Linnenkamp, U.; Shaw, J. Global estimates of diabetes prevalence for 2013 and projections for 2035. *Diabetes Res. Clin. Pract.* **2014**, *103*, 137–149. [CrossRef] [PubMed]
4. Devi, H.; Mazumder, P. Methanolic Extract of Curcuma caesia Roxb. Prevents the Toxicity Caused by Cyclophosphamide to Bone Marrow Cells, Liver and Kidney of Mice. *Pharmacogn. Res.* **2016**, *8*, 43–49. [CrossRef]
5. Panjeshahin, M.R.; Azadbakht, M.; Akbari, N. Antidiabetic Activity of Different Extracts of Myrtus Communis in Streptozotocin Induced Diabetic Rats. *Rom. J. Diabetes Nutr. Metab. Diseases* **2016**, *23*, 183–190. [CrossRef]

6. Mirzaee, F.; Hosseini, A.; Jouybari, H.B.; Davoodi, A.; Azadbakht, M. Medicinal, biological and phytochemical properties of Gentiana species. *J. Tradit. Complement. Med.* **2017**, *7*, 400–408. [CrossRef] [PubMed]
7. Gharaghani, A.; Solhjoo, S.; Oraguzie, N. A review of genetic resources of pome fruits in Iran. *Genet. Resour. Crop Evol.* **2016**, *63*, 151–172. [CrossRef]
8. Rop, O.; Sochor, J.; Jurikova, T.; Zitka, O.; Skutkova, H.; Mlcek, J.; Salas, P.; Krska, B.; Babula, P.; Adam, V.; et al. Effect of five different stages of ripening on chemical compounds in medlar (*Mespilus germanica,* L.). *Molecules* **2011**, *16*, 74–91. [CrossRef] [PubMed]
9. Baharvand-Ahmadi, B.; Bahmani, M.; Tajeddini, P.; Naghdi, N.; Rafieian-Kopaei, M. An ethno-medicinal study of medicinal plants used for the treatment of diabetes. *J. Nephropathol.* **2016**, *5*, 44. [CrossRef] [PubMed]
10. Tabatabaei-Yazdi, F.; Alizadeh-Behbahani, B.; Zanganeh, H. The Comparison among Antibacterial Activity of Mespilus germanica Extracts and Number of Common Therapeutic Antibiotics "In Vitro". *Zahedan J. Res. Med. Sci.* **2015**, *17*, 29–34. [CrossRef]
11. Avram, M.; Stoica, A.; Dobre, T.; Stroescu, M. Extraction of vegetable oil from ground seeds by percolation techniques. *UPB Sci. Bull. B* **2014**, *76*, 13–22. [CrossRef]
12. Do, Q.; Angkawijaya, A.; Tran-Nguyen, P.; Huynh, L.; Soetaredjo, F.; Ismadji, S.; Ju, Y.H. Effect of extraction solvent on total phenol content, total flavonoid content, and antioxidant activity of Limnophila aromatica. *J. Food Drug Anal.* **2014**, *22*, 296–302. [CrossRef] [PubMed]
13. Shokri, G.; Fathi, H.; Jafari Sabet, M.; Nasri Nasrabadi, N.; Ataee, R. Evaluation of anti-diabetic effects of hydroalcoholic extract of green tea and cinnamon on streptozotocin-induced diabetic rats. *Pharm. Biomed. Res.* **2015**, *1*, 20–29. [CrossRef]
14. Kabir, M.; Al Noman, M.; Rahman, M.; Ara, J.; Hossain, M.; Hasanat, A.; Zaheed, F. Antibacterial activity of organic and aqueous extracts of Hopea odorata Roxb. leaves and their total flavonoid content. *Br. Microbiol. Res. J.* **2015**, *9*, 1–7. [CrossRef]
15. Khuwaja, G.; Khan, M.; Ishrat, T.; Ahmad, A.; Raza, S.; Ashafaq, M.; Javed, H.; Khan, M.B.; Khan, A.; Vaibhav, K.; et al. Neuroprotective effects of curcumin on 6-hydroxydopamine-induced Parkinsonism in rats: Behavioral, neurochemical and immunohistochemical studies. *Brain Res.* **2011**, *1368*, 254–263. [CrossRef] [PubMed]
16. Shaki, F.; Hosseini, M.-J.; Ghazi-Khansari, M.; Pourahmad, J. Depleted uranium induces disruption of energy homeostasis and oxidative stress in isolated rat brain mitochondria. *Metallomics* **2013**, *5*, 736–744. [CrossRef] [PubMed]
17. Kharouta, M.; Miller, K.; Kim, A.; Wojcik, P.; Kilimnik, G.; Dey, A.; Steiner, D.F.; Hara, M. No mantle formation in rodent islets—The prototype of islet revisited. *Diabtes Res. Clin. Pract.* **2009**, *85*, 252–257. [CrossRef] [PubMed]
18. Hatice, B.; Mine, G.; Lale, G.; Galip, M.D.; Dogukan, C.; Halis, S.; Zekai, H.; Nurcan, K.B. Effects of Aqueous Extract of *Myrtus Communis,* L. Leaves on Streptozotocin-Induced Diabetic Rats. *J. Res. Med. Dent. Sci.* **2016**, *4*. [CrossRef]
19. Li, S.; Brault, A.; Sanchez Villavicencio, M.; Haddad, P.S. *Rhododendron groenlandicum* (Labrador tea), an antidiabetic plant from the traditional pharmacopoeia of the Canadian Eastern James Bay Cree, improves renal integrity in the diet-induced obese mouse model. *Pharm. Biol.* **2016**, *54*, 1998–2006. [CrossRef] [PubMed]
20. Shantha, T.; Patchaimal, P.; Reddy, M.P.; Kumar, R.K.; Tewari, D.; Bharti, V.; Venkateshwarlu, G.; Mangal, A.K.; Padhi, M.M.; Dhiman, K.S. Pharmacognostical Standardization of *Upodika-Basella alba,* L.: An Important Ayurvedic Antidiabetic Plant. *Anc. Sci. Life* **2016**, *36*, 35–40. [CrossRef] [PubMed]
21. Moradi-Afrapoli, F.; Asghari, B.; Saeidnia, S.; Ajani, Y.; Mirjani, M.; Malmir, M.; Bazaz, R.D.; Hadjiakhoondi, A.; Salehi, P.; Hamburger, M.; et al. In vitro α-glucosidase inhibitory activity of phenolic constituents from aerial parts of Polygonum hyrcanicum. *DARU J. Pharm. Sci.* **2012**, *20*, 37. [CrossRef] [PubMed]

medicines

MDPI

Article

The Lipid Lowering and Cardioprotective Effects of *Vernonia calvoana* Ethanol Extract in Acetaminophen-Treated Rats

Godwin Eneji Egbung *, Item Justin Atangwho, Ochuole Diana Odey and Victor Ndubuisi Ndiodimma

Department of Biochemistry, University of Calabar, P.M.B 1115, Calabar 540, Nigeria; dratangwho@gmail.com (I.J.A.); diianer12@yahoo.com (O.D.O.); ndiodimmavictor@gmail.com (V.N.N.)

* Correspondence: eneji.egbung@unical.edu.ng or eneji6@gmail.com; Tel.: +234-803-837-5557

Academic Editors: Gema Nieto and Gerhard Litscher

Received: 22 October 2017; Accepted: 6 December 2017; Published: 12 December 2017

Abstract: Background: Paracetamol overdose/abuse as a result of self-medication is a common occurrence amongst people living in low/middle income countries. The present study was designed to investigate the hypolipidemic and cardioprotective potentials of *Vernonia calvoana* (VC) ethanol extract in acetaminophen (paracetamol)-treated rats. **Methods:** Thirty-five Wistar rats weighing 100–150 g were randomly assigned into five groups of seven rats each. Groups 2–5 received high doses of paracetamol to induce liver damage, while group 1 was used as normal control. Afterwards, they were allowed to receive varying doses of VC (group 3 and 4) or vitamin E (group 5), whilst groups 1 and 2 were left untreated. The treatment period lasted for twenty one days after which sera were harvested and assayed for serum lipid indices using standard methods. **Results:** Groups 3 to 5 treated animals indicated significant decrease ($p < 0.001$) in low density lipoprotein cholesterol (LDL-c), total cholesterol (TC) and triacylglycerol (TG) levels relative to the normal and acetaminophen-treated controls, the atherogenic index showed a significant decrease ($p < 0.001$) in all treated groups compared with normal and acetaminophen-treated controls. However, the VC- and vitamin E-treated groups showed significant ($p < 0.001$) increase in high density lipoprotein cholesterol (HDL-c) relative to the controls. **Conclusions:** Data from our study suggest that ethanol leaf extract of VC possesses probable hypolipidemic and cardioprotective effects.

Keywords: Acetaminophen; *Vernonia calvoana*; serum lipid indices; hypolipidemic activity and antioxidants

---

1. Introduction

Acetaminophen, also known as paracetamol, is most often classified as a mild, over-the-counter analgesic used in the treatment of pains/headaches. It is mostly intentionally abused. The drug is generally safe when taken in recommended doses, though even a very small overdose could be deleterious. In the United States of America, paracetamol overdose has been reported to account for more calls to the poison control center than an overdose of any other pharmacological substance [1]. It is the number one drug of choice in managing pains globally. However, its mechanism of action in relieving pain is yet to be fully elucidated but suggested to be implicated in a number of pain pathways [2].

Paracetamol metabolism in the liver could result in the formation of a highly toxic metabolite, *N*-acetyl-*p*-benzoquinone imine (NAPQI) by the cytochrome P_{450} enzyme system [3]. Further detoxification to eliminate the metabolite is accomplished by its conjugation with glutathione, but in cases of overdose or abuse, glutathione stores are depleted resulting in the accumulation of the metabolite and eventual toxicity [3]. Abuse of the drug may lead to toxicity which could result in hepatocellular necrosis and kidney damage [4]. Oxidative stress mediated action of NAPQI accumulation has been implicated in the pathogenesis of paracetamol-induced liver and renal damage in experimental animals [4]. Paracematol abuse in third world countries has been on the increase since a greater proportion of the population tends to resort to self-medication. The non-availability of standard health facilities poses another challenge of the arbitrary use of ethno botanicals instead of synthetic drugs to treat complications of paracetamol abuse.

Medicinal plants have played an important role in the abatement of toxic substances in the human body. They also function as vital hypolipidemic agents [5]. *Vernonia calvoana* (Hook.F) is an asteraceae with local name "Ekeke leaf" by the indigenes of the central senatorial district of Cross-River State of Nigeria [6]. The plant is distributed in the upper Guinea Cameroun mountains, South-West Cameroun and South-Eastern Nigeria [7]. It is consumed by natives based on the belief that the plant remedies heart diseases, diabetes, malaria, stomach aches and can be used as a vermifuge [6]. Igile et al. and Egbung et al. [6,8], respectively, reported that the leaves and the inflorescents of *Vernonia calvoana* contained flavonoids in appreciable amounts thus responsible for its antioxidant properties. Iwara et al. [9] also reported its hepatoprotective, hypolipidemic and antidiabetic activity in Steptozotocin-induced rats. Folklore medicine and ethno botanicals application when not developed could go into extinction [10]. Most medicinal plants have outstanding therapeutic effects and are better tolerated than some synthetic drugs, and as such produce fewer allergic reactions [11]. However, a good number of these herbal formulations may exert some toxic effect as well [12].

Vernonia amygdalina, a member of the same genus like *Vernonia calvoana* has been exploited in the management of certain disease conditions like diabetes and obesity thus exerting anti-diabetic, anti-bacterial, anti-malarial, anti-fungal, antioxidant, hepatoprotective, and non-cytotoxic properties [13]. However, there is scanty information on the probable lipid lowering and cardio protective potentials of *Vernonia calvoana* extracts in acetaminophen-treated Wistar rats. This study was therefore designed to investigate this information gap and recommend its use as alternative therapy in acetaminophen toxicities.

2. Materials and Methods

2.1. Procurement of Leaves, Rat Chow and Acetaminophen

Fresh *Vernonia calvoana* leaves were purchased from a local market in Ugep town in Yakurr Local Government Area of Cross-River State, Nigeria. The rat chow was bought from Pfizer Livestock Feeds, Aba, Abia State, Nigeria. The leaves were authenticated by Pastor Frank Aposeye, a botanist in the Department of Botany, University of Calabar, Calabar, Cross-River State, Nigeria, and voucher number BOT/VC/2/2015 deposited in the herbarium of the same department. Paracetamol manufactured by Emzor pharmaceuticals was purchased from Anijah Pharmacy, Etta Agbor Road, Calabar, Cross River State, Nigeria.

2.2. Preparation of Extract

The leaves were washed thoroughly to remove dust and other forms of dirt, and afterwards, air dried at room temperature (27 °C ± 2 °C) for seven days to remove moisture until completely dry. The dried leaves were blended to a fine powder using a dry Moulinex super blender and stored in air-tight containers. 1.5 kg of the powder was weighed using an electronic scale and afterwards soaked in 2000 mL of 98% ethanol (*v*/*v*) in a ratio of 3:4, i.e., (powder/solvent). To allow for proper mixing of the powder and the solvent, the mixture was agitated and then put in air-tight containers. The containers holding the mixtures were kept in the refrigerator at a temperature of 4 °C for 48 h. Filtration of the mixture was accomplished first by using a cheesecloth, followed by the Whatman No. 1 filter paper (24 cm). The filtrate was concentrated using a rotary evaporator (model RE52A, Zhengzhou, China) to 10% of its original volume at a temperature of 37–40 °C. It was then concentrated to complete dryness in a water bath. The extract was afterwards refrigerated at 2–8 °C until when required for administration.

2.3. Experimental Animals

Thirty-five male albino Wistar rats weighing between 100 and 150 g were obtained from a disease-free stock of the animal house, Department of Zoology, University of Calabar, Calabar. The animals were acclimatized for two weeks on pelletized rat chow and water provided *ad libitum*. The experiment was conducted in accordance with the internationally accepted principles for laboratory animal use and care [14]. Permission and approval (009BC20816) for the use of the animals to carry out the study were obtained from the Faculty Animal Research Ethics Committee, Faculty of Basic Medical Sciences (FAREC-FBMS) University of Calabar on 20 August 2016. The animals were distributed randomly into five groups of seven animals each based on weight as shown in Table 1.

Table 1. Experimental treatment groups.

Group	Number of Animals	Treatment
Group 1	7	Normal saline
Group 2	7	2 g/kg paracetamol only
Group 3	7	2 g/kg paracetamol + 200 mg/kg b.w. VC
Group 4	7	2 g/kg paracetamol + 400 mg/kg b.w. VC
Group 5	7	2 g/kg paracetamol + 100 mg/kg b.w. Vit. E

VC = Extract of *Vernonia calvoana*; Vit. E = Vitamin E; b.w. = body weight.

Hepatic damage was induced with paracetamol (2 g/kg b.w.) prepared in normal saline and administered per orals once a day to all the groups except the normal control for four days. Three days after paracetamol administration, one animal was selected at random from all the groups and sacrificed under anesthesia. Whole blood was collected, centrifuged and sera obtained used for the estimation of serum enzymes (aspartate aminotransferase, alanine aminotransferase and alkaline phosphatase) to confirm toxicity.

2.4. Extract and Drug Administration

The doses (200 mg/kg and 400 mg/kg) used were based on the predetermined LD_{50} values obtained using Lorke's method [15]. The extract was diluted in normal saline, which acted as the vehicle and administered orally through gastric intubation accordingly after hepatic damage had been established. The control animals received 0.2 mL of normal saline. VC treatment lasted 21 days. The animals were fasted 12 h overnight prior to the time of sacrifice. The animals were euthanised with chloroform and blood samples collected via cardiac puncture.

2.5. Preparation of Serum for Biochemical Assays

Whole blood was collected from each experimental animal through cardiac puncture and put into to sterile non heparinized sample tubes which were allowed to stand for 2–4 h before centrifugation. The serum was carefully taken out using a syringe and needle down the side of the tube, leaving the clot behind. The serum gotten was subjected to further separation by centrifugation, using an MSE table top centrifuge (Buckinghamshire, England), set at 8000 rpm (revolutions per minute) for 15 min to ensure clear supernatant devoid of traces of red cells The serum samples collected were stored in a refrigerator at 4 °C for subsequent biochemical assays.

2.6. Assay of Selected Lipid Parameters

Triacylglycerol (TG), total cholesterol (TC), and high density lipoprotein cholesterol (HDL-c) were determined with analytical kits from Randox laboratories Ltd. (Admore Diamond Road, Crumlin, Co., Antrim, UK). Very low density lipoprotein cholesterol (VLDL-c), low density lipoprotein—cholesterol

(LDL-c) and atherogenic index were estimated by modification of Friedewald formula as described by [16].The assays were conducted according to the manufacturer's instructions.

2.7. Statistical Analysis

Data obtained were expressed as mean ± standard error of mean (SEM). One-way analysis of variance was used to determine the differences between means, followed by posthoc multiple comparisons. Data were considered significant at $p < 0.05$. Computer software SPSS version 17.0 and Microsoft Excel (2007 version) analyzer were used for analysis.

3. Results

Results of the effects of *V. calvoana* leaf extract on some selected lipid biomarkers in paracetamol-treated rats are presented in Figures 1–5.

3.1. Effects of V. calvoana on Total Cholesterol (TC) Concentration

The mean total cholesterol values for the different experimental groups (control group, hepatotoxic untreated group, 400 mg/kg bwt *V. calvoana* treated group, 200 mg/kg bwt *V. calvoana* treated groups and vitamin E-treated group namely groups 1, 2, 3, 4 and 5 respectively) are 104.45 ± 1.86, 177.52 ± 4.72, 93.27 ± 5.08, 86.80 ± 1.32 and 135.78 ± 1.95 respectively. The mean total cholesterol value for the hepatotoxic untreated group significantly increased at $p < 0.001$ when compared to the normal control group. The group treated with 200 mg/kg bwt of the extract had a significantly lower TC value at $p < 0.005$ compared to the normal control and a significantly lower value at $p < 0.001$ when compared to the hepatotoxic untreated group. The group treated with 400 mg/kg bwt of the extract showed a much more reduced value significant at $p < 0.001$ when compared with the normal control and the hepatotoxic untreated group. The vitamin E-treated group significantly reduced at $p < 0.001$ when compared with the hepatotoxic untreated group, but had a higher value than the normal control and the *V. calvoana* treated groups, significant at $p < 0.001$ respectively. The result obtained above is represented in Figure 1.

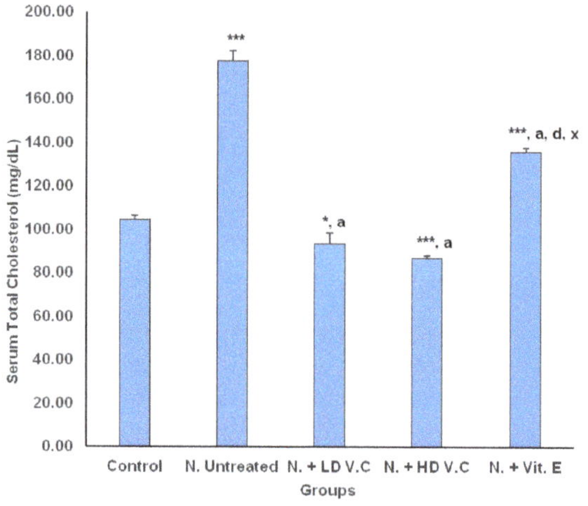

Figure 1. Effect of *V. calvoana* extract on serum total cholesterol in paracetamol-treated rats. Values are presented as mean ± SEM, $n = 5$. * $p < 0.05$, *** $p < 0.001$ vs. control, a = $p < 0.001$ vs. N. untreated, d = $p < 0.001$ vs. N + LD VC, x = $p < 0.001$ vs. N + HD VC. Where N = hepatotoxic.

3.2. *Effect of V. calvoana on Triacylglycerol Concentration*

Triacylglycerol mean values for the groups are 53.09 ± 3.88, 125.97 ± 5.12, 55.95 ± 1.51, 55.75 ± 1.15, and 56.62 ± 1.24 respectively. The mean value for group 2 was significantly higher at $p < 0.001$ when compared with the normal control. The *V. calvoana* treated groups (200 mg/kg b.wt and 400 mg/kg b.wt) and vitamin E-treated showed significantly lower values than the untreated hepatotoxic group ($p < 0.001$). The result as presented in Figure 2.

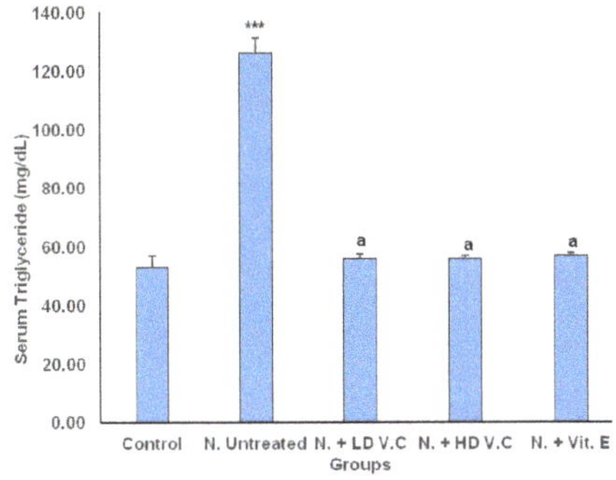

Figure 2. Effect of *V. calvoana* extract on serum triacylglycerol in paracetamol treated rats. Values are presented as mean ± SEM, $n = 5$. *** $p < 0.001$ vs. control, a = $p < 0.001$ vs. N. untreated. Where N = hepatotoxic.

3.3. *Effect of Treatment on High-Density Lipoprotein Cholesterol*

The high density lipoprotein cholesterol (HDL-c) values for the groups are 55.13 ± 0.71, 21.23 ± 1.21, 54.38 ± 1.38, 57.02 ± 2.23 and 75.16 ± 0.82 respectively. The mean HDL-c value of the hepatotoxic untreated group was significantly ($p < 0.001$) lower than the normal control group. The *V. calvoana* treated groups (200 mg/kg b.wt and 400 mg/kg b.wt) have significantly higher HDL-c values than the untreated hepatotoxic group at $p < 0.001$. The vitamin E-treated group has a significantly higher value at $p < 0.001$, compared to the normal control, untreated hepatotoxic group and the *V. calvoana* treated groups. The result as presented in Figure 3.

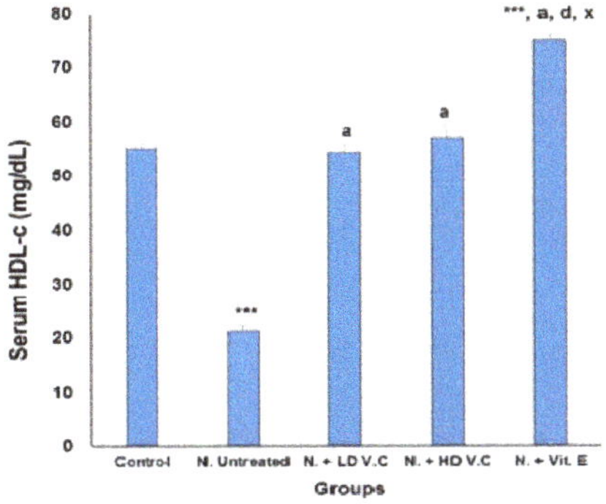

Figure 3. Effect of *V. calvoana* extract on serum high density lipoprotein cholesterol in paracetamol treated rats. Values are presented as mean ± SEM, $n = 5$. *** $p < 0.001$ vs. control, a = $p < 0.001$ vs. N. untreated, d = $p < 0.001$ vs. N. + LD V.C., x = $p < 0.001$ vs. N. + HD V.C. Where N = hepatotoxic.

3.4. *Effect of Treatment on the Low-Density Lipoprotein Cholesterol*

The mean LDL-c values for all the groups are 38.70 ± 2.12, 131.09 ± 5.07, 27.70 ± 4.04, 18.63 ± 1.43 and 49.30 ± 1.68. Group 2 has a significantly higher value at $p < 0.001$ when compared to the normal control. Mean LDL-c value for group 3 showed a significant decrease at $p < 0.05$ and $p < 0.001$ compared to the normal control (group 1) and group 2 respectively. Compared to group 1 and 2, group 4 showed a significant decrease at $p < 0.001$ respectively, while the mean value for group 5 was significantly lower at $p < 0.05$ compared to group 1. However, compared to group 3 and 4, the mean LDL-c value of group 5 was significantly higher at $p < 0.001$. The mean value of group 5 dropped significantly ($p < 0.001$) compared to group 2. The result as presented in Figure 4.

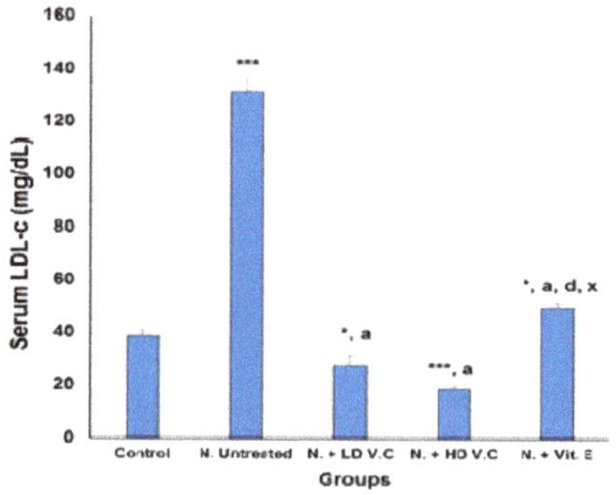

Figure 4. Effect of *V. calvoana* extract on serum low density lipoprotein cholesterol (LDL-c) in paracetamol treated rats. Values are presented as mean ± SEM, $n = 5$. * $p < 0.05$, *** $p < 0.001$ vs. control, a = $p < 0.001$ vs. N. untreated, d = $p < 0.001$ vs. N. + LD V.C., x = $p < 0.001$ vs. N. + HD V.C. Where N = hepatotoxic.

3.5. *Effect of Treatment on Atherogenic Index*

Figure 5 shows that group 2 has a significantly ($p < 0.001$) higher atherogenic index of plasma compared to the normal control (group 1). Group 3 has a significantly lower value at $p < 0.001$ compared to group 2. Similarly, group 4 has a significantly lower atherogenic index compared to group 2 at $p < 0.001$, and a lower value also compared to group 2 at $p < 0.001$. However, group 5 has a significantly lower value as well compared to group 2 at $p < 0.001$, but a significantly higher value than group 4 at $p < 0.01$.

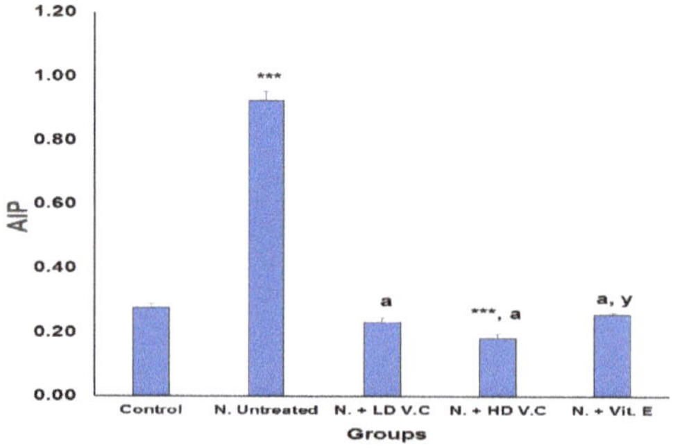

Figure 5. Effect of *V. calvoana* extract on the atherogenic index in paracetamol treated rats. Values are presented as mean ± SEM, $n = 5$. *** $p < 0.001$ vs. control, a = $p < 0.001$ vs. N. untreated, y = $p < 0.01$ vs. N. + HD V.C. Where N = hepatotoxic.

4. Discussion

The prevalence of drug abuse as a result of overdose has been increasing, especially in economically deprived communities in the developing countries where there is little or no access to standard health facilities and the majority of the population resort to self-medication [17]. In this study, we reported the effect of *V. calvoana* leaf extract on some selected lipid biomarkers in paracetamol-treated Wistar rats. The 400 mg/kg body weight extracts of *V. calvoana* exert more potent lipid lowering activity which is similar to the pattern in a study by Iwara et al. [9]. Acetaminophen poisoning may be due to ingestion of excessive/repeated or too frequent doses [18]. Obu et al. [19] reported that most administration of paracetamol to children was done through self-prescription with possible tendency of abuse. The paracetamol treated rat model used was to mimic a situation where persons especially involved in unskilled labor practice will walk into patent medicine stores to purchase paracetamol for treating pains due to a hard day's labor at construction/building sites. The trend continues for about three to four days in a week. *V. calvoana* is safe because its dose at above 5000 mg/kg body weight in mice showed no toxicity from our preliminary studies. The animal model groups treated with 200 mg/kg b.wt and 400 mg/kg b.wt of the *V. calvoana* (groups 3 and 4) showed significantly lower LDL-C, TC and atherogenic index, as well as increased HDL-C levels. This finding is in agreement with the report of [9], where the extract was administered to diabetic rats and it exhibited a lipid lowering effect. Oxidative stress conditions will often trigger lipid peroxidation as represented by increased levels of malondialdehyde concentrations. The metabolite of acetaminophen has been known to be a depleting agent of the glutathione pool, the body's antioxidants defense system. The administration of ethanol extracts of *V. calvoana* mimics the replenishing potentials of glutathione, thus, preventing free radical generation following overdose of paracetamol.

The increased HDL-C levels noticed in groups 3 and 4 indicates a possibly lower risk of developing coronary heart diseases and other related cardiovascular events. Nichols et al. [20] reported that a moderate rise in HDL-C levels, resulting from the use of statin drugs, has been linked to a corresponding decline in the risk of developing coronary atherosclerosis. Stocker et al. [21] also reported that lowering LDL-C was a more effective method of reducing the risk of developing cardiovascular diseases than surgical methods. However, the abundance of antioxidants in the plant (*V. calvoana*) could prevent the oxidation of LDL-C within the blood vessels. It is a known fact that LDL-C is virtually harmless till it is oxidized by reactive species in the blood vessels, resulting in atherosclerosis [22]. The reduced atherogenic indices of the extract-treated groups implies a decreased risk of developing atherosclerosis since the atherogenic index of plasma is considered a reliable indicator of the onset of cardiovascular events [23,24]. Our finding is in agreement with the hypolipidemic effect of *V. calvoana* extracts in a diabetic rat model as reported by Iwara et al. [9] which implicated flavonoids and other bioactive principles for the effects. They are also in agreement with the report of Johnson et al. [25] where *V. amygdalina* decreased levels of MDA and prevented peroxidation of lipids in PC-3 cells.

5. Conclusions

From the results obtained in this study, it is safe to further confirm that the ethanolic leaf extract of *V. calvoana* possesses a lipid-lowering and cardioprotective effects and is a candidate in the management of paracetamol-induced toxicities, however, further studies on the molecular mechanism underlying the effect of *V. calvoana* on functional lipids is being investigated in our laboratory.

Acknowledgments: The authors are grateful to Victor Udo Nna of the Department of Physiology for his critical suggestions during the manuscript preparation.

Author Contributions: G.E.E. designed and supervised the work, O.D.O. carried out the work, I.J.A. and V.N.N. provided some literature information and also read and approved the final manuscript.

Conflicts of Interest: The authors declare no conflict of interest.

References

1. Lee, W.M. Acetaminophen and the US. Acute Liver Failure Study Group: Lowering the risks of hepatic failure. *Hepatology* **2004**, *40*, 6–9. [CrossRef] [PubMed]
2. Sharma, C.V.; Mehta, V. Paracetamol: Mechanisms and updates. *Contin. Educ. Anaesth. Crit. Care Pain* **2014**, *14*, 153–158. [CrossRef]
3. Kaplowitz, N. Acetaminophen hepatotoxic: What we know, what don't we know, and what do we do next? *Hepatology* **2004**, *40*, 23–26. [CrossRef] [PubMed]
4. Ramadan, B.K.; Schaalan, M.F. The renoprotective effect of honey on paracetamol—Induced Hepatotoxicity in Adult Male Albino Rats. *Life Sci. J.* **2011**, *8*, 589–596.
5. Luo, Q.; Cai, Y.; Yan, J.; Sun, M.; Corke, H. Hypoglycemic and hypolipidemic effects and antioxidant activity of fruit extracts from lyceum barbarum. *Life Sci.* **2004**, *76*, 137–149. [CrossRef] [PubMed]
6. Igile, G.O.; Iwara, I.A.; Mgbeje, B.A.; Uboh, F.E.; Ebong, P.E. Phytochemical, proximate and nutrient composition of *Vernonia calvoana* hook (Asterecea). A Green-Leafy vegetable in Nigeria. *J. Food Res.* **2013**, *2*, 6.
7. Ejoh, R.A.; Djuikwo, V.N.; Gouado, I.; Mbofung, C.M. Nutritional components of some non-conventional leafy vegetables consumed in Cameroon. *Pak. J. Nutr.* **2007**, *6*, 712–717. [CrossRef]
8. Egbung, G.E.; Atangwho, I.J.; Kiasira, Z.B.; Iwara, A.I.; Igile, G.O. Antioxidant activity of the inflorescents of *Vernonia calvoana* growing in Yakurr Local Government Area of Cross River State, Nigeria. *Glob. J. Pure Appl. Sci.* **2016**, *22*, 141–146. [CrossRef]
9. Iwara, I.A.; Igile, G.O.; Uboh, F.E.; Eyong, E.U.; Ebong, P.E. Hypoglycemic and hypolipidemic potentials of extract of *Vernonioa Calvoana* on alloxan-induced diabetic albino Wistar rats. *Eur. J. Med. Plant* **2015**, *8*, 78–86. [CrossRef]
10. Hostettmann, K.; Martson, A.; Ndjoko, K.; Wolfender, J.L. The potential of African Medicinal plants as a source of drugs. *Curr. Org. Chem.* **2000**, *4*, 937–1010. [CrossRef]
11. Lovkora, M.Y.; Buzuk, G.V.; Sokolova, S.M.; Kliment'era, N.I. Chemical features of medicinal plants (Review). *Appl. Biochem. Microbiol.* **2001**, *37*, 229–237. [CrossRef]
12. Bnouham, M.; Ziyyat, A.; Mekhfi, H.; Tahri, A.; Legssyer, A. Medicinal plants with potential antidiabetic activity–A review of 10 years of herbal medicine research (1990–2000). *Int. J. Diabetes Metab.* **2006**, *6*, 1–25.
13. Yeap, S.W.; Hol, W.Y.; Beh, B.K.; Liang, W.S.; Ky, H.; Yousr, H.N.; Alitheen, N.B. *Vernonia amygdalina*, an ethnoveterinary and ethnomedical used green vegetable with multiple bio-activities. *J. Med. Plants Res.* **2010**, *4*, 2787–2812.
14. NIH Guide. *Revised Guide for the Care and Use of Laboratory Animals*; The National Academies Press: Washington, DC, USA, 1996.
15. Lorke, D. A new approach to practical acute toxicity testing. *Arch. Toxicol.* **1983**, *53*, 275–287. [CrossRef]
16. Rotimi, O.A.; Olayiwola, I.O.; Ademuyiwa, O.; Balogun, E.A. Effects of fibre-enriched diets on tissue lipid profiles of MSG obese rats. *Food Chem. Toxicol.* **2012**, *50*, 4062–4067. [CrossRef] [PubMed]
17. Bennadi, D. Self-medication: A current challenge. *J. Basic Clin. Pharm.* **2014**, *5*, 19–23. [CrossRef] [PubMed]
18. Kett, D.H.; Breitmeyer, J.B.; Ang, R.; Royal, M.A. A randomized study of the efficacy and safety of intravenous acetaminophen vs. intravenous placebo for the treatment of fever. *Clin. Pharm. Ther.* **2011**, *90*, 32–39. [CrossRef] [PubMed]
19. Obu, H.A.; Chinawa, J.M.; Ubesie, A.C.; Eke, C.B.; Ndu, I.K. Paracetamol use (and/or misuse) in children in Enugu, South-East, Nigeria. *BMC Pediatr.* **2012**, *12*, 103. [CrossRef] [PubMed]
20. Nichols, S.J.; Tuzcu, E.M.; Sipahi, I. Statins, HDL-C, and regression of coronary atherosclerosis. *J. Am. Med. Assoc.* **2007**, *297*, 499–508. [CrossRef] [PubMed]
21. Stocker, R.; Keaney, J.F. Role of oxidative modification in atherosclerosis. *Physiol. Rev.* **2004**, *84*, 1381–1478. [CrossRef] [PubMed]
22. William, E.; Boden, M.D. Optimal medical therapy with or without PCI for stable coronary disease. *N. Engl. J. Med.* **2007**, *356*, 1503–1516.
23. Dobiasova, M.; Frohlich, J. The plasma parameter log (TG/HDL-C) as an atherogenic index: Correlation with lipoprotein particle size and esterification rate in apoB-lipoprotein-depleted plaoma (FER_{HDL}). *Clin. Biochem.* **2001**, *34*, 583–588. [CrossRef]

24. Tan, M.H.; Johns, D.; Glazer, N.B. Pioglitazone reduces artherogenic index of plasma in patient with type 2diabetes. *Clin. Biochem.* **2004**, *50*, 1184–1188.
25. Johnson, W.; Tchounwou, P.B.; Yedjou, C.G. Therapeutic mechanisms of *Vernonia amygdalina* Delile in the treatment of prostate cancer. *Molecules* **2017**, *22*, 1594. [CrossRef] [PubMed]

medicines

MDPI

Article

Anti-Lipase Potential of the Organic and Aqueous Extracts of Ten Traditional Edible and Medicinal Plants in Palestine; a Comparison Study with Orlistat

Nidal Jaradat *, Abdel Naser Zaid, Fatima Hussein, Maram Zaqzouq, Hadeel Aljammal and Ola Ayesh

Department of Pharmacy, Faculty of Medicine and Health Sciences, An-Najah National University, P.O. Box 7, Nablus 00970, Palestine; anzaid@najah.edu (A.N.Z.); f.huseen@najah.edu (F.H.); maram-zaqzouq@hotmail.com (M.Z.); hadeeljawad133@outlook.com (H.A.); oayesh@najah.edu (O.A.)

* Correspondence: nidaljaradat@najah.edu; Tel.: +970-599739476

Academic Editor: Gema Nieto
Received: 21 October 2017; Accepted: 6 December 2017; Published: 8 December 2017

Abstract: Background: Herbs have played a fundamental and essential role in the humans life since ancient times, especially those which are used as food and/or folk medicinedue to both their nutritive and curative properties.This study aimed to investigate new antilipase agents from tentraditional Palestinian edible and medicinal plants through inhibition of the absorption of dietary lipids. **Methods:** The anti-lipase activity for ten plants was evaluated and compared with the reference compound Orlistat by using the porcine pancreatic lipase inhibitory test which was conducted by using a UV-visible spectrophotometer. **Results:** The aqueous extracts of *Vitis vinifera* and *Rhus coriaria* had the highest antilipase effects with IC_{50} values 14.13 and 19.95 mcg/mL, respectively. Meanwhile, the organic extract of *Origanum dayi* had an IC_{50} value 18.62 mcg/mL. *V. vinifera* showed the highest porcine pancreatic lipase inhibitory effects when compared with Orlistat, which has an IC_{50} value 12.38 mcg/mL. **Conclusions:** According to the obtained results, *V. vinifera*, *R. coriaria*, and *O. dayi* can be considered a natural inhibitors of the pancreatic lipase enzyme as well as new players in obesity treatment. In fact, these plants can be freely and safely consumed in a daily diet or can be prepared as nutraceutical formulations to treat or prevent of obesity.

Keywords: anti-obesity; anti-lipase; traditional medicine; folkloric food

1. Introduction

The results from the WHO global survey on traditional, complementary/alternative, and herbal medicines showed that the market for these kinds of medicines is growing steadily worldwide. In fact, the usage of phytopharmaceuticals and nutraceuticals is rapidly and continuously expanding. Recently, many people have been using these formulations in the treatment or prevention of various diseases and disorders in different national healthcare systems. Moreover, many patients often use herbal medicines to complement treatment with conventional medicines [1–3]. Herbals and phytopharmaceuticals for the treatment of excess weightand obesity were among the most used remedies, especially in developing and developed countries, since these metabolic disorders became very prominent [4,5]. In fact, obesity poses a worldwide concern, not only for the harm which excess weight alone may cause, but also due to associated health problems such as endocrine, metabolic, and cardiovascular disorders [6–8].

Accordingly, various therapeutic protocols are utilized globally to control excess body weight and hyperlipidemia in obese patients. In fact, many drugs which have recently become available in pharmaceutical markets are recommended for use hand-in-hand with diet and exercise changes for the reduction of body weight and decreasing lipid levels in the plasma [6,9].

Orlistat is prototype weight loss drug. It is a gastrointestinal lipase inhibitor that competes with dietary fats for sites on the lipase molecules and has been shown to block the absorption of around 30% of dietary fat at a therapeutic oral dose of 120 mg, three times a day. Orlistat inhibits the hydrolysis of dietary triglycerides and thus reduces the subsequent intestinal absorption of the products of lipolysis (monoglycerides and free fatty acids), and does not demonstrate any efficient effect on appetite [10].Therefore, one of the most important screening strategies in the discovery of anti-obesity formulations is to search for potent lipase inhibitors from natural plant extracts [10].

Traditional medicinal plants have been used for obesity and body weight control in many countries. In fact, their consumption, along with appropriate dietary changes, is becoming one of the most popular complementary and alternative medicine strategies for the control of obesity and weight gain [11,12].

In this study, the organic and the aqueous extracts of various edible and traditional medicinal plants, which were collected from different regions of Palestine, were screened as potential anti-obesity agents by monitoring their anti-lipase activity. A total of 10 plants belonging to nine families from Palestine, which are used both as folk medicine and food, were studied, including: *Arum palaestinum* Boiss., *Crataegus azarolus* L., *Malva parviflora* L., *Taraxacum syriacum* Boiss., *Rhus coriaria* L., *Rosmarinus officinalis* L., *Psidium guajava* L., *Origanum dayi* Post, *Brassica nigra* (L.) K. Koch, and *Vitis vinifera* L. The first nine plants grow wildly in the mountains of Palestine and most of them are used in folk medicine to control weight gain [13,14].

In this study, the tested plants were evaluated for their antilipase activity by using a simple, fast, efficient, and reliable spectrophotometric method, in an attempt to investigate these new agents for their ability to impair the of digestion and assimilation of dietary fats. In addition, they were compared with Orlistat in order to assess their potential use as an alternative to this chemical agent.

2. Materials and Methods

2.1. Instrumentation

Shaker device (Memmert shaking incubator, Buchenbach, Germany), UV-visible spectrophotometer (Jenway 7135, Staffordshire, UK), grinder (Moulinex, model LM2211, UNO, Shanghai, China), balance (Rad wag, AS 220/c/2, Radom, Poland), freeze-dryer (Mill rock technology, model BT85, Danfoss, Shanghai, China), filter paper (Machrery-Nagel, Bethlehem, PA, USA; MN 617 and Whatman no.1), and rotary evaporator (Heidolph OB2000, VV2000, Schwabach, Germany).

2.2. Chemicals

From Sigma-Aldrich (Schnelldorf, Germany) the following were purchased: dimethyl sulfoxide, p-nitrophenyl butyrate, Orlistat, and tris-HCl buffer; while from Sigma (St. Louis, MO, USA) we purchased porcine pancreatic lipase type II (100–500 units/mg protein (using olive oil (30 min incubation))) and 30–90 units/mg protein (using triacetin)); from Lobachemie (Mumbai, India). We purchased ethanol, acetone, hexane and acetonitrile from SPF (Gurugram, India).

2.3. Preparation of Plants Extracts

The required parts from *A. palaestinum*, *C. azarolus*, *M. parviflora*, *T. syriacum*, *R. coriaria*, *R. officinalis*, *P. guajava*, *O. dayi*, *B. nigra*, and *V. vinifera* were collected in May 2016 from different regions of Palestine during the flowering time, except *C. azarolus* fruits which were gathered during the fruiting period of the plant. Botanical identification was carried out at the Pharmacognosy and Herbal Products Laboratory at An-Najah National University, and three samples of each plant were taken for the identification process as well as the voucher specimen codes, including: Pharm-PCT-246, Pharm-PCT-712, Pharm-PCT-1506, Pharm-PCT-2396, Pharm-PCT-2037,

Pharm-PCT-2732, Pharm-PCT-2720, Pharm-PCT-1727, Pharm-PCT-408, and Pharm-PCT-2665, respectively. The required parts used from the 10 plants were washed and then dried in the shade at a controlled temperature (25 ± 2 °C) and humidity (55 ± 5 RH). It took about two weeks until all the plant parts became well dried. After drying, the plant materials were well ground into a fine powder by using a mechanical blender and transferred into airtight containers with proper labeling for future use.

2.4. Preparation of Plant Extracts for Pancreatic Lipase Inhibition Assay

A total of 25 g of the powdered plant was weighed and then exhaustively extracted by adding 100 mL of n-hexane and 150 mL of 50% ethanol into triply-distilledwater. The mixture was then shaken for 48 h at room temperature using a shaker that was set at 200 rpm. Afterwards, the mixture was filtered using a suction flask and Buchner funnel filtration. The obtained filtrate was separated individually by a separatory funnel into 2 phases—a lower aqueous phase representing the first aqueous extract and an upper organic phase representing the organic extract. The aqueous extract was dried using a freeze-dryer for 48 h. Meanwhile, the organic extracts were placed in a hood at 25 °C to evaporate leftover organic solvents until completely dried. The crude organic and aqueous extracts were stored at 4 °C for further use [1].

2.5. Pancreatic Lipase Inhibition

The porcine pancreatic lipase inhibitory assay was adapted from Zheng et al., 2010, and Bustanji et al., (2010) [2,3], with some modifications. 1 mg/mL (1000 µg/mL) plant extract stock solution in 10% DMSO was used, from which five different solutions were prepared with the following concentrations: 50, 100, 200, 300, and 400 µg/mL. 1 mg/mL stock solution of pancreatic lipase enzyme was prepared immediately before being used. This procedure was carried for the ten studied plants species. A stock solution of PNPB (p-nitrophenyl butyrate) was prepared by dissolving 20.9 mg of PNPB in 2 mL of acetonitrile. 0.1 mL of porcine pancreatic lipase (1 mg/mL) was added to test tubes containing 0.2 mL of the various concentrations (50, 100, 200, 300, 400 µg/mL) of plant extract. The resulting mixtures were then made up to 1 mL by adding Tri-HCl solution (pH 7.4) and incubated at 25 °C for 15 min. After the incubation period, 0.1 mL of PNPB solution was then added to each test tube. The mixture was again incubated for 30 min at 37 °C. Pancreatic lipase activity was determined by measuring the hydrolysis of p-nitrophenyl butyrate to p-nitrophenol at 405 nm using a UV-visible spectrophotometer. The same procedure was repeated for the aqueous and organic extracts and for Orlistat (a positive control) using the same concentrations as mentioned above.The established tests were performed in triplicates.

3. Results

Twenty crude aqueous and organic extracts were prepared from ten plant species found in the West Bank area of Palestine and their anti-lipase activity was investigated at a concentration of 1000 µg/mL for porcine pancreatic lipase inhibition. The inhibitory activities towards pancreatic lipase are reported in Table 1.

The inhibitory effects of the reference drug (Orlistat) and plant extracts aredose-dependent. Different solutions of the Orlistat and plant extracts were prepared in escalating doses as shown in Table 1. The activity of lipase decreased by increasing the concentration of Orlistat and the plant extracts. TheIC_{50} values for the drug and plant extracts were calculated and the degree of lipase inhibition was plotted as shown in Figures 1–10. The IC_{50} values represent the concentration of the inhibitors at which 50% of the enzyme is inhibited and it is generally used to express the inhibitory effect of the lipase enzyme.

Table 1. Porcine pancreatic lipase inhibitory properties, expressed as IC_{50} (μg/mL), and yield percentages of the aqueous and organic extracts of 10 plant species that were collected from different regions in Palestine.

Aqueous Extract Yield,%	IC_{50} of the Aqueous Extract, μg/mL	Organic Extract Yield,%	IC_{50} of the Organic Extract, μg/mL	Parts Used	Family	Local Name	Studied Plants' Latin Names
18.8	107.2 ± 2	2.7	147.9 ± 2	Leaves	Araceae	Loof	*A. palaestinum*
9.8	83.2 ± 1.9	1.8	40.7 ± 1.8	Leaves	Rosaceae	Zaaror	*C. azarolus*
6.2	28.2 ± 2.4	0.6	23.7 ± 3	Leaves	Malvaceae	Khobeze Baladi	*M. parviflora*
18.6	39.8 ± 1.8	0.7	74.1 ± 2.2	Leaves	Compositae	Ejr Alasad	*T. syriacum*
14.4	19.95 ± 2.8	2.8	30.2 ± 1.5	Fruits	Anacardiaceae	Sumak	*R. coriaria*
7.2	51.3 ± 2.4	7.2	65 ± 2	Leaves	Lamiaceae	Hasaa Alban	*R. officinalis*
9.8	87.1 ± 1.4	9	64.6 ± 2	Leaves	Myrtaceae	Jawafa	*P. guajava*
19.9	26.9 ± 2	1.5	18.6 ± 2.6	Leaves	Lamiaceae	Albardaqosh	*O. dayi*
26	47.9 ± 2.4	1.4	66.1 ± 2.1	Leaves	Brassicaceae	Khardal	*B. nigra*
12.5	14.1 ± 1.9	0.6	28.8 ± 2.5	Leaves	*Vitaceae*	Anab	*V. vinifera*

Among the 20 plant extractsexamined, seven crude extracts at a concentration 100 µg/mL significantly inhibited porcine pancreatic lipase activity in vitro as demonstrated using a p-nitrophenyl butyrate-based assay. Throughout the investigated results, the aqueous extracts of *V. vinifera* and *R. coriaria*, with IC_{50} values of 14.13 and 19.95 µg/mL, respectively, showed the highest porcine pancreatic lipase inhibitory effects of all the studied aqueous extracts. Meanwhile, the organic extract of *O. dayi*, with an IC_{50} value of 18.62 µg/mL, showed the highest porcine pancreatic lipase inhibitory effects of all studied organic extracts.

In addition to that, the studied extracts' IC_{50} values were compared with the standard antilipase compound Orlistat, which has an IC_{50} value of 12.38 ± 2.3 µg/mL. These results, and the results of all of the 10 studied plants, are well clarified in Table 1 and in Figures 1–10.

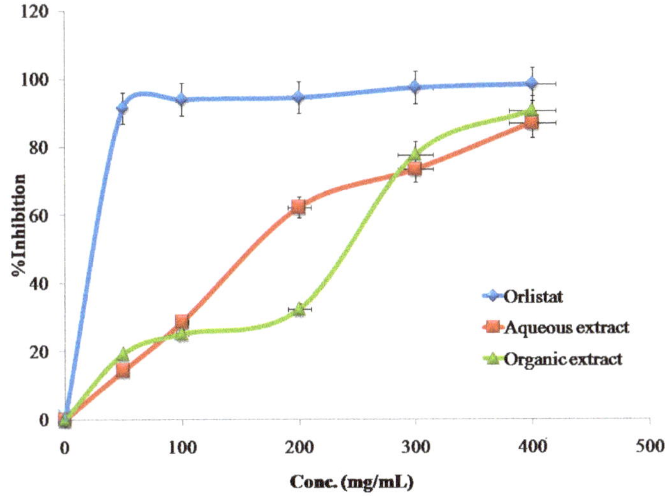

Figure 1. The inhibitory effects of the aqueous and organic extracts of *A. palaestinum* and Orlistat on the activity of porcine pancreatic lipase.

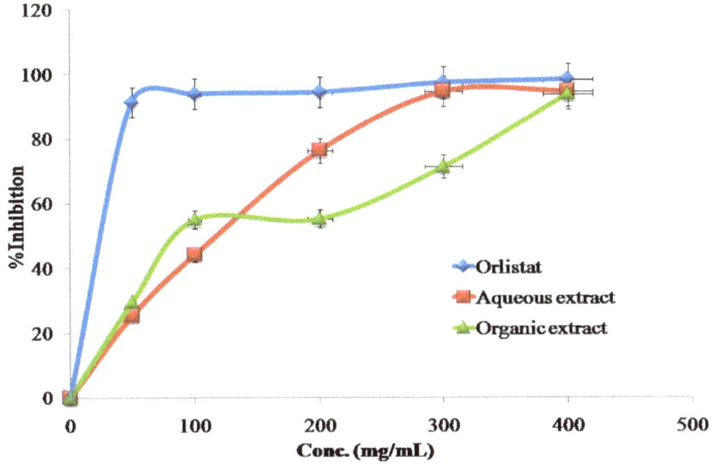

Figure 2. The inhibitory effects of the aqueous and organic extracts of *B. nigra* and Orlistat on the activity of porcine pancreatic lipase.

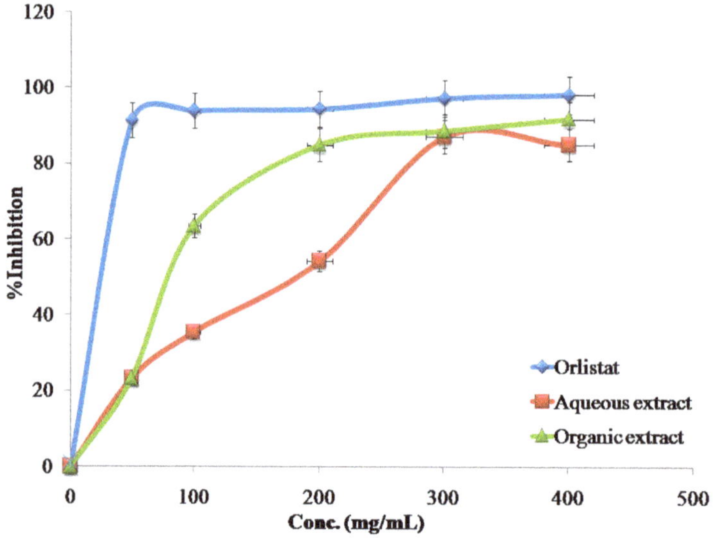

Figure 3. The inhibitory effects of the aqueous and organic extracts of *C. azarolus* and Orlistat on the activity of porcine pancreatic lipase.

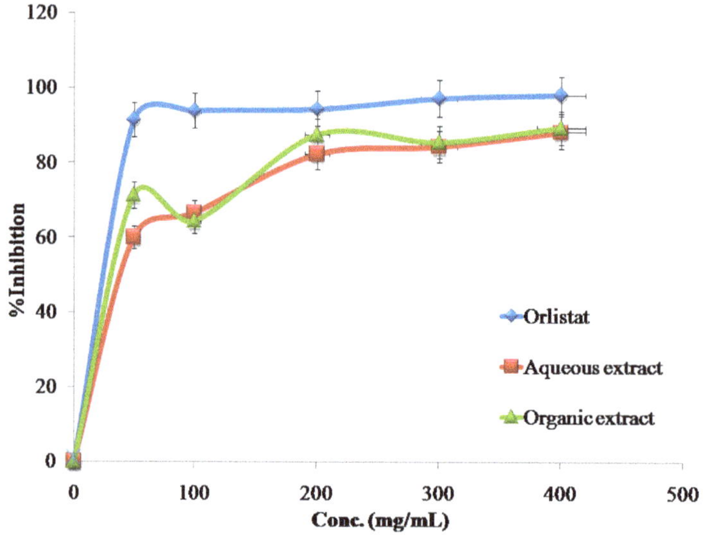

Figure 4. The inhibitory effects of the aqueous and organic extracts of *M. parviflora* and Orlistat on the activity of porcine pancreatic lipase.

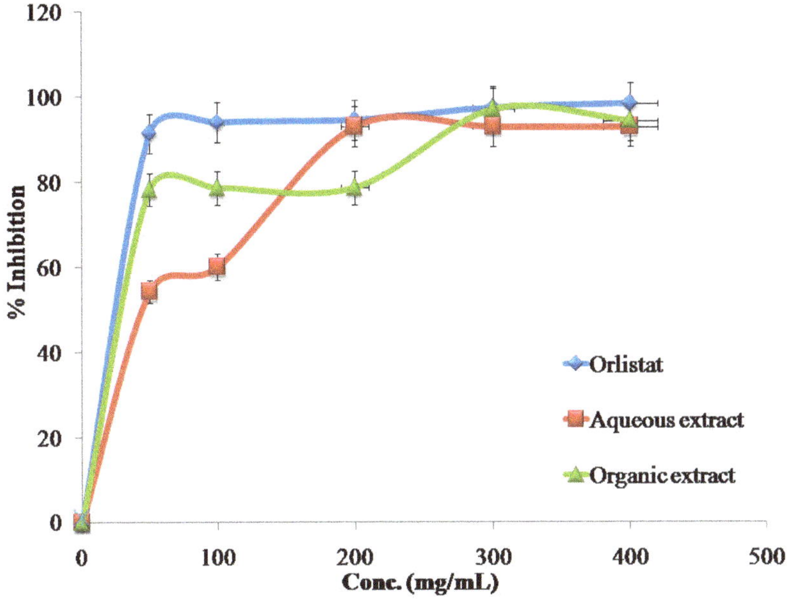

Figure 5. The inhibitory effects of the aqueous and organic extracts of *O. dayi* and Orlistat on the activity of porcine pancreatic lipase.

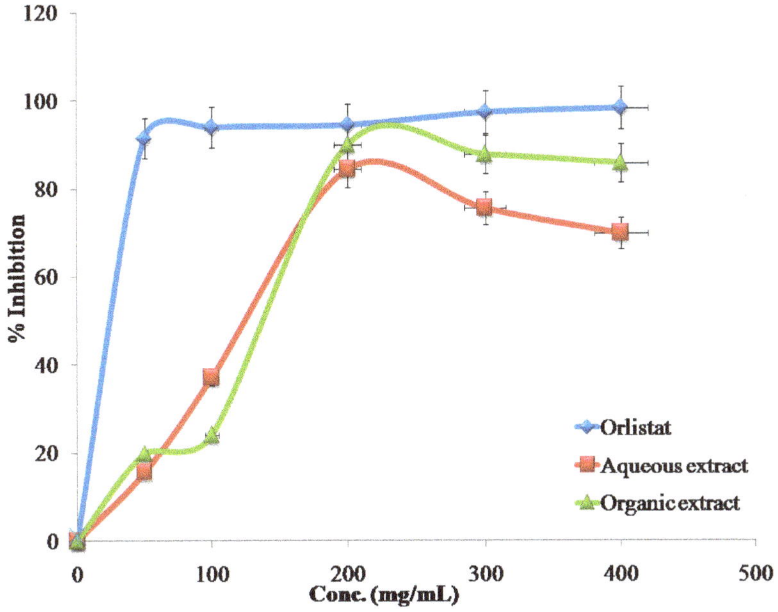

Figure 6. The inhibitory effects of the aqueous and organic extracts of *P. guajava* and Orlistat on the activity of porcine pancreatic lipase.

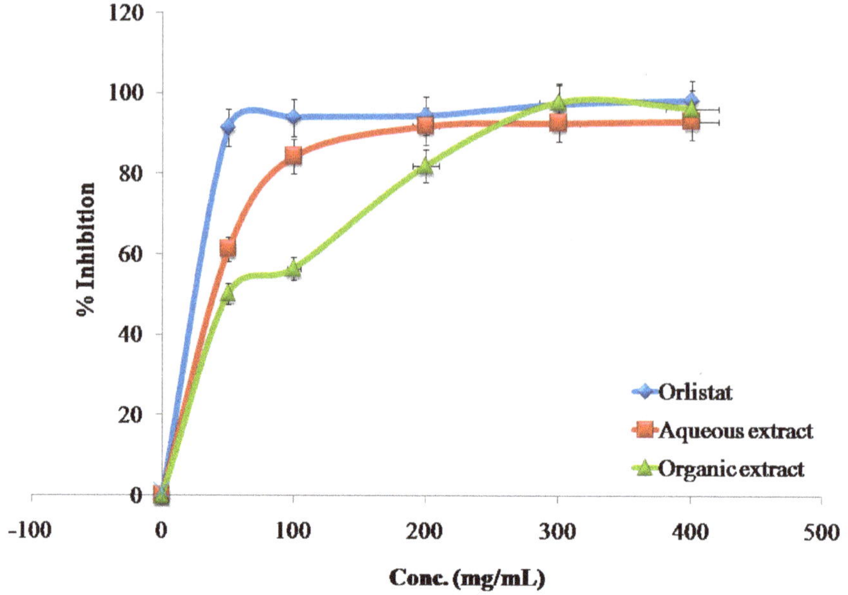

Figure 7. The inhibitory effects of the aqueous and organic extracts of *R. coriaria* and Orlistat on the activity of porcine pancreatic lipase.

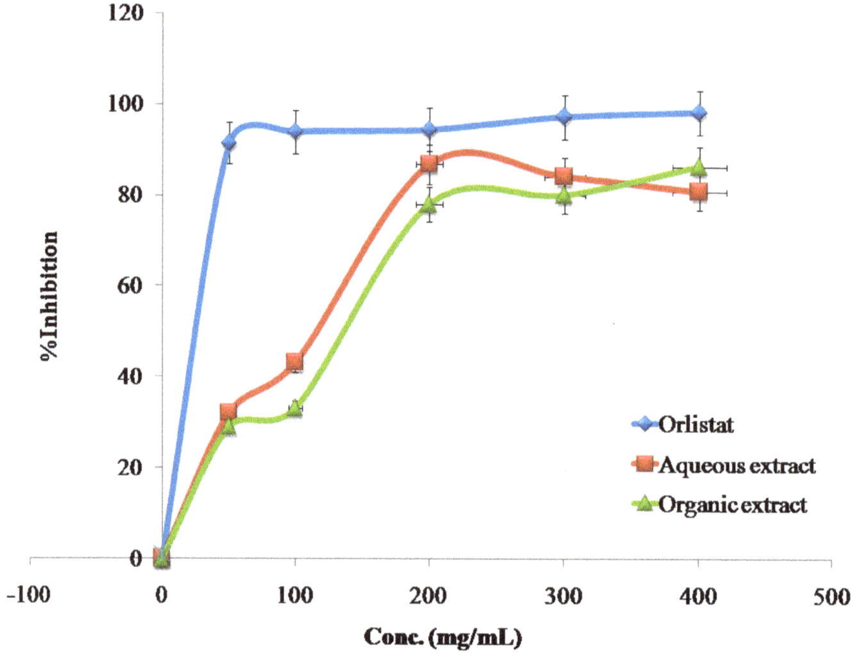

Figure 8. The inhibitory effects of the aqueous and organic extracts of *R. officinalis* and Orlistat on the activity of porcine pancreatic lipase.

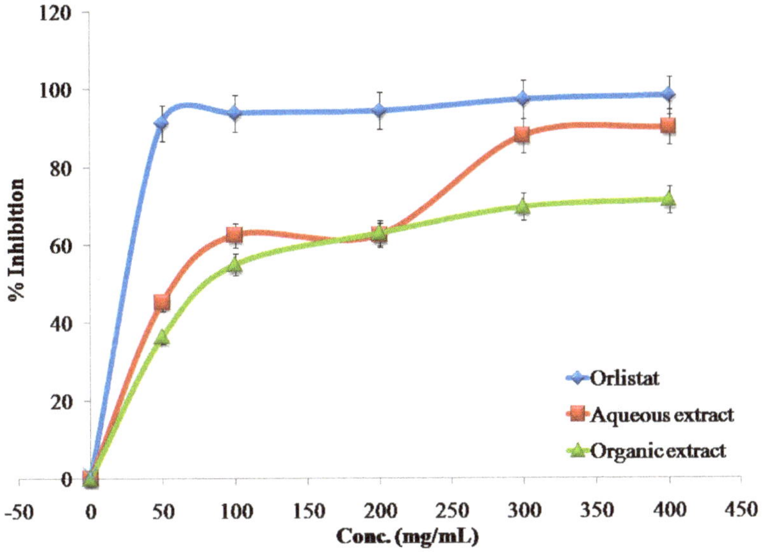

Figure 9. The inhibitory effects of the aqueous and organic extracts of *T. syriacum* and Orlistat on the activity of porcine pancreatic lipase.

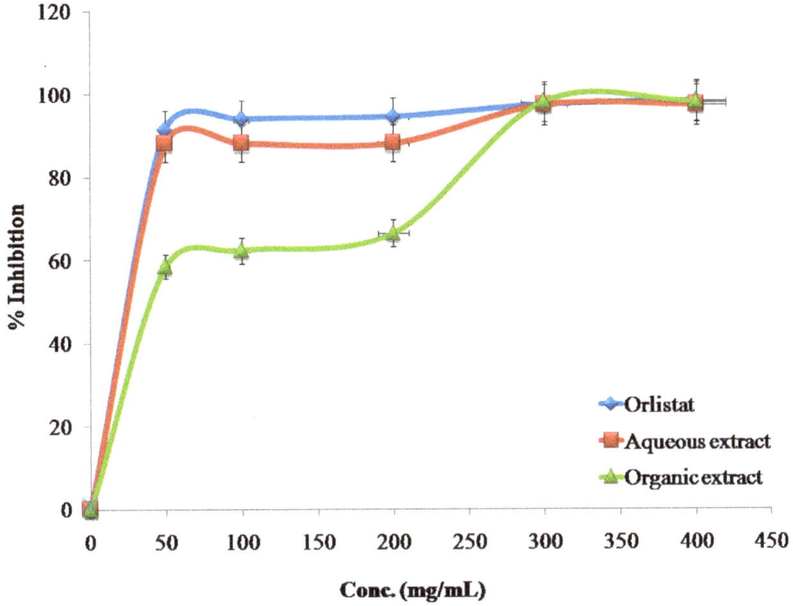

Figure 10. The inhibitory effects of the aqueous and organic extracts of *V. vinifera* and Orlistat on the activity of porcine pancreatic lipase.

4. Discussion

In this study, ten traditional edible medicinal plants, including *T. syriacum, O. dayi, M. parviflora, B. nigra, V. vinifera, C. azarolus, R. coriaria, A. palaestinum, P. guajava*, and *R. officinalis*, were assessed for their activity as porcine pancreatic lipase inhibitors. In many countries such as Palestine, Jordan, Iraq, Greece, and Pakistan, most of these plants were reported as being used as traditional medicines for the treatment of obesity [4–16].

Obesity is a chronic metabolic disorder caused by an imbalance between energy intake and expenditure. It is a major risk factor for cancer as well as endocrine, metabolic, and cardiovascular disorders [17–19]. Accordingly, the use of functional foods, such as the consumption of edible plants, would be a great and safe medicinal alternative in the treatment of obesity. They have been targeted to promote beneficial health effects, especially for the prevention of pathophysiological conditions such as obesity, dyslipidemia, diabetes, hypertension, and cancer [20,21].

The lipolytic pancreatic lipase enzyme is synthesized and secreted by the pancreas, plays a key role in the efficient digestion of lipids, and is responsible for the hydrolysis of 50–70% of total dietary lipids. The anti-lipase effect is one of the most widely studied mechanisms in determining the potential efficacy of natural products as anti-obesity agents [22,23].

Recently, global attention has been focused on the effects of plants, especially those that classified as traditional medicinal and edible types for the treatment of obesity and for controlling of overweight due to their safety issue, as well as these plants have been consumed from ancient times and their toxic and other side effects have been observed and documented if present [24].

In addition to this, Palestinian territory is covered with a huge number of plants and from this huge biodiversity, there are large numbers of them considered traditional medicines or foodssinceancient times [25]. From these plants, *A. palaestinum*, *C. azarolus*, *M. parviflora*, *T. syriacum*, *R. coriaria*, *R. officinalis*, *P. guajava*, *O. dayi*, *B. nigra*, and *V. vinifera* were investigated for their efficacy as natural anti-obesity products and compared with Orlistat, which considered the anti-lipase drug of choice [26].

Orlistatis a potent inhibitor of pancreatic lipase enzyme isolated from bacteria *Streptomyces toxytricini*. This prescription drug is designed to treat obesity by lowering lipid digestion and is produced under the trade name Xenical® by Roche [27].

Our obtained results showed that the IC_{50} values of the aqueous extracts of *V. vinifera* and *R. coriaria* have high porcine pancreatic lipase inhibition potential with IC_{50} values of 14.13 and 19.95 μg/mL, respectively. The IC_{50} value of the organic extract of *O. dayi* was 18.62 μg/mL, in comparison with the reference compound (positive control) Orlistat which has an IC_{50} of 12.38 μg/mL.

Moreover, the *R. coriaria* (Sumac) fruit's aqueous extract showed potential antilipase effects with an IC_{50} value 19.95 μg/mL, and this plant is an edible one and grows wildly in tropical and temperate regions worldwide, often growing in agriculturally-in viable regions. *R. coriaria* belongs to the Anacardiaceae family and is used in Turkey as a folk medicine for the treatment of diabetes due to its ability to cure various diabetes complications [28].

A study performed by Golzadeh et al., (2012), showed that Sumac reduced total cholesterol, triglyceride, low-density lipoprotein, and blood sugar levels in animal studies [29].

Accordingly, these results were confirmed in our in-vitro study which confirmed its activity as an anti-lipase agent.

In addition to these results, the organic extract of *O. dayi* also showed potential anti-lipase effects with an IC_{50} value 18.62 μg/mL. It is a perennial, endemic, culinary plant, and is considered a desert plant that is mainly distributed in African and Mediterranean regions [30,31]. It is used as a tea, a spice, and boiled with meat also used in salads in many countries, reflecting its therapeutic effect of reducing lipid absorption in the gastrointestinal tract [32,33].

Vitis vinifera belongs to the Vitaceae family, whose origin is Mediterranean, and is considered one of most common plant species cultivated worldwide and one of the most important economical plants because it is used to produce wine, table grape juice, and raisins [34,35].

The leaves of *V. vinifera* consumed with rice and meat and considered one of the most popular culinary dishes in Arabian countries, as well as other countries such as Turkey and Italy [36–38].

This plant's leaves showed a powerful anti-lipase effect in comparison with Orlistat and have an IC_{50} value 14.13 μg/mL.

In a study which was conducted on the aqueous extract of *V. vinifera* leaves by Fernandes et al., (2013), it was found that the plant's leaves are rich in phenolic compounds, including phenolic acids and flavonoids such as trans-caffeoyl tartaric acid, trans-coumaroyl tartaric acids, myricetin-3-*O*-glucoside, quercetin-3-*O*-glucoside, quercetin, kaempferol-3-*O*-glucoside, quercetin-3-*O*-galactoside, kaempferol, and isorhamnetin [34].

In addition, *R. coriaria* fruits have high concentrations of phenolic compounds, including caffeoylquinic acid, quercetin, rhamnetin, myricetin, kaempferol, gallic acid, ellagic acid, methyl gallate, m-digallic acid, amenthoflavone, agathisflavone, hinokiflavone, and sumaflavone [39,40].

Origanum dayi is an endemic subshrub plant species that grows in the West Bank area of Palestine. The leaves of *O. dayi* contain a mixture of volatile oils such as terpinen-4-ol, α-terpineol, 1,8-cineole, (E)-sabinene hydrate, (E)-sabinene hydrate acetate, and linalyl acetate [30,31]. To the best of the authors' knowledge, there were no previous studies in the literature about the chemical constituents of *O. dayi*, except on the volatile oils. However, many phenolic compounds were isolated from other species of *Origanum* (*O. vulgare*), including protocatechuic acid, caffeic acid, 2-caffeoyloxy-3-[2-(4-hydroxybenzyl)-4,5-dihydroxy]phenylpropionic acid, and phenyl glucoside [41].

In fact, in many previous studies, it was reported that flavonoids and other phenolic compounds act as porcine pancreatic lipase enzyme inhibitors by binding to the enzyme−substrate complex, reducing the lipid absorption [42,43].

To the best of the authors' knowledge, there were no previous studies on the effects of the aqueous and organic extracts of *V. vinifera*, *R. coriaria* and *O. dayi* on the lipase enzyme and our study is the first one on these plants. Further pharmacological in-vivo studies are required to confirm these findings and to identify the key chemical elements in these plants, using chromatographical isolation of the bioactive molecules, responsible for these pharmacological effects.

5. Conclusions

Obesity has reached epidemic proportions and is becoming a public health concern of the highest order. Several methods are now available to treat obesity and Orlistat is the most used one. Several plants are used in folk medicine to treat obesity and the use of edible plants is of great importance since they have few of the adverse effects that may be encountered with chemical or drug treatments. Our obtained results showed that some edible plants could replace Orlistat in the treatment of obesity. According to the obtained results, *V. vinifera*, *R. coriaria*, and *O. dayi* can be used as natural inhibitors of pancreatic lipase and so are new players in obesity treatment. In fact, these plants can be freely and safely consumed in the daily diet, be prepared as natural supplements to treat or prevent obesity and control weight gain, and can be used for the treatment of hyperlipidemia.

Acknowledgments: The authors acknowledge the assistance of the technicians Mohamad Arar and Linda Isa.

Author Contributions: N.J. wrote the manuscript. N.J., A.N.Z., F.H., M.Z., and H.A. carried out the experiments. N.J., A.N.Z., and F.H. supervised research work and O.A. drafted the manuscript. All authors read and approved the final manuscript.

Conflicts of Interest: The authors declare that they have no financial and/or non-financial competing interests.

References

1. Jaradat, N.A. Evaluation of the Exhaustive Extraction Yields for *Teucrium polium* L. from Different Regions of the West Bank-Palestine. *Inter. J. Pharm. Pharm. Sci.* **2014**, *7*, 511–513.
2. Bustanji, Y.; Issa, A.; Mohammad, M.; Hudaib, M.; Tawah, K.; Alkhatib, H.; Almasri, I.; Al-Khalidi, B. Inhibition of hormone-sensitive lipase and pancreatic lipase by *Rosmarinus officinalis* extract and selected phenolic constituents. *J. Med. Plants Res.* **2010**, *4*, 2235–2242.

3. Zheng, C.-D.; Duan, Y.-Q.; Gao, J.-M.; Ruan, Z.-G. Screening for anti-lipase properties of 37 traditional Chinese medicinal herbs. *J. Chin. Med. Assoc.* **2010**, *73*, 319–324. [CrossRef]
4. Afifi, F.U.; Abu-Irmaileh, B. Herbal medicine in Jordan with special emphasis on less commonly used medicinal herbs. *J. Ethnopharmacol.* **2000**, *72*, 101–110. [CrossRef]
5. Al-Qudah, M.M. Histological and Biochemical Studies on Liver of Female Rats Treated with Different Concentrations of Ethanolic Extract of *Arum palaestinum*. *J. Appl. Environ. Biol. Sci.* **2016**, *6*, 7–16.
6. Abu-Irmaileh, B.E.; Afifi, F.U. Herbal medicine in Jordan with special emphasis on commonly used herbs. *J. Ethnopharmacol.* **2003**, *89*, 193–197. [CrossRef]
7. Al–Douri, N.A. Some important medicinal plants in Iraq. *Int. J. Adv. Herb. Altern. Med.* **2014**, *2*, 10–20.
8. Ali-Shtayeh, M.S.; Jamous, R.M.; Jamous, R.M. Complementary and alternative medicine use amongst Palestinian diabetic patients. *Complement. Ther. Clin. Pract.* **2012**, *18*, 16–21. [CrossRef] [PubMed]
9. Hudaib, M.; Mohammad, M.; Bustanji, Y.; Tayyem, R.; Yousef, M.; Abuirjeie, M.; Aburjai, T. Ethnopharmacological survey of medicinal plants in Jordan, Mujib Nature Reserve and surrounding area. *J. Ethnopharmacol.* **2008**, *120*, 63–71. [CrossRef] [PubMed]
10. Jaradat, N. Ethnopharmacological survey of natural products in Palestine. *An-Najah Univ. J. Res. (N. Sc.)* **2005**, *19*, 13–67.
11. Afifi-Yazar, F.U.; Kasabri, V.; Abu-Dahab, R. Medicinal plants from Jordan in the treatment of diabetes: Traditional uses vs. in vitro and in vivo evaluations—Part 2. *Planta Med.* **2011**, *77*, 1210–1220. [CrossRef] [PubMed]
12. Marrelli, M.; Loizzo, M.R.; Nicoletti, M.; Menichini, F.; Conforti, F. Inhibition of key enzymes linked to obesity by preparations from Mediterranean dietary plants: Effects on α-amylase and pancreatic lipase activities. *Plant Foods Hum. Nutr.* **2013**, *68*, 340–346. [CrossRef] [PubMed]
13. Tareen, R.B.; Bibi, T.; Khan, M.A.; Ahmad, M.; Zafar, M. Indigenous knowledge of folk medicine by the women of Kalat and Khuzdar regions of Balochistan, Pakistan. *Pak. J. Bot.* **2010**, *42*, 1465–1485.
14. Gutierrez, R.M.P. Evaluation of hypoglycemic activity of the leaves of *Malva parviflora* in streptozotocin-induced diabetic rats. *Food Funct.* **2012**, *3*, 420–427. [CrossRef] [PubMed]
15. Hanlidou, E.; Karousou, R.; Kleftoyanni, V.; Kokkini, S. The herbal market of Thessaloniki (N Greece) and its relation to the ethnobotanical tradition. *J. Ethnopharmacol.* **2004**, *91*, 281–299. [CrossRef] [PubMed]
16. Giancarlo, S.; Rosa, L.M.; Nadjafi, F.; Francesco, M. Hypoglycaemic activity of two spices extracts: *Rhus coriaria* L. and *Bunium persicum* Boiss. *Nat. Prod. Res.* **2006**, *20*, 882–886. [CrossRef] [PubMed]
17. De Pergola, G.; Silvestris, F. Obesity as a major risk factor for cancer. *J. Obes.* **2013**, *2013*, 291546. [CrossRef] [PubMed]
18. Melmed, S.; Polonsky, K.S.; Larsen, P.R.; Kronenberg, H.M. *William's Textbook of Endocrinology*; Elsevier Health Sciences: Toronto, ON, Canada, 2015.
19. Keihani, S.; Hosseinpanah, F.; Barzin, M.; Serahati, S.; Doustmohamadian, S.; Azizi, F. Abdominal obesity phenotypes and risk of cardiovascular disease in a decade of follow-up: The Tehran Lipid and Glucose Study. *Atherosclerosis* **2015**, *238*, 256–263. [CrossRef] [PubMed]
20. Abete, I.; Astrup, A.; Martínez, J.A.; Thorsdottir, I.; Zulet, M.A. Obesity, and the metabolic syndrome: The role of different dietary macronutrient distribution patterns and specific nutritional components on weight loss and maintenance. *Nutr. Rev.* **2010**, *68*, 214–231. [CrossRef] [PubMed]
21. Dhurandhar, N.; Schoeller, D.; Brown, A.; Heymsfield, S.; Thomas, D.; Sørensen, T.; Speakman, J.; Jeansonne, M.; Allison, D. Energy balance measurement: When something is not better than nothing. *Int. J. Obes.* **2015**, *39*, 1109–1113. [CrossRef] [PubMed]
22. Mukherjee, M. Human digestive and metabolic lipases—A brief review. *J. Mol. Catal. B Enzym.* **2003**, *22*, 369–376. [CrossRef]
23. Abumrad, N.A.; Nassi, F.; Marcus, A. Digestion and absorption of dietary fat, carbohydrate, and protein. In *Sleisenger & Fordtran's Gastrointestinal and Liver Disease*, 10th ed.; Elsevier Saunders: Philadelphia, PA, USA, 2016.
24. Chen, N.N. *Food, Medicine, and the Quest for Good Health: Nutrition, Medicine, and Culture*; Columbia University Press: New York, NY, USA, 2007.
25. Jaradat, N.A.; Shawahna, R.; Eid, A.M.; Al-Ramahi, R.; Asma, M.K.; Zaid, A.N. Herbal remedies use by breast cancer patients in the West Bank of Palestine. *J. Ethnopharmacol.* **2016**, *178*, 1–8. [CrossRef] [PubMed]

26. Del Castillo-Santaella, T.; Maldonado-Valderrama, J.; Cabrerizo-Vílchez, M.A.N.; Rivadeneira-Ruiz, C.; Rondon-Rodriguez, D.; Gálvez-Ruiz, M.A.J. Natural Inhibitors of Lipase: Examining Lipolysis in a Single Droplet. *J. Agric. Food Chem.* **2015**, *63*, 10333–10340. [CrossRef] [PubMed]
27. Amin, H.M.; Tawfek, N.S.; Abo-El Hussein, B.K.; El-Ghany, M.S.A. Anti-Obesity Potential of Orlistat and Amphetamine in Rats Fed on High Fat Diet. *Sciences* **2015**, *5*, 453–461.
28. Doğan, A.; Çelik, İ. Healing effects of sumac (*Rhus coriaria*) in streptozotocin-induced diabetic rats. *Pharm. Biol.* **2016**, *54*, 2092–2102. [CrossRef] [PubMed]
29. Golzadeh, M.; Farhoomand, P.; Daneshyar, M. Dietary *Rhus coriaria* L. powder reduces the blood cholesterol, VLDL-c and glucose, but increases abdominal fat in broilers. *S. Afr. J. Anim. Sci.* **2012**, *42*, 398–405. [CrossRef]
30. Dudai, N.; Larkov, O.; Chaimovitsh, D.; Lewinsohn, E.; Freiman, L.; Ravid, U. Essential oil compounds of *Origanum dayi* Post. *Flavour Fragr. J.* **2003**, *18*, 334–337. [CrossRef]
31. Solowey, E.; Lichtenstein, M.; Sallon, S.; Paavilainen, H.; Solowey, E.; Lorberboum-Galski, H. Evaluating medicinal plants for anticancer activity. *Sci. World J.* **2014**, *2014*, 721402. [CrossRef] [PubMed]
32. Atkins, R.D.; Gare, M. *Dr. Atkins' New Diet Cookbook*; M. Evans and Company Inc.: Lanham, MD, USA, 1995.
33. Dudai, N.; Yaniv, Z. Endemic Aromatic Medicinal Plants in the Holy Land Vicinity. In *Medicinal and Aromatic Plants of the Middle-East*; Yaniv, Z., Dudai, N., Eds.; Springer: Dordrecht, The Netherlands, 2014; pp. 37–58.
34. Fernandes, F.; Ramalhosa, E.; Pires, P.; Verdial, J.; Valentão, P.; Andrade, P.; Bento, A.; Pereira, J.A. *Vitis vinifera* leaves towards bioactivity. *Ind. Crops Prod.* **2013**, *43*, 434–440. [CrossRef]
35. Rattanakan, S.; George, I.; Haynes, P.A.; Cramer, G.R. Relative quantification of phosphoproteomic changes in grapevine (*Vitis vinifera* L.) leaves in response to abscisic acid. *Hortic. Res.* **2016**, *3*, 16029–16038. [CrossRef] [PubMed]
36. Rivera, D.; Obon, C.; Heinrich, M.; Inocencio, C.; Verde, A.; Fajardo, J. *Gathered Mediterranean Food Plants-Ethnobotanical Investigations and Historical Development*; Karger Publishers: Basel, Switzerland, 2006; Volume 59, pp. 18–74.
37. Dogan, Y.; Nedelcheva, A.; Łuczaj, Ł.; Drăgulescu, C.; Stefkov, G.; Maglajlić, A.; Ferrier, J.; Papp, N.; Hajdari, A.; Mustafa, B. Of the importance of a leaf: The ethnobotany of sarma in Turkey and the Balkans. *J. Ethnobiol. Ethnomed.* **2015**, *11*, 26. [CrossRef] [PubMed]
38. Lentini, F.; Venza, F. Wild food plants of popular use in Sicily. *J. Ethnobiol. Ethnomed.* **2007**, *3*, 15. [CrossRef] [PubMed]
39. Abu-Reidah, I.M.; Ali-Shtayeh, M.S.; Jamous, R.M.; Arráez-Román, D.; Segura-Carretero, A. HPLC–DAD–ESI-MS/MS screening of bioactive components from *Rhus coriaria* L. (Sumac) fruits. *Food Chem.* **2015**, *166*, 179–191. [CrossRef] [PubMed]
40. Shabbir, A. *Rhus coriaria* linn, a plant of medicinal, nutritional and industrial importance: A review. *J. Anim. Plant Sci.* **2012**, *22*, 505–512.
41. Kikuzaki, H.; Nakatani, N. Structure of a new antioxidative phenolic acid from oregano (*Origanum vulgare* L.). *Agric. Biol. Chem.* **1989**, *53*, 519–524. [CrossRef]
42. Villa-Ruano, N.; Zurita-Vásquez, G.G.; Pacheco-Hernández, Y.; Betancourt-Jiménez, M.G.; Cruz-Durán, R.; Duque-Bautista, H. Anti-lipase and antioxidant properties of 30 medicinal plants used in Oaxaca, México. *Biol. Res.* **2013**, *46*, 153–160. [CrossRef] [PubMed]
43. Sergent, T.; Vanderstraeten, J.; Winand, J.; Beguin, P.; Schneider, Y.-J. Phenolic compounds and plant extracts as potential natural anti-obesity substances. *Food Chem.* **2012**, *135*, 68–73. [CrossRef]

medicines

Review

Antioxidant and Antimicrobial Properties of Rosemary (*Rosmarinus officinalis*, L.): A Review

Gema Nieto [1], Gaspar Ros [1] and Julián Castillo [2,*]

[1] Department of Food Technology and Human Nutrition, Veterinary Faculty, University of Murcia, Espinardo, 30071 Murcia, Spain; gnieto@um.es (G.N.); gros@um.es (G.R.)
[2] Research and Development Department of Nutrafur-Frutarom Group, Camino Viejo de Pliego s/n, Alcantarilla, 80320 Murcia, Spain
* Correspondence: j.castillo@Nutrafur.com

Received: 1 June 2018; Accepted: 31 August 2018; Published: 4 September 2018

Abstract: Nowadays, there is an interest in the consumption of food without synthetic additives and rather with the use of natural preservatives. In this regard, natural extracts of the *Lamiaceae* family, such as rosemary, have been studied because of its bioactive properties. Several studies have reported that rosemary extracts show biological bioactivities such as hepatoprotective, antifungal, insecticide, antioxidant and antibacterial. It is well known that the biological properties in rosemary are mainly due to phenolic compounds. However, it is essential to take into account that these biological properties depend on different aspects. Their use in foods is limited because of their odour, colour and taste. For that reason, commercial methods have been developed for the preparation of odourless and colourless antioxidant compounds from rosemary. Owing to the new applications of natural extracts in preservatives, this review gives a view on the use of natural extract from rosemary in foods and its effect on preservative activities. Specifically, the relationship between the structure and activity (antimicrobial and antioxidant) of the active components in rosemary are being reviewed.

Keywords: rosemary; phenolic compounds; antioxidant; antimicrobial

1. Introduction

Because consumers are concerned about the negative effect of synthetic chemicals in food, there is a need to find "clean label products". Therefore, there is a growing interest in using natural extracts as alternatives for synthetic additives because of (a) their synergy with other preservation methods (b) they are considered safe, and (c) their specific properties as antioxidant, antidiabetic, antimutagenic, antitoxigenic and antibacterial [1].

In general, herbs and plants are rich in compounds with antioxidant properties, such as vitamins (E and C), glutathione, enzymes and phenolic compounds [2]. Several spice extracts have shown their properties to prevent the autoxidation of unsaturated triacylglycerols [3]. Specifically, the natural extract from the *Lamiaceae* family (thyme, sage and rosemary) has been reported in several studies for its antioxidative activity [1,4].

Rosmarinus officinalis, L. originating from the Mediterranean region is an aromatic plant from the *Lamiaceae* family. The province of Murcia (Southeast Spain) is one of the major processors and importers of rosemary. In the United States and Europe, rosemary is a unique spice commercially available for use as an antioxidant [5]. Rosemary extracts have been used in the treatment of diseases, due to its hepatoprotective potential [6], therapeutic potential for Alzheimer's disease [7] and its antiangiogenic effect [8]. On the other hand, they have been used in food preservation, because they prevent oxidation and microbial contamination [9–13]. Therefore, rosemary extract could be useful for replacing or even decreasing synthetic antioxidants in foods. As preservatives, rosemary extracts offer several technological advantages and benefits to consumers.

EFSA (European Food Safety Authority) has reviewed the safety of rosemary extracts [14]. It concluded that there are high-intake estimates ranging from 0.09 (the elderly) to 0.81 (children) mg/kg per day of carnosol and carnosic acid. Nowadays, in the European Union, rosemary extracts are added to food and beverages at levels of up to 400 mg/kg (as the sum of carnosic acid and carnosol).

2. Preparation of Antioxidants from Rosemary

When a new rosemary extract is tested, the most important aspect to take into account is the method of extraction and the sort of solvent used, as this will affect the antioxidant properties.

Various extraction methods for the selective extraction of rosemary leaves have been identified in the scientific literature. This includes both solvent extraction using vegetable oil or animal fat, mechanical pressing methods, water at alkaline pH and organic solvents (e.g. hexane, ethyl ether, chloroform, ethanol, methanol, dioxane and ethylene dichloride).

Previous extraction processes are obsolete and unusual in the industry. Chang et al. [15] and Bracco et al. [16] demonstrated the possibility of separating an active fraction of the rosemary extract by molecular distillation. The process realized by Chang et al. [15] for the extraction of antioxidant involves the extraction with ethyl ether under refluxing conditions. The crude material is washed with water and the solvent is removed. The crude material is dissolved in methanol and activated with carbon at 60 °C for 15 min. Another process reported by Bracco [16], involves reducing the particle size to 600 µL and suspending in peanut oil. The finely antioxidant components have a molecular weight range lower than the triglyceride components of the oil used (peanut oil) and can therefore be physically separated by molecular distillation on either a fall-film or centrifugal system.

Nowadays, rosemary extracts are usually prepared from dried rosemary leaves. In all the new methods, the extraction process is often accompanied by a step involving partial deodorisation and/or extract decolourisation. Considering the methods used, in general, the yield of rosemary extract indicated by various authors varies between 2% and 26% based on the raw material used.

3. Composition of Rosemary Extract and Essential Oil

The polyphenolic profile of rosemary has been widely described in the scientific literature [17–20]. The polyphenolic profile of these plants is characterized by the presence of carnosic acid, carnosol, rosmarinic acid and hesperidin, as major components [21].

Among the most effective antioxidant constituents of rosemary, the cyclic diterpene diphenols, carnosolic acid and carnosol have been identified. In addition, its extract contains carnosic acid, epirosmanol, rosmanol, methylcarnosate and isorosmanol [21–23].

Rosemary oils are obtained by steam distillation of twigs and fresh leaves. Sienkiewicz et al. [24] reported that rosemary essential oil contains mainly 1,8-cineole (46.4%), camphor (11.4%) and α-pinene (11.0%). The composition of the rosemary essential oil used by Jiang et al. [25], was composed mainly by 1,8-cineole (26.54%) and α-pinene (20.14%). Bendeddouche et al. [26], observed that the main constituents of the tested essential oil were camphor (37.6%), 1,8-cineole (10.0%), p-cymene-7-ol (7.8%) and borneol (5.4%).

Rosmarinus officinalis, L. is a rich source of phenolic compounds and their properties are derived from its extracts [27] and essential oils [28]. Both are used for the treatment of illnesses and in the food preservation.

In addition to the volatile constituents, extracts of rosemary also contain several antioxidant components, which belong mainly to the classes of phenolic acids, flavonoids, and diterpenoids. Del Baño et al. [2] studied the composition of seven flavonoids in rosemary leaves, flower, roots and steam. They studied the presence of 7-*O*-glucoside, hispidulin, diosmin, hesperidin, 3′-O-β-D-glucuronide, genkwanin and isoscutellarein 7-*O*-glucoside. These authors concluded significant presence of diosmin and hesperidin in the vascular system. Of the other identified compounds found in extracts of rosemary, rosmarinic acid and hydroxyhydrocaffeic acid, also exhibit some complementary antioxidant activity.

The extract of rosemary also contains other caffeic acid derivates. These compounds react with present metal ions, so chelates are formed; they consequently react with peroxide radicals and in that way, stabilise these free radicals.

Rosemary oil is used as a food seasoning [29], due to its chemical compound constituents responsible for the antibacterial, antifungal and antioxidant properties. Traditionally, rosemary oil has been shown to possess a number of applications in managing or curing many diseases such as inflammatory diseases [30] and diabetes mellitus [31].

On the other hand, the bioactivities of rosemary extracts include properties such as anti-inflammatory [32], antidiabetic [33], hepatoprotective [34] and antimicrobial activity [35]. These bioactivities are related to the phenolic compound constituents (mainly caffeic acid, rosmarinic acid and carnosic acid).

4. Mechanism of Antioxidant Action

The mechanism of action of these compounds has been widely covered in several publications. For example, Höulihan et al. [36] and Wu et al. [37] determined that the antioxidant properties of rosemary are attributed to its richness in isoprenoid quinones, which act as chain terminators of free radicals, and as chelators of reactive oxygen species (ROS). In addition, Gordon [38] indicated that the phenolic compounds existing in the commercial extracts of rosemary act as primary antioxidants when reacting with the lipid and hydroxyl radicals to turn them into stable products. Subsequently, Fang and Wada [39] pointed out that these compounds could act as metal ion chelators (Fe^{+2} fundamentally), therefore reducing the formation ratio of the reactive species derived from oxygen.

According to Löliger [40], carnosic acid and carnosol act as potent scavengers of peroxyl radicals. This fact explains the conclusions obtained by Chen et al. [41], who confirmed that the effect of both compounds on peroxidation of membrane lipids is higher than the effect reported by artificial antioxidants such as BHA, BHT and propyl gallate [42].

The antioxidative activity of rosemary extracts has been evaluated using different solvents. In this regard, Inatani et al. [43] reported that rosmanol, showed an antioxidant capacity four times higher than BRT and BRA (synthetic antioxidants) in both linoleic acid and lard. In addition, this study reported the antioxidant activity of carnosol and rosmanol by TBA and ferric thiocyanate methods. They reported the correlation between activity and chemical structure as an antioxidant. Aruoma et al. [44] studied the antioxidant and pro-oxidant properties of rosemary. The main constituents with antioxidant properties are carnosic acid and carnosol that are responsible for 90% of the properties. Both are inhibitors of lipid peroxidation in liposomal and microsomal systems, they are good scavengers of CCl_3O_2 (peroxyl radicals), reduce cytochrome c and scavenge hydroxyl radicals. Specifically, carnosic acid scavenges H_2O_2, but could also act as a substrate for the peroxidase system.

The antioxidant properties depend on fruiting stages: the increase in concentration of polyphenols, which include carnosol, rosmarinic acid and hesperidin, during the fruiting stage, is directly related to the improvement of the extract antioxidant capacity. This statement is supported by scientific papers previously published by Cui et al. [45] and Kontogianni et al. [20], who consider lactone carnosol (Figure 1) as the main property responsible for this activity. Likewise, rosmarinic acid and hesperidin have been cited in literature as important free radical scavengers [46,47].

One of the most significant aspects of the antioxidant activity of rosemary is the relationship between diterpenes and radical-scavenging activity. In this regard, the study by Munné-Bosch and Alegre [48] describes the antioxidant capacity of diterpenes in rosemary. The most important elements in the rosemary structure are the aromatic ring (C_{11}–C_{12}) in the catechol group together with the conjugation of the three basic rings.

The catechol group is responsible for scavenging the radical electron formed as result of oxidation. The skeleton formed by the three rings allows the delocalization of the charge. The presence of the carboxylic group (in the case of carnosic acid) increases this conjugation, especially in aqueous systems. However, in slightly polar media, such as fats, it is the lactone structure that seems to confer greater stability.

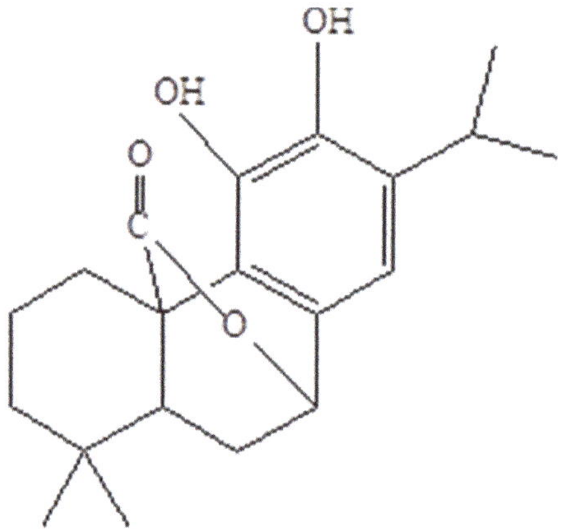

Figure 1. The chemical structure of carnosol.

Moreover, activation of redox-dependent signalling pathways such as Nrf2-dependent transcriptional regulation is known to take part in the antioxidant response of rosemary. The main metabolites carnosol and carnesolic acid have been reported to mediate antioxidant activities by differential mechanisms. Carnosic acid, carnosol, rosmanol and epirosmanol are the major phenolic diterpenes responsible for the antioxidant properties of rosemary (the first proposed oxidation pathway of carnosic acid was reported by Wenkert et al. [49] as shown in Figure 2). In the same way, Wijeratne and Cuppett [50] suggest that the antioxidant activities of carnosic acid are due to their ability to increase or maintain superoxide dismutase and glutathione peroxidase activities. These authors reported that carnosic acid and carnosol inhibited lipid peroxidation by 88–100% and 38–89%, respectively, under oxidative stress conditions.

Generally, the antioxidant effectiveness of natural extracts is higher than synthetic antioxidants, independent of the medium, which is different in water or oil. Table 1 shows the relative antioxidant effectiveness of spices and herbs.

Table 1. Antioxidant effectiveness of herbs and spices, evaluated as complete plant materials in different foods.

Spice, Herb	Food	Antioxidant Effectiveness
Marjoram, black pepper, white pepper, sage, rosemary, nutmeg, corianda	Bacon	Rosemary > sage > nutmeg > white pepper > marjoram [51]
Materials of 32 different plants	Bacon	Rosemary > sage > oreganum > nutmeg > thyme [52]
Materials of 32 different plants	Emulsion oil in water	Clove > turmeric > Jamaica pepper > Rosemary [53]
Materials of 15 different plants	Sausages	Sage > Rosemary > paprika > marjoram > Anís [54]

For reasons explained in past years, the use of new rosemary extracts, mainly refined extracts with antioxidant properties, is an interesting strategy as a food preservative, especially those with animal and/or vegetable fats [16].

There are different applications of rosemary in foods. For example, it has been added to animal products and oils. Different studies have demonstrated the potent activity of rosemary by reducing the colour loss of carotenoids and delaying lipid oxidation in oils [55] and meat products [56–58].

Several studies have shown rosemary properties to achieve good sensory results and the reduction of lipid oxidation after addition into foods: Stoick et al. [59] used 500–1000 ppm of rosemary extracts in beef; Shahidi et al. [60] used rosemary at 200 and 1000 ppm in different foods; Huisman et al. [61] used a concentration of 0.05% in pork; Sánchez-Escalante et al. [62] used a combination of 500 ppm vitamin C and 1000 ppm of rosemary in beef burgers; Formanek et al. [63] used 0.25% of rosemary in beef burgers. In general, all these authors showed that rosemary inhibited the formation of hydroperoxides [64].

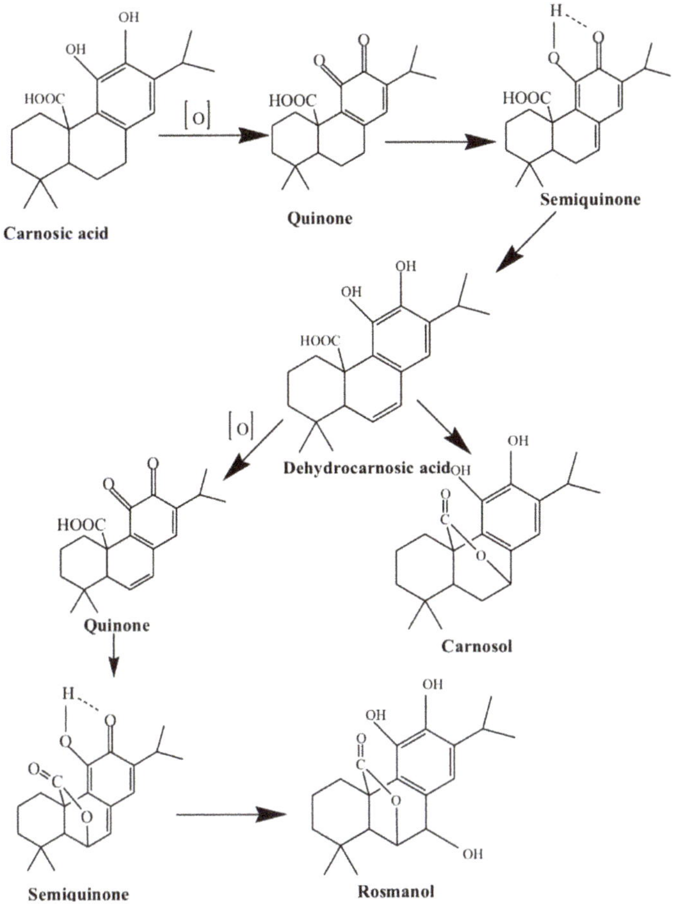

Figure 2. The first proposed oxidation pathway of carnosic acid. Reproduced from [49]. Copyright 1965, American Chemical Society, Washington, DC, USA.

On the other hand, rosemary extract could be applied through animal diet. In this regard, delayed lipid oxidation was reported in broilers with the administration of sage and rosemary [65]. This agreed with the results of Moñino et al. [66], indicating that antioxidant stability improved with 10% of rosemary leaves into the ewes feed.

The antioxidant activity of rosemary through animal diet has been reported in additional studies by: Lopez Bote et al. [65] with 500 mg kg^{-1} in broiler diets; Descalzo et al. [67] in feed of cattle; Petron et al. [68] in lamb, in pork meat [69,70], turkey meat products [71,72], chicken meat [65], hen's meat [73,74], cooked sausages [75]. Generally, the addition of rosemary extract into the meat products or through animal feed improved the meat lipid stability. On the contrary, O'Grady et al. [76] and Galobart et al. [77] concluded that feeding animals with rosemary did not improve the lipid stability of meat or eggs.

As previously reported, the antioxidant effect of rosemary is due to the polyphenols present in the leaves (mainly rosmarinic acid, carnosol and carnosic acid), which accumulate in the fatty membranes of cells where the antioxidant effect is required [72].

Other studies reported the effectiveness of rosemary oil to control oxidation in frankfurters [78] and to protect protein oxidation of meat patties [79]. This behaviour is very important to control colour changes of meat products mainly caused when the haem pigments are oxidized. In this regard, lipid oxidation and their consequences are reduced through the addition of rosemary.

In addition, rosemary has been added as an antioxidant in oils: Tohma et al. [80] studied the effect of the rosemary plant, its alcoholic extracts and essential oil on the oxidative stability of hazelnut oil during deep frying. This study showed that rosemary plant, or its extracts, could be used to extend the usage life of hazelnut oil for frying. The rosemary additives considerably inhibited the formation of oxidation products. The total phenolic compounds and profile of the enriched oils might cause increased frying stability. In addition, Reblova et al. [3] and Taha et al. [81] reported that rosemary extracts improved the sensory characteristic of fries, increased the oxidative stability of the oil, inhibited the decomposition of polyunsaturated triacylglycerols and the formation of polar substances in rape-seed oil. Urbancic et al. [82] reported that rosemary extract reduced acrylamide formation during potato frying. This effect was due to the transfer of phenolic compounds from rosemary into the oil.

5. Mechanism of Antimicrobial Action and Food Applications

The antibacterial activity of rosemary has been determined in various assay types based on either MIC or MBC. In this regard, Sienkiewicz et al. [24], demonstrated the antibacterial activities of basil (*Ocimum basilicum*, L.) and rosemary (*Rosmarinus officinalis*, L.) These authors reported the inhibition of microbial growth by both essential oils, presented as MIC values. Antibiotic susceptibility was carried out using disc diffusion. The results showed that both essential oils tested are active against all the clinical strains from *Escherichia coli*. Mihajilov-Kristev et al. [83], showed that essential oils containing mainly carvacrol (67.0%) and γ-terpinene (15.3%) were effective against Gram-negative strains, including *Escherichia coli*, with MIC values from 0.025 μL/mL to 0.78 μL/mL according to the broth microdilution method. Probuseenivasan et al. [84], confirmed that rosemary essential oil strongly inhibits *E. coli* ATCC 25922. The minimal inhibitory concentration for rosemary oil against *E. coli* was >6.4 mg/L.

Other studies have shown the antibacterial activity of rosemary oil against *E. coli*, *Bacillus cereus*, *Staphylococcus aureus* [85], *Staphylococcus aureus*, *Clostridium perfringens*, *Aeromonas hydrophila*, *Bacillus cereus* and *Salmonella choleraesuis*. This essential oil was incorporated into meat reporting antibacterial activity against *Brochothrix thermosphacta and Enterobacteriaceae* [86].

The inhibitory effect of rosemary is the result of the action of rosmarinic acid, rosmaridiphenol, carnosol, epirosmanol, carnosic acid, rosmanol and isorosmanol. They interact with the cell membrane, causing changes in genetic material and nutrients, altering the transport of electrons, leakage of cellular components and production changes in fatty acid. In addition, it also produced an interaction with the membrane of proteins that produced the loss of membrane functionality and its structure [87].

Vegara et al. [88] reported that the effectiveness of carnosic acid against pathogenic bacteria is superior to that of any other major extract component, including rosmarinic acid. In contrast, several scientific publications disagree about the possible relationships that may exist between the composition of the polyphenolic extract and its antimicrobial activity. Such is the case of Moreno et al. [89] and Ivanovic et al. [90] who demonstrated that the effectiveness of rosemary is related to a possible synergy between the rosmarinic phenolic acid and the carnosic acid diterpene. Bernardes et al. [91], however, state that there is a close relationship between the concentration levels of the carnosic acid, carnosol diterpenes and the antimicrobial activity of these extracts.

Zaouali et al. [92] reported that, compared with *S. aureus*, antimicrobial activity improves with the presence of α-pinene as a major component. This effect can be correlated with the fact that terpenes can disorganize the cell membrane, and therefore promote the lysis, as stated by Bjapai et al. [93]. The effectiveness of the essential oil of rosemary against *E. coli*, is related to the combined action of the different minority components present in its volatile fraction and should not be associated with the action of any particular component, agreeing with the conclusions published by Zaouali et al. [94]. There are numerous authors who claim that *E. coli*, *L. monocytogenes* and *S. aureus*, are very resistant bacteria and highlight the importance of chemical composition and proportion between the oil components on their antimicrobial efficacy [94,95].

The antibacterial effect of rosemary has been widely demonstrated in several food studies: beef meatballs [96], cooked beef [97] and in pork sausage [98]. Gomez-Estaca et al. [99] reported that rosemary oil inhibited the growth of common food bacteria contributing to food spoilage. Burt [85] also showed the antibacterial activity of rosemary essential oil against *E. coli*, *Bacillus cereus* and *S. aureus*. In addition, Sirocchi et al. [86] showed that rosemary essential oil inhibited the growth of *Brochothrix thermosphacta* and *Enterobacteriaceae*. Govaris et al. [72] reported an inhibitory effect of dietary supplementation of turkeys with rosemary (5 and 10 g/kg) on the growth of bacteria responsible for spoilage (psychrotrophs, mesophilics, enterobacteria and lactic acid bacteria). Camo et al. [56] also observed an inhibitory effect of the use of rosemary extract added to lamb meat packed in a modified atmosphere in the growth of psychrotrophic bacteria, compared with control meat. This same effect was observed by Quattara et al. [100], however these authors studied pure rosemary essential oil. On the contrary, Ismail et al. [101] showed that rosemary had no antibacterial effect in chicken.

Fernández-López et al. [96], evaluated the antibacterial activity of rosemary extracts in veal meatballs. The results showed a higher antibacterial activity in rosemary extracts, compared to other extracts studied. Only rosemary extracts were able to inhibit the 11 bacteria tested (such as *Lb. lactis FMRD*, *Br. thermosphacta CRA*, *Lb. carnosum*, *Br. thermosphacta CRA*, *L. innocua*, *Lb. sake*, *Br. thermosphacta CRA*, *Lc. mesenteroides* subsp *mesenteroides*, *L. monocytogenes*, *Lc. mesenteroides* subsp *dextranicum*, *Lb. curvatus*).

6. Synergistic Effect

It is important to note the possible synergistic effect between rosemary extract and other natural antioxidants. The results shown in the scientific literature offer contradictory conclusions. Resurreccion and Reynolds [102], observed that the joint addition of rosemary extract and tocopherols in meat products failed to increase the antioxidant efficacy of these individually used compounds. On the contrary, Wong et al. [103], concluded that the components of rosemary participate in the regeneration of α-tocopherol, which can be used as substitutes for vitamin C to enhance the stability of vitamin E. Wada and Fang [104], proposed that the synergism between both antioxidants is due to the capacity of the rosemary extract to yield hydrogen atoms to the tocopheryl radicals. This fact justifies the results obtained by Fang and Wada [37], who observed that the antioxidant activity of the α-tocopherol-rosemary mixture on a model fish system was significantly higher than that exhibited by the individually added products. In addition, these authors found that the α-tocopherol molecule remained stable for 10 more days when administered together with rosemary extract.

In this same line, Lai et al. [105] and Stoick et al. [59] showed the existence of a synergistic effect between sodium tripolyphosphate (STTP) and rosemary oleoresin (OR). The combination of OR/STTP was as effective as the application of the BHT-BHA or STPP/TBHQ mixtures during the prevention of WOF (warmed-over flavor) in pre-cooked beef and pork meats respectively [58].

7. Conclusions

The health problems derived from lipid oxidation have attracted the attention of consumers and researchers. Numerous diseases, such as aging, cancer, ischemia and atherosclerosis are linked to dietary and biological lipid oxidation products. In this regard, antioxidant compounds present in rosemary extracts and essential oils, delay lipid oxidation in biological systems and food. However, it is essential to consider that the antioxidant and antimicrobial activity of rosemary depend on the fruiting stage, nature of the extracts, mode of extraction, presence of an inhibitor, presence of a synergistic effect with other components, and the concentration of active extract components. If these aspects are taken into account, the application of this natural extract can be complimented in different food systems such as meat, oils and dressing. In view of its application, rosemary extracts could be used in functional foods, pharmaceutical products, plant products and food preservation. Because rosemary is a cheap, available, and a non-toxic herb, these considerations warrant the introduction of rosemary extracts or essential oils, with high phenolic compound contents, into the food industry.

Author Contributions: G.N., G.R. and J.C. wrote the article.

Funding: This research received no external funding.

Conflicts of Interest: The authors declare no conflict of interest.

References

1. Nieto, G.; Huvaere, K.; Skibsted, L.H. Antioxidant activity of rosemary and thyme by-products and synergism with added antioxidant in a liposome system. *Eur. Food Res. Technol.* **2011**, *233*, 11–18. [CrossRef]
2. Del baño, M.J.; Lorente, J.; Castillo, J.; Benavente-Garcia, O.; Marín, P.; Del Río, J.A.; Ortuó, A.; Ibarra, I. Flavoid distribution during the development of leaves flowers, stems and roots of Rosmarinus officinalis postulation of the Biosynthetic pathway. *J. Agric. Food Chem.* **2004**, *52*, 4987–4992. [CrossRef] [PubMed]
3. Reblova, Z.; Kudrnova, J.; Trojakova, L.; Pokorny, J. Effect of rosemary extracts on the stabilization of frying oil during deep fat frying. *J. Food Lipids* **1999**, *6*, 13–23. [CrossRef]
4. Botsoglou, N.A.; Christaki, E.; Fletouris, D.J.; Florou-Paneri, P.; Spais, A.B. The effect of dietary oregano essential oil on lipid oxidation in raw and cooked chicken during refrigerated storage. *Meat Sci.* **2002**, *62*, 259–265. [CrossRef]
5. Cuvelier, M.E.; Richard, H.; Berset, C. Antioxidative activity and phenolic composition of pilot-plant and commercial extracts of sage and rosemary. *J. Am. Oil Chem. Soc.* **1996**, *73*, 645–652. [CrossRef]
6. Rašković, A.; Milanović, I.; Pavlović, N.; Ćebović, T.; Vukmirović, S.; Mikov, M. Antioxidant activity of rosemary (*Rosmarinus officinalis* L.) essential oil and its hepatoprotective potential. *BMC Complement. Altern. Med.* **2014**, *14*, 225. [CrossRef] [PubMed]
7. Habtemariam, S. The therapeutic potential of rosemary (*Rosmarinus officinalis*) diterpenes for Alzheimer's disease. *Evid. Based Complement. Altern. Med.* **2016**, *2016*, 2680409. [CrossRef] [PubMed]
8. Kayashima, T.; Matsubara, K. Antiangiogenic effect of carnosic acid and carnosol, neuroprotective compounds in rosemary leaves. *Biosci. Biotechnol. Biochem.* **2012**, *76*, 115–119. [CrossRef] [PubMed]
9. Djenane, D.; Sánchez-Escalante, A.; Beltrán, J.A.; Roncalés, P. Ability of α-tocopherol, taurine and rosemary, in combination with vitamin C, to increase the oxidative stability of beef steaks displayed in modified atmosphere. *Food Chem.* **2002**, *76*, 407–415. [CrossRef]
10. Nieto, G.; Díaz, P.; Bañón, S.; Garrido, M.D. Dietary administration of ewe diets with a distillate from rosemary leaves (*Rosmarinus officinalis* L.): Influence on lamb meat quality. *Meat Sci.* **2010**, *84*, 23–29. [CrossRef] [PubMed]
11. Nieto, G.; Bañon, S.; Garrido, M.D. Incorporation of thyme leaves in the diet of pregnant and lactating ewes: Effect on the fatty acid profile of lamb. *Small Rumin. Res.* **2012**, *105*, 140–147. [CrossRef]
12. Nieto, G.; Estrada, M.; Jordán, M.J.; Garrido, M.D.; Bañon, S. Effects in ewe diet of rosemary by-product on lipid oxidation and the eating of cooked lamb under retail display conditions. *Food Chem.* **2011**, *124*, 1423–1429. [CrossRef]
13. Nieto, G.; Bañon, S.; Garrido, M.D. Administration of distillate Thyme leaves into the diet of Segureña ewes: Effect on lamb meat quality. *Animal* **2012**, *6*, 2048–2056. [CrossRef] [PubMed]

14. Aguilar, F.; Autrup, H.; Barlow, S.; Castle, L.; Crebelli, R.; Dekant, W.; Engel, K.H.; Gontard, N.; Gott, D.; Grilli, S.; et al. Use of rosemary extracts as a food additive–scientific opinion of the panel on food additives, flavourings, processing aids and materials in contact with food. *EFSA J.* **2008**, *721*, 1–29.
15. Chang, S.S.; Ostric-Matijasevic, B.; Hosieh, O.A.L.; Huang, C.L. Natural antioxidants from rosemary and sage. *J. Food Sci.* **1977**, *42*, 1102–1106. [CrossRef]
16. Bracco, U.; Loliger, J.; Viret, J.-L. Production and use of natural antioxidants. *J. Am. Oil Chem. Soc.* **1981**, *58*, 686–690. [CrossRef]
17. Zegura, B.; Dobnik, D.; Niderl, M.H.; Filipi, M. Antioxidant and antigenotoxic effects of rosemary (*Rosmarinus officinalis* L.) extracts in Salmonella Typhimurium TA98 and HepG2 cells. *Environ. Toxicol. Pharmacol.* **2011**, *32*, 296–305. [CrossRef] [PubMed]
18. Visentin, A.; Rodríguez-Rojo, S.; Navarrete, A.; Maestri, D.; Cocero, M.J. Precipitation and encapsulation of rosemary antioxidants by supercritical antisolvent process. *J. Food Eng.* **2012**, *109*, 9–15. [CrossRef]
19. Sasaki, K.; El Omri, A.; Kondo, S.; Han, J.; Isoda, H. Rosmarinus officinalis polyphenols produce anti-depressant like effect through monoaminergic and cholinergic functions modulation. *Behav. Brain Res.* **2013**, *238*, 86–94. [CrossRef] [PubMed]
20. Kontogianni, V.G.; Tomic, G.; Nikolic, I.; Nerantzaki, A.; Sayyad, A.; Stosic-Grujicic, N.; Stojanovic, S.; Gerothanassis, I.P.; Tzakos, A.G. Phytochemical profile of Rosmarinus officinalis and Salvia officinalis extracts and correlation to their antioxidant and anti-proliferative activity. *Food Chem.* **2013**, *136*, 120–129. [CrossRef] [PubMed]
21. Tai, J.; Cheung, S.; Wu, M.; Hasman, D. Antiproliferation effect of Rosemary (*Rosmarinus officinalis*) on human ovarian cancer cells in vitro. *Phytomedicine* **2012**, *19*, 436–443. [CrossRef] [PubMed]
22. Hölihan, C.M.; Ho, C.T.; Chang, S.S. Elucidation of the chemical structure of a novel antioxidant, rosmaridiphenol, isolated from rosemary. *J. Am. Oil Chem. Soc.* **1984**, *61*, 1036–1039. [CrossRef]
23. Bozin, B.; Mimica-Dukic, N.; Samojlik, I.; Jovin, E. Antimicrobial and Antioxidant properties of Rosemary and Sage (*Rosmarinus officinalis* L. and *Salvia officinalis* L., Laminaceae) essential oils. *J. Agric. Food Chem.* **2007**, *55*, 7879–7885. [CrossRef] [PubMed]
24. Sienkiewicz, M.; Lysakowska, M.; Pastuszka, M.; Bienias, W.; Kowalczyk, E. The potential of use Basil and Rosemary essential oils as effective antibacterial agents. *Molecules* **2013**, *18*, 9334–9351. [CrossRef] [PubMed]
25. Jiang, Y.; Wu, N.; Fu, Y.-J.; Wang, W.; Luo, M.; Zhao, C.J.; Zu, Y.G.; Liu, X.L. Chemical composition and antimicrobial activity of the essential oil of Rosemary. *Environ. Toxicol. Pharmacol.* **2011**, *32*, 63–68. [CrossRef] [PubMed]
26. Bendeddouche, M.S.; Benhassaini, H.; Hazem, Z.; Romane, A. Essential oil analysis and antibacterial activity of Rosmarinus tournefortii from Algeria. *Nat. Prod. Commun.* **2011**, *6*, 1511–1514. [PubMed]
27. Gao, M.; Feng, L.; Jiang, T.; Zhu, J.; Fu, L.; Yuan, D.; Li, J. The use of rosemary extract in combination with nisin to extend the shelf life of pompano (*Trachinotus ovatus*) fillet during chilled storage. *Food Control* **2014**, *37*, 1–8. [CrossRef]
28. Olmedo, R.H.; Nepote, V.; Grosso, N.R. Preservation of sensory and chemical properties in flavoured cheese prepared with cream cheese base using oregano and rosemary essential oils. *LWT-Food Sci. Technol.* **2013**, *53*, 409–417. [CrossRef]
29. Lo Presti, M.; Ragusa, S.; Trozzi, A.; Dugo, P.; Visinoni, F.; Fazio, A.; Dugo, G.; Mondello, L. A comparison between different techniques for the isolation of rosemary essential oil. *J. Sep. Sci.* **2005**, *28*, 273–280. [CrossRef] [PubMed]
30. Arranz, E.; Jaime, L.; García-Risco, M.R.; Fornari, T.; Reglero, G.; Santoyo, S. Anti-inflammatory activity of rosemary extracts obtained by supercritical carbon dioxide enriched in carnosic acid and carnosol. *Int. J. Food Sci. Technol.* **2015**, *50*, 674–681. [CrossRef]
31. Kültür, S. Medicinal plants used in Kirklareli Province (Turkey). *J. Endocrinol.* **2007**, *111*, 341–364. [CrossRef] [PubMed]
32. Arraz, E.; Mes, J.; Wichers, H.J.; Jaime JL Mendiola, A.; Reglero, R.; Santoyo, S. Anti-inflammatory activity of the basolateral fraction of Caco-2 cells exposed to a rosemary supercritical extract. *J. Funct. Foods* **2013**, *13*, 384–390. [CrossRef]
33. Bakiral, T.; Bakirel, U.; Keles, O.U.; Ulgen, S.G.; Yardibi, H. In vivo assessment of antidiabetic and antioxidant activities of rosemary (*Rosmarinus officinalis*) in alloxan-diabetic rabbits. *J. Ethnopharmacol.* **2008**, *116*, 64–73. [CrossRef] [PubMed]

34. Al-Attar, A.; Shawush, N.A. Influence of olive and rosemary leaves extracts on chemically induced liver cirrhosis in male rats. *Saudi J. Biol. Sci.* **2015**, *22*, 157–163. [CrossRef] [PubMed]
35. Laham, S.A.A.; Fadel, F.M. Antibacterial efficacy of variety plants against the resistant streptococcus which cause clinical mastitis cows. *AJPRHC* **2013**, *5*, 32–41.
36. Hölihan, C.M.; Ho, C.T.; Chang, S.S. The structure of rosmariquinone—A new antioxidant isolated from *Rosmarinus officinalis* L. *J. Am. Oil Chem. Soc.* **1985**, *61*, 1036–1039. [CrossRef]
37. Wu, J.W.; Lee, M.-H.; Ho, C.-T.; Chan, S.S. Elucidation of the chemical structures of natural antioxidants isolated from rosemary. *J. Am. Oil Chem. Soc.* **1982**, *59*, 339–345. [CrossRef]
38. Gordon, M.H. The mechanism of antioxidant action in vitro. In *Food Antioxidants*; Hudson, B.J.F., Ed.; Elsevier Science Publishing: New York, NY, USA, 1990; pp. 1–18.
39. Fang, X.; Wada, S. Enhancing the antioxidant effect of α-tocopherol with rosemary in inhibiting catalyzed oxidation caused by Fe^{2+} and hemoprotein. *Food Res. Int.* **1993**, *26*, 405–411. [CrossRef]
40. Löliger, J. The use of antioxidants in foods. In *Free Radicals and Food Additives*; Aruoma, O.I., Halliwell, B., Eds.; Taylor & Francis: London, UK, 1991; pp. 121–150.
41. Chen, C.H.; Pearson, A.M.; Gray, J.I. Effects of synthetic antioxidants (BHA, BHT and PG) on the mutagenicity of IQ-like compounds. *Food Chem.* **1992**, *43*, 177–183. [CrossRef]
42. Aruoma, O.I. Antioxidant actions of plant foods, use of oxidative DNA damage as a tool for studying antioxidant efficacy. *Free Radic. Res.* **1999**, *30*, 419–427. [CrossRef] [PubMed]
43. Inatani, R.; Nakatani, N.; Fuwa, H. Antioxidative effect of the constituents of Rosemary (*Rosmarinus officinalis* L.) and their derivatives. *Agric. Biol. Chem.* **1983**, *47*, 521–528. [CrossRef]
44. Aruoma, O.I.; Halliwell, B.; Aeschbach, R.; Lolingers, J. Antioxidant and pro-oxidant properties of active rosemary constituents: Carnosol and carnosic acid. *Xenobiotica* **1992**, *22*, 257–268. [CrossRef] [PubMed]
45. Cui, L.; Kim, M.O.; Seo, J.H.; Kim, I.S.; Kim, N.Y.; Lee, S.H.; Park, J.; Kim, J.; Lee, H.S. Abietane diterpenoids of Rosmarinus officinalis and their diacylglycerolacyltransferase-inhibitory activity. *Food Chem.* **2012**, *132*, 1775–1780. [CrossRef]
46. Souza, L.C.; de Gomes, M.G.; Goes, A.T.R.; Del Fabbro, L.; Filho, C.B.; Boeira, S.P.; Jesse, C.R. Evidence for the involvement of the serotonergic 5-HT1A receptors in the 2 antidepressant-like effect caused by hesperidin in mice Q13. *Prog. Neuro-Psychopharmacol. Biol. Psychiatry* **2012**, *40*, 103–109. [CrossRef] [PubMed]
47. Yang, S.Y.; Hong, C.O.; Lee, G.P.; Kim, C.T.; Lee, W.W. The hepatoprotectionof caffeic acid and rosmarinic acid, major compounds of Perilla frutescens, against t-BHP-induced oxidative liver damage. *Food Chem. Toxicol.* **2013**, *55*, 92–99. [CrossRef] [PubMed]
48. Munné Bosch, S.; Alegre, L. Subcellular compartmentation of the diterpene carnosic acid and its dervivatives in the leaves of rosemary. *Plant Physiol.* **2001**, *125*, 1094–1102. [CrossRef] [PubMed]
49. Wenkert, E.; Fuchs, A.; McChesney, J. Chemical artifacts from the family Labiatae. *J. Org. Chem.* **1965**, *30*, 2932–2934. [CrossRef]
50. Wijeratne, S.S.; Cuppett, S.L. Potential of rosemary (*Rosmaninus officinalis* L.) diterpenes in preventing lipid hydroperoxide-mediated oxidative stress in Caco-2 cells. *J. Agric. Food Chem.* **2007**, *55*, 1993–1999. [CrossRef] [PubMed]
51. Palitzsc, A.; Schulte, H.; Metzl, F.; Baas, H. Effect of natural spices, spice extracts, essential oil, extraction residues, and synthetic antioxidants on the descomposition of pork fat and model lipids I. Effect of natural spices and spice extracts on pork fat. *Fleischwirtschaft* **1969**, *49*, 1349–1354.
52. Chipault, J.R.; Mizuno, G.R.; Hawkins, J.M.; Lundberg, W.O. The antioxidant properties of natural spices. *Food Res.* **1952**, *17*, 46–55. [CrossRef]
53. Chipault, J.R.; Mizuno, G.R.; Hawkins, J.M.; Lundberg, W.O. Antioxidant properties of spices in oil-in-water emulsion. *Food Res.* **1955**, *20*, 443–448. [CrossRef]
54. Gerhardt, U.; Böhm, T. Redox behaviour of spices in meat products. *Fleischwirtschaft* **1980**, *60*, 1523–1526.
55. Madsen, H.L.; Andersen, L.; Christiansen, L.; Brockhoff, P.; Bertelsen, G. Antioxidant activity of summer savory (*Satureja hortensis.* L) and rosemary (*Rosmarinus officinalis.* L) in minced, cooked pork meat. *Z. Lebensm. Unters. Forsch.* **1996**, *203*, 303–338. [CrossRef]
56. Camo, J.; Beltrán, J.A.; Roncalés, P. Extension of the display life of lamb with an antioxidant active packaging. *Meat Sci.* **2008**, *80*, 1086–1091. [CrossRef] [PubMed]
57. Formanek, Z.; Kerry, J.P.; Buckley, D.J.; Morrissey, P.A.; Farkas, J. Effects of dietary vitamin E supplementation and packaging on the quality of minced beef. *Meat Sci.* **1998**, *50*, 203–210. [CrossRef]

58. Murphy, A.; Kerry, J.P.; Buckley, D.J.; Gray, I. The antioxidative properties of rosemary oleoresin and inhibition of off-flavours in precooked roast beef slices. *J. Sci. Food Agric.* **1998**, *77*, 235–243. [CrossRef]
59. Stoick, S.M.; Gray, J.I.; Booren, A.M.; Buckley, D.J. Oxidative stability of restructured beef steaks processed with oleoresin rosemary, tertiary butylhydroquinone and sodium tripolyphospahte. *J. Food Sci.* **1991**, *56*, 597–600. [CrossRef]
60. Shahidi, F.; Wanasundara, P.; Janhita, P.K. Phenolic antioxidants. *Crit. Rev. Food Sci. Nutr.* **1992**, *32*, 67–103. [CrossRef] [PubMed]
61. Huisman, M.; Madsen, H.L.; Skibsted, L.H.; Bertelsen, G. The combined effect of rosemary (*Rosmarinus officinalis*, L.) and modified atmosphere packaging as protein against warmed over flavour in cooked minced meat. *Z. Lebensm. Unters. Forsch.* **1994**, *198*, 57–59. [CrossRef]
62. Sánchez-Escalante, A.; Djenane, D.; Torrescano, G.; Beltrán, J.A.; Roncalés, P. The effects of ascorbic acid, taurine, carnosine and rosemary powder on colour and lipid stability of beef patties packaged in modified atmosphere. *Meat Sci.* **2001**, *58*, 421–429. [CrossRef]
63. Formanek, Z.; Lynch, A.; Galván, K.; Farkas, J.; Kerry, J.P. Combined effects of irradiation and the use of natural antioxidants on the shelf-life stability overwrapped minced beef. *Meat Sci.* **2003**, *63*, 433–440. [CrossRef]
64. Frankel, E.N.; Huang, S.W.; Aeschbach, R.; Prior, E. Antioxidant activity of rosemary extract and its constituents, carnosic acid, carnosol, and rosmarinic acid, in bulk oil and oil-in water emulsion. *J. Agric. Food Chem.* **1996**, *44*, 131–135. [CrossRef]
65. López-Bote, C.J.; Gray, J.I.; Gomaa, E.A.; Flegal, C.J. Effect of dietary administration of oil extracts from rosemary and sage on lipid oxidation in broiler meat. *Br. Poult. Sci.* **1998**, *39*, 235–240. [CrossRef] [PubMed]
66. Moñino, M.I.; Martínez, C.; Sotomayor, J.A.; Lafuente, A.; Jordán, M.J. Polyphenolic transmission to segureño lamb meat from ewes dietary supplemented with the distillate from rosemary (*Rosmarinus officinalis*) leaves. *J. Agric. Food Chem.* **2008**, *56*, 3363–3367. [CrossRef] [PubMed]
67. Descalzo, A.M.; Insani, E.M.; Violatto, A.; Sancho, A.M.; García, P.T.; Pensel, N.A.; Josifovich, J.A. Influence of pasture or grain-based diets supplemented with vitamin E on antioxidant/oxidative balance of Argentine beef. *Meat Sci.* **2005**, *70*, 35–44. [CrossRef] [PubMed]
68. Petron, M.J.; Raes, K.; Claeys, E.; Lourenço, M.; Fremaut, D.; De Smet, S. Effect of grazing pastures of different botanical composition on antioxidant enzyme activities and oxidative stability of lamb meat. *Meat Sci.* **2007**, *75*, 737–745. [CrossRef] [PubMed]
69. Mc Carthy, T.L.; Kerry, J.P.; Kerry, J.F.; Lynch, P.B.; Buckley, D.J. Assessment of the antioxidant potential of natural food and plant extracts in fresh and previously frozen pork patties. *Meat Sci.* **2001**, *57*, 177–184. [CrossRef]
70. Janz, J.A.M.; Morel, P.C.H.; Wilkinson, B.H.P.; Purchas, R.H. Preliminary investigation of the effects of low-level dietary inclusion of fragrant essential oils and oleoresins on pig performance and pork quality. *Meat Sci.* **2007**, *75*, 360–365. [CrossRef] [PubMed]
71. Yu, L.; Scanlin, L.; Wilson, J.; Schmidt, G. Rosemary extracts as inhibitors of lipid oxidation and color cahnge in cooked turkey products during refrigerated storage. *J. Food Sci.* **2002**, *67*, 582–585. [CrossRef]
72. Govaris, A.; Florou-Paneri, P.; Botsoglou, E.; Giannenas, I.; Amvrosiadis, I.; Botsoglou, N. The inhibitory potential of feed supplementation with rosemary and/or α-tocopheryl acetate on microbial growth and lipid oxidation of turkey breast during refrigerated storage. *LWT-Food Sci. Technol.* **2007**, *40*, 331–337. [CrossRef]
73. Parpinello, G.P.; Meluzzi, A.; Sirri, F.; Tallarico, N.; Versari, A. Sensory evaluation of egg products and eggs laid from hens fed diets with different fatty acid composition and supplemented with antioxidants. *Food Res. Int.* **2006**, *39*, 47–52. [CrossRef]
74. Florou-Paneri, P.; Dotas, D.; Mitsopoulos, I.; Dotas, V.; Botsoglou, E.; Nikolakakis, I.; Botsoglou, N. Effect of feeding rosemary and α-tocoferol acetate on hen performance and egg quality. *J. Poult. Sci.* **2006**, *43*, 143–149. [CrossRef]
75. Sebranek, J.G.; Sewalt, V.J.H.; Robbins, K.L.; Houser, T.A. Comparison of a natural rosemary extract and BHA/BHT for relative antioxidant effectiveness in pork sausage. *Meat Sci.* **2005**, *69*, 289–296. [CrossRef] [PubMed]
76. O'Grady, M.N.; Maher, M.; Troy, D.J.; Moloney, A.P.; Kerry, J.P. An assessment of dietary supplementation with tea catechins and rosemary extract on the quality of fresh beef. *Meat Sci.* **2006**, *73*, 132–143. [CrossRef] [PubMed]

77. Galobart, J.; Barroeta, A.C.; Baucells, M.D.; Codony, R.; Ternes, W. Effect of dietary supplementation with rosemary extract and α-tocoferol acetate on lipid oxidation in eggs enriched with w3-fatty acids. *Poult. Sci.* **2001**, *80*, 460–467. [CrossRef] [PubMed]
78. Estévez, M.; Cava, R. Effectiveness of rosemary essential oil as an inhibitor of lipid and protein oxidation: Contradictory effects in different types of frankfurters. *Meat Sci.* **2006**, *72*, 348–355. [CrossRef] [PubMed]
79. Nieto, G.; Jongberg, S.; Andersen, M.L.; Skibsted, L.H. Thiol oxidation and protein cross-link formation during chill storage of pork patties added essential oil of oregano, rosemary, or garlic. *Meat Sci.* **2013**, *95*, 177–184. [CrossRef] [PubMed]
80. Tohma, S.; Turan, S. Rosemary plant (*Rosmarinus officinalis* L.), solvent extract and essential oil can be used to extend the usage life of hazelnut oil during deep frying. *Eur. J. Lipid Sci. Technol.* **2015**, *117*, 1978–1990. [CrossRef]
81. Taha, E.; Abouelhawa, S.; El-Geddawy, M.; Sorour, M.; Aladedunye, F.; Matthäus, B. Stabilization of refined rapeseed oil during deep-fatfrying by selected herbs. *Eur. J. Lipid Sci. Technol.* **2014**, *116*, 771–779. [CrossRef]
82. Urbancic, S.; Kolar, M.H.; Dimitrijevic, D.; Demsar, L.; Vidrih, R. Stabilization of sunflower oil and reductionof acrylamide formation of potato with rosemary extractduring deep-fat frying. *LWT-Food Sci. Technol.* **2014**, *57*, 671–678. [CrossRef]
83. Mihajilov-Kristev, T.; Radnovic, D.; Kitic, D.; Stajnovic-Radic, Z.; Zlatkovic, B. Antimicrobial activity of *Satureja hortensis* L. essential oil against pathogenic microbial strains. *Bioterchnol. Biotechnol. Equip.* **2009**, *23*, 1492–1496. [CrossRef]
84. Probuseenivasan, S.; Jayakumar, M.; Ignacimuthu, S. In vitro antibacterial activity of some plant essential oils. *BMC Complement. Altern. Med.* **2006**, *6*, 39. [CrossRef] [PubMed]
85. Burt, S. Essential oils: Their antibacterial properties and potential applications in foods—A review. *Int. J. Food Microbiol.* **2004**, *94*, 223–253. [CrossRef] [PubMed]
86. Sirocchi, V.; Caprioli, G.; Cecchini, C.; Coman, M.M.; Cresci, A.; Maggi, F.; Papa, F.; Ricciutelli, M.; Vittori, S.; Sagratini, G. Biogenic amines as freshness index of meat wrapped in a new active packaging system formulated with essential oils of Rosmarinus officinalis. *Int. J. Food Sci. Nutr.* **2013**, *64*, 921–928. [CrossRef] [PubMed]
87. Fung, D.Y.C.; Taylor, S.; Kahan, J. Effect of butylated hydroxyanisole (BHA) and buthylated hydroxytoluebe (BHT) on growth and aflatoxin production of *Aspergillus flavus*. *J. Food Saf.* **1977**, *1*, 39–51. [CrossRef]
88. Vegara, S.; Funes, L.; Martí, N.; Saura, D.; Micol, V.; Valero, M. Bactericidal activities against pathogenic bacteria by selected constituents of plant extracts in carrot broth. *Food Chem.* **2011**, *128*, 872–877. [CrossRef]
89. Moreno, S.; Scheyer, T.; Romano, C.S.; Vojnov, A.A. Antioxidant and antimicrobial activities of rosemary extracts linked to their polyphenol composition. *Free Radic. Res.* **2006**, *40*, 223–231. [CrossRef] [PubMed]
90. Ivanovic, J.; Misic, D.; Zizovic, I.; Ristic, M. In vitro control of multiplication of some food-associated bacteria by thyme, rosemary and sage isolates. *Food Control* **2012**, *25*, 110–116. [CrossRef]
91. Bernardes, W.A.; Lucarini, R.; Tozatti, M.G.; Souza, M.G.M.; Silva, M.L.; Filho, A.A.; Gomes Martin, C.H.; Crotti, A.E.M.; Pauletti, P.M.; Groppo, M.; et al. Antimicrobial Activity of Rosmarinus officinalisagainst OralPathogens: Relevance of Carnosic Acid and Carnosol. *Chem. Biodivers.* **2010**, *7*, 1835–1840. [CrossRef] [PubMed]
92. Zaouali, Y.; Bouzaine, T.; Boussaid, M. Essential oils composition in two *Rosmarinus officinalis* L. varieties and incidence for antimicrobial and antioxidant activities. *Food Chem. Toxicol.* **2010**, *48*, 3144–3152. [CrossRef] [PubMed]
93. Bajpai, V.K.; Kwang-Hyun Baek, K.; Kang, S.C. Control of Salmonella in foods by using essential oils: A review. *Food Res. Int.* **2012**, *45*, 722–734. [CrossRef]
94. Tornuk, F.; Cankurt, H.; Ozturk, I.; Sagdic, O.; Bayram, O.; Yetim, H. Efficacy of various plant hydrosols as natural food sanitizers in reducing *Escherichia coli* O157:H7 and Salmonella Typhimurium on fresh cut carrots and apples. *Int. J. Food Microbiol.* **2011**, *148*, 30–35. [CrossRef] [PubMed]
95. Teixeira, B.; Marques, A.; Ramos, C.; Neng, N.R.; Nogueira, J.M.F.; Saraiva, J.A.; Nunes, M.L. Chemical composition and antibacterial and antioxidant properties of commercial essential oils. *Ind. Crops Prod.* **2013**, *43*, 587–595. [CrossRef]
96. Fernández-López, J.; Zhi, N.; Aleson-Carbonell, L.; Pérez-Álvarez, J.A.; Kuri, V. Antioxidant and antibacterial activities of natural extracts: Application in beef meatballs. *Meat Sci.* **2005**, *69*, 371–380. [CrossRef] [PubMed]

97. Ahn, J.; Grün, I.U.; Mustapha, A. Effects of plant extracts on microbial growth, color change and lipid oxidation in cooked beef. *Food Microbiol.* **2007**, *24*, 7–14. [CrossRef] [PubMed]
98. Pandit, V.A.; Shelef, L.A. Sensitivity of Listeria monocytogenes to rosemary (*Rosmarinus officinalis* L.). *Food Microbiol.* **1994**, *11*, 57–63. [CrossRef]
99. Gómez-Estaca, J.; López de Lacey, A.; López-Caballero, M.E.; Gómez-Guillén, M.C.; Montero, P. Biodegradable gelatin–chitosan films incorporated with essential oils as antimicrobial agents for fish preservation. *Food Microbiol.* **2010**, *27*, 889–896. [CrossRef] [PubMed]
100. Ouattara, B.; Sabato, S.F.; Lacroix, M. Combinated effect of antimicrobial coating and gamma irradiation on shelf life extension of pre-cooked shrimp (*Penaus* spp.). *Int. J. Food Microbiol.* **2001**, *68*, 1–9. [CrossRef]
101. Ismail, A.A.; Pierson, M.D. Effect of sodium nitrite and origenum oil on growth and toxin production of *Clostridium botulinum* in TYG broth and ground pork. *J. Prot.* **1990**, *53*, 958–960.
102. Resurreccion, A.V.A.; Reynold, A.E., Jr. Evaluation of Natural Antioxidants in Frankfurters containing Chicken and Pork. *J. Food Sci.* **1990**, *55*, 629–631. [CrossRef]
103. Wong, J.W.; Hashimoto, K.; Shibamoto, T. Antioxidant activities of rosemary and sage extracts and vitamin E in a model system. *J. Agric. Food Chem.* **1995**, *43*, 2707–2712. [CrossRef]
104. Wada, S.; Fang, X. The synergistic antioxidant effect of rosemary extract and α-tocopherol in sardine oil model system and frozen-crushed fish meat. *J. Food Process. Preserv.* **1992**, *16*, 263–274. [CrossRef]
105. Lai, S.H.; Gray, J.I.; Smith, D.M.; Booren, A.M.; Crackel, R.L.; Buckley, D.J. Effects of oleoresin rosemary, tertiary butylhydroquinone, and sodium tripolyphsphate on the development of oxidative rancidity in restructed chicken nuggets. *J. Food Sci.* **1991**, *56*, 616–620. [CrossRef]

medicines

MDPI

Review

Bioactive Compounds and Extracts from Traditional Herbs and Their Potential Anti-Inflammatory Health Effects

Antonio Serrano, Gaspar Ros * and Gema Nieto

Department of Food Technology, Nutrition and Food Science, Veterinary Faculty University of Murcia, Campus de Espinardo, Espinardo, 30100 Murcia, Spain; antonio.serrano5@um.es (A.S.); gnieto@um.es (G.N.)
* Correspondence: gros@um.es

Received: 10 May 2018; Accepted: 11 July 2018; Published: 16 July 2018

Abstract: The inflammatory processes associated with several chronic illnesses like cardiovascular disease and cancer have been the focus of mechanistic studies of the pathogenicity of these diseases and of the use of different pharmacological and natural methods to prevent them. In this study we review the current evidence regarding the effectiveness of natural extracts from as-yet little-studied traditional botanical species in alleviating the inflammation process associated with several chronic diseases. Additionally, the intention is to expose the known pathways of action and the potential synergistic effects of the constituent compounds of the discussed extracts. It is noted that the here-studied extracts, which include black garlic rich in S-allylcystein, polyphenols from cat's claw (*Uncaria tomentosa*), devil's claw (*Harpagophytum procumbens*), camu-camu (*Myrciaria dubia*), and blackcurrant (*Ribes nigrum*), and citrus fruit extracts rich in hesperidin, have similar or greater effects than other, more extensively studied extracts such as tea and cocoa. The combined use of all of these extracts can give rise to synergetic effects with greater biological relevance at lower doses.

Keywords: anti-inflammatory; medicinal plants; chronic diseases; *Uncaria tomentosa*; *Harpagophytum procumbens*; *Myrciaria dubia*; *Ribes nigrum*; hesperidin

1. Introduction

Inflammation represents a biological response of the organism to a series of mechanical, chemical, or infectious stimuli. Its mission is to isolate, destroy, or dilute, as a form of localized protection. Inflammation can be chronic or acute depending on the characteristics of humoral response and the molecules involved. When inflammatory balance is altered, with excessive pro inflammatory signals (for example in the cyclooxygenase pathway), physiological damage can occur [1].

Chronic inflammation is a status derived from physiopathogenic situations such as metabolic syndrome or inflammatory bowel diseases that involve prolonged exposition to a number of potential pathogenic substances. Those substances are mainly inflammatory mediators like tumor necrosis factor alpha (TNF-α), and are linked to cancer initiation [2]. The combination of these factors leads to an unbalanced inflammatory status with an increment in markers like inflammatory cytokines, including TNF-α, interleukin (IL)-6, and IL-1β, which are also associated with cardiometabolic diseases [3].

Thus, a way to prevent inflammation which can lead to carcinogenesis or cardiovascular diseases is through the use of botanic extracts of spices and herbs which show both antioxidant and anti-inflammatory properties. For this reason, anti-inflammatory phytochemicals could represent an exogenous aid crucial for the prevention of chronic diseases mediated by inflammatory processes.

2. Natural Extracts and Compounds with Anti-Inflammatory Properties

2.1. *Allium nigrum (Black Garlic)*

Garlic is a commonly used condiment with many biological activities due to its sulfur compounds [4] which have antioxidant and antimicrobial properties [5]. Black garlic is obtained through fermentation at a controlled high temperature (60–90 °C) and high humidity (80–90%). It has distinct bioactivity with respect to fresh garlic, conferring numerous benefits like anti-inflammatory, anticancer, and antiobesity activity [6]. This nutritional variation is characterized by a decrease in fructan, which is linked to an increase of fructose due to a Maillard reaction that subsequently impacts the color and taste [7]. Changes in the profile of volatile compounds provide black garlic with higher concentrations of S-alk(en)-yl-L-cysteine derivatives, while the quantity of ascorbic acid decreases due to thermal treatment [8]. Meanwhile, the concentrations of some flavonoids, pyruvate, total phenol, and the main antioxidant compound of black garlic, S-allylcystein, are increased [9] (Figure 1).

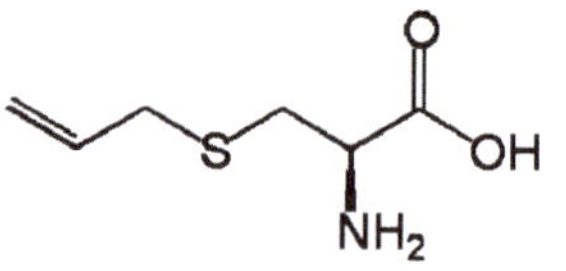

Figure 1. Chemical structure of S-allylcystein.

Some studies have isolated bioactive compounds from black garlic in order to evaluate their bioactivity. When black garlic aqueous extract is compared to raw garlic aqueous extract at similar dose range (between 31.25 µg/mL and 250 µg/mL), higher inhibition of tumor necrosis factor alpha (TNF-α) and prostaglandin E2 (PGE2) is reported for the aged garlic extract [10]. Kim et al. [11] demonstrated that even concentrations as low as between 5 µg/mL and 10 µg/mL of black garlic ethanol extract have anti-inflammatory effects as they inhibit nitric oxide (NO) and PGE2 production in lipopolysaccharide-stimulated (LPS-stimulated) RAW264.7 cells, and also decrease nitric oxide synthases and prostaglandin-endoperoxide synthase 2 expression. Choi et al. [12] showed that antioxidant power increased between day 0 and 21 of fermentation, reaching its limit at day 21 and keeping most of its properties at day 35 even though the levels of ascorbic acid were lower, as shown by Martínez-Casas et al. [8].

2.2. *Uncaria tomentosa ("Cat's Claw")*

Uncaria tomentosa (UT) is a climbing vine from Peru commonly known as cat's claw from the Spanish "*Uña de Gato*" because of its thorns. It has been used over time in traditional medicine to treat diseases like rheumatism and cancer [13]. It has up to 32 phenolic compounds, including hydroxybenzoic acids, hydroxycinnamic acids, flavan-3-ols monomers, procyanidin dimers and trimers, flavalignans, and propelargonidin dimers [14]. One of the major bioactive compounds of UT is mitraphylline (Figure 2), which was isolated and evaluated by Rojas-Duran et al. [15] using a dose of 30 mg/kg/day for 3 days in mice, resulting in cytokine modulation providing fewer inflammatory signals.

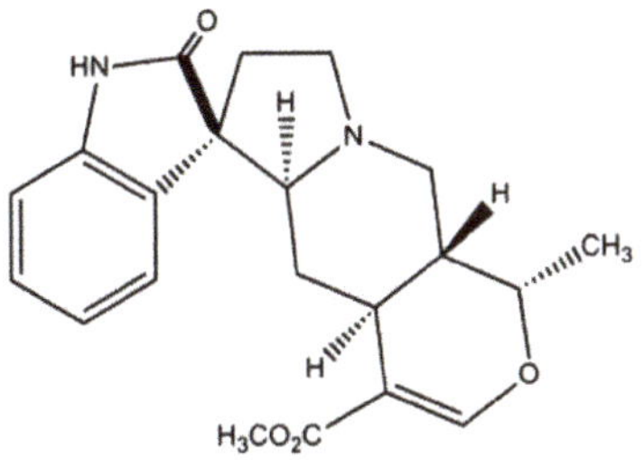

Figure 2. Chemical structure of mitraphylline.

The anticancer properties of UT are due to the synergistic activity of alkaloids with its non-polar compounds [16] like isopteropodine, pteropodine, isomitraphylline, uncarine F, and mitraphylline. These compounds also have exhibited anti-apoptotic properties in lymphoblastic leukemia [17]. The antioxidant properties of UT are attributed to its capacity to scavenge radicals such as superoxide anions and hydroxyl radicals, and also prevent lipid membrane oxidation [18]. Allen-Hall et al. [19] used human THP-1 monocytes (human monocytic cell line derived from an acute monocytic leukemia patient), reporting how UT affects the nuclear factor kappa-light-chain-enhancer of activated B cells (NF-κB) pathway, inhibiting inflammatory cytokines such as TNF-α and interleukin 1 beta (IL-1β). UT aqueous ethanol extract also has the potential to treat T-helper 1 immuno-mediated disorders with no cytotoxic or immunotoxicity at concentrations of 100 μg/mL and 500 μg/mL on murine splenocytes [20]

Another study suggested that both aqueous and alkaloid-enriched extract of UT act over the wnt-signaling pathway which influences degenerative diseases, diabetes, and cancer, modulating it to a less pathogenic environment [21].

2.3. *Harpagophytum procumbens (Devil's Claw)*

Harpagophytum procumbens (HP), commonly named devil's claw because of its fruits, is a perennial herbaceous plant which has roots that are traditionally used as anti-inflammatory agents for symptomatic treatment in arthritis and rheumatism. It grows mainly in the Kalahari Desert in the south of Africa. It had been linked with healthy properties like antimalarial, anticancer and uterotonic activities [22].

Its bioactivity is conferred by iridoids, a family of monoterpenoids. The glycoside fraction (containing mainly harpagoside; Figure 3) in devil's claw has been proven to be antimutagenic against environmental injury [23].

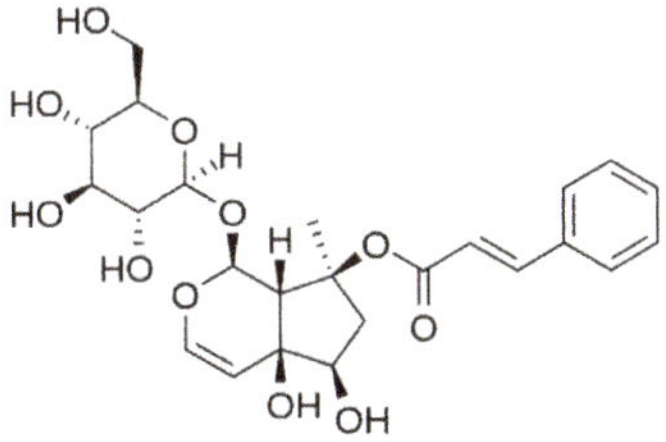

Figure 3. Chemical structure of harpagoside.

In addition, anti-inflammatory properties have been widely evaluated. The extract of HP influences the synthesis and release of pro-inflammatory factors, inhibiting transcription factor activator protein 1 (AP-1) activity in murine macrophages and cytokine expression such as TNF-α and interleukin 6 (IL-6) when used at concentrations between 100 μg/mL and 200 μg/mL. It decreases

COX-2 mRNA levels at concentrations between 50 μg/mL and 200 μg/mL [24]. In any case, devil's claw's effectiveness is not only based on its harpagosides but also on synergistic activity with other compounds, as seen by Hostanska et al. [25], who observed less cytokine TNF-α, IL-6, and interleukin 8 (IL-8) production at concentrations of 250 μg/mL of HP ethanolic extract.

Hapargophytum extract also exhibits the capacity to prevent oxidative stress or loss of cell viability against common oxidants [26]. The phytochemicals responsible for these effects are primarily verbascosides, followed by phenylethanoid-containing fractions from methanolic extract [27].

2.4. *Myrciaria dubia* (Camu Camu)

Myrciaria dubia (MD) is a shrub from the Amazon rainforest which produces a round red-colored berry with a strong acid flavor. It is characterized by its content in vitamin C and polyphenols which confer it antioxidant, anti-inflammatory, and antimicrobial activities [28]

Camu camu juice, due to its vitamin C content, has been demonstrated to have physiological antioxidant power, decreasing total reactive oxygen species and anti-inflammatory activity and reducing circulating C reactive protein in human at a dose of 70 mL/day [29]. However, polyphenols present in camu camu such as proanthocyanidins, ellagitannins, and ellagic acid derivatives also have antioxidant and anti-inflammatory activities [30]. Separately, higher antioxidant activities were reported for stachyurin and casuarinin together with other tannins present in the fruit [31]. Other authors focused on antigenotoxic effects linked to the antioxidant capacity of the compound mixture present in camu camu, demonstrating that regardless of whether the processes are acute, sub-acute, or chronic, the administration of juice at a concentration of 25%, 50%, and 100% by injection of 0.1 mL/10 g reduces significantly genotoxic damage induced by hydrogen peroxide in mice blood cells [32].

2.5. Citrus Fruits Rich in Hesperidin

Hesperidin (Figure 4) is a flavanone from the flavonoid family and is mainly found in the epicarp, mesocarp, and endocarp of oranges, lemon, lime, and other citrus fruits [33].

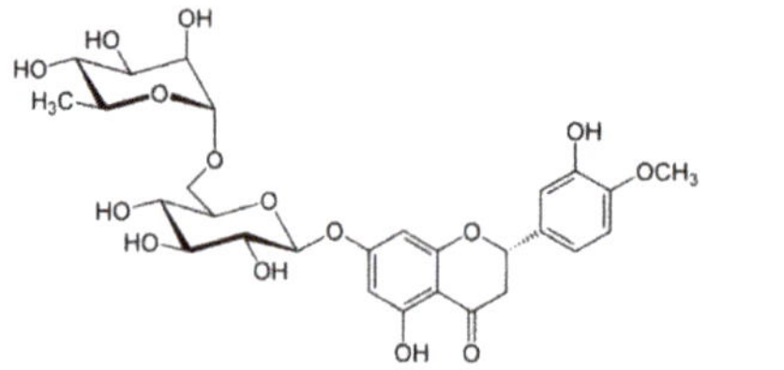

Figure 4. Chemical structure of hesperidin.

Hesperidin has been widely studied due to its health benefits against cardiovascular diseases and cancer through its anti-inflammatory properties. It induces apoptotic cell death in gastric, colon, breast, lung, and liver cancer [34]. Its presence at a dose of 25 mg/kg a week before colon carcinogenesis induction and during the next 3 weeks in mice has been proven to enhance antioxidant-inhibiting reactive oxygen species and downregulate expression of inflammatory markers such as NF-κB, iNOS (a gene on chromosome 17q11.2-q12 that encodes inducible nitric oxide synthase), and COX-2 [35]. At a dose of 50 mg/kg 1 h before carrageenan injection it also exhibits antioxidative potential, enhancing endogenous antioxidants and decreasing inflammatory markers such as TNF-α, total leukocytes, neutrophils, lymphocytes, and nitrite concentrations [36]. Hesperidin's anti-inflammatory properties have been observed in mice with induced cognitive impairment, showing that a pretreatment of 100 mg/kg to 200 mg/kg administered intraperitoneal once daily for 15 days modulates neuronal cell death, inhibiting the overexpression of inflammatory markers and providing neuroprotective effects [37].

Similar studies were conducted in rats. Those rats that were supplemented with doses of 50 mg/kg, 100 mg/kg, and 200 mg/kg prior to lipopolysaccharide-induced endotoxicity showed an improvement in endothelial status with respect to those that were not treated [38]. The capacity of hesperidin to down-regulate inflammatory status has been reported to improve rat postoperative ileus in a dose-dependent manner between 5 and 80 mg/kg [39]. A dose of 160 mg/kg in rats reduced lipid peroxidation and improved the activity of endogenous antioxidant enzymes, palliating effects of rheumatoid arthritis [40].

Clinical assays performed in 75 patients with myocardial infarction at a dose of 600 mg/day for four days showed an improvement in inflammatory markers and lipid profiles [41].

2.6. *Ribes nigrum* (Blackcurrant)

Ribes nigrum (RN) is a woody shrub natural from central and Eastern Europe. Its fruit, the blackcurrant, is traditionally used for the treatment of rheumatic disease. It contains significant concentrations of vitamin C and some polyphenols, mostly anthocyanins. As seen in other extracts, synergistic activities are key in natural extracts but in the blackcurrant, the most remarkable compounds are prodelphinidins [42]. Rutinosides and glucosides of delphinidin and cyaniding are the major compounds in blackcurrant extract, but also other compounds have also been found, such as myiricetin and quercentin glucosides, at lower concentrations [43]. Considering the presence of those compounds, it is not surprising that different studies found anti-inflammatory and antioxidant activities in blackcurrants.

Blackcurrant extract obtained from freeze-dried blackcurrants at a concentration of 1 mg/mL applied to cell culture supernatant down-regulates the expression of inflammatory mediators through the action of intestinal cells and macrophages stimulated with lipopolysaccharides [44]. Another study which also used RAW264.7 macrophages stimulated with LPS showed a reduction in mRNA levels of TNF-α, IL-1β, and iNOS when blackcurrant extract was added at a concentration of 0.2 mg/mL to cultured supernatant. [45]. Further studies with a mix of berries (blueberries, blackberries, and blackcurrants) support these results, using lower concentrations of between 10 and 20 μg/mL in cell cultures and obtaining lower levels of IL-1β messenger RNA [46].

Proanthocyanin-enriched blackcurrant extract suppressed IL-4 and IL-13 secretion from alveolar epithelial cells in a study performed with concentrations of 0.5–10 mg/mL total blackcurrant polyphenolic extract [47]. Concentrations of 5 μg/mL to 25 μg/mL of blackcurrant extract and cyanidin-3-O-glucoside on supernatant were used with monocyte-derived macrophages (U937), showing higher cell viability against nicotine and lower levels of IL-6 secretion when inflammation was induced through lipopolysaccharides [48].

Animal studies were also performed, obtaining anti-inflammatory results due to a depletion in the contents of TNF-α, IL-1β, IL-6, and IL-10 on Wistar rats pretreated with an intraperitoneal administration of proanthocyanidins from RN leaves at concentrations of 10 mg/kg, 30 mg/kg, 60 mg/kg, and 100 mg/kg [49]. In addition, the chemopreventive effects of anthocyanins from RN were tested against hepatic carcinogenesis in Sprague–Dawley rats using a dose between 100 mg/kg and 500 mg/kg of extract during four weeks, obtaining as a result antihepatocarcinogenic effects [50].

3. Comparing Emergent Extracts with Classics

There is a great complexity in the modes of action of the phytochemical species present in the extracts described above, and while most are used traditionally to palliate a broad spectrum of diseases, just a few natural extracts have been widely popularized.

One of these is green tea (*Camellia sinensis*) for which its phytocompounds have been proven to have anticancer properties [51]. It provides protection against environmental factors that affect homeostasis, such as genotoxic substances and free radicals [52]. Green coffee also exhibits a number of health benefits, such as protection of hepatic cells from oxidative damage [53]. Its chlorogenic acids inhibit LDL (low-density lipoprotein) peroxidation and COX-2 production, helping to prevent colon cancer and cardiovascular diseases [54], and down-regulate cytokines and proliferative factors [55]. Cocoa, from *Theobroma cacao*, has also been studied because of its antioxidant and anti-inflammatory characteristics [56]. The fruit from *Vitis vinifera*, commonly named grape, is also a source of antioxidant and anti-inflammatory compounds in both the seeds and the skin [57,58]. It is widely studied due to its involvement in wine production, which also gives rise to the presence of stilbenoids [59].

World famous foods such as tea, coffee, and cocoa have been studied extensively due to interest not only as foods that promote health but also for their commercial potential given high levels of production and exportation. For this reason, other botanical species potentially beneficial for health have been relegated to the background and should be studied more thoroughly

4. Conclusions

Nowadays, cardiovascular disease and different types of cancers represent major challenges to public health, and because identification is crucial. Growing interest in health can be an incentive when producing food and nutraceuticals that promote research in this field.

In this review, which includes a summary of the dose–response activity of selected extracts, we can see how different lesser-known extracts have an effectiveness similar to those of more widely used extracts. It is important to bear in mind that botanical species such as UT and HT at low doses have anti-inflammatory, anti-oxidant, and anti-carcinogenic effects when evaluated in cell and animal studies. Even species such as *Allium nigrum* are able to enhance their beneficial effects or add new ones after processing. Hesperidin has also been studied as a representative of citrus fruits given its anti-inflammatory and cardioprotective effects. To conclude, MD and RN suppose a source of antioxidants that are present in the fruit of these botanical species that can not only act as such but also enhance the beneficial effect of the extracts described above.

As we have seen in the selected extracts, synergistic activity is one of the factors that potentiates the effects of natural extracts against purified compounds. This way, it is assumable that the joint use of different sources of bioactive compounds could lead to higher effectiveness. However, the safety of these mixtures should be evaluated and the action pathways identified.

Funding: This research received no external funding.

Conflicts of Interest: The authors declare no conflict of interest.

References

1. Wang, M.; Honn, K.; Nie, D. Cyclooxygenases, prostanoids, and tumor progression. *Cancer Metastasis Rev.* **2007**, *26*, 525–534. [CrossRef] [PubMed]
2. Balkwill, F. TNF-α in promotion and progression of cancer. *Cancer Metastasis Rev.* **2006**, *25*, 409–416. [CrossRef] [PubMed]
3. Minihane, A.; Vinoy, S.; Russell, W.; Baka, A.; Roche, H.; Tuohy, K.; Teeling, J.; Blaak, E.; Fenech, M.; Vauzour, D.; et al. Low-grade inflammation, diet composition and health: Current research evidence and its translation. *Br. J. Nutr.* **2015**, *114*, 999–1012. [CrossRef] [PubMed]
4. Block, E.; Naganathan, S.; Putman, D.; Zhao, S. Allium chemistry: HPLC analysis of thiosulfinates from onion, garlic, wild garlic (ramsoms), leek, scallion, shallot, elephant (great-headed) garlic, chive, and Chinese chive. Uniquely high allyl to methyl ratios in some garlic samples. *J. Agric. Food Chem.* **1992**, *40*, 2418–2430. [CrossRef]
5. Horita, C.; Farías-Campomanes, A.; Barbosa, T.; Esmerino, E.; da Cruz, A.; Bolini, H.; Meireles, M.; Pollonio, M. The antimicrobial, antioxidant and sensory properties of garlic and its derivatives in Brazilian low-sodium frankfurters along shelf-life. *Food Res. Int.* **2016**, *84*, 1–8. [CrossRef]
6. Kimura, S.; Tung, Y.; Pan, M.; Su, N.; Lai, Y.; Cheng, K. Black garlic: A critical review of its production, bioactivity, and application. *J. Food Drug Anal.* **2017**, *25*, 62–70. [CrossRef] [PubMed]
7. Yuan, H.; Sun, L.; Chen, M.; Wang, J. An analysis of the changes on intermediate products during the thermal processing of black garlic. *Food Chem.* **2018**, *239*, 56–61. [CrossRef] [PubMed]

8. Martínez-Casas, L.; Lage-Yusty, M.; López-Hernández, J. Changes in the Aromatic Profile, Sugars, and Bioactive Compounds When Purple Garlic Is Transformed into Black Garlic. *J. Agric. Food Chem.* **2017**, *65*, 10804–10811. [CrossRef] [PubMed]
9. Ryu, J.; Kang, D. Physicochemical Properties, Biological Activity, Health Benefits, and General Limitations of Aged Black Garlic: A Review. *Molecules* **2017**, *22*, 919. [CrossRef] [PubMed]
10. Kim, M.; Yoo, Y.; Kim, H.; Shin, S.; Sohn, E.; Min, A.; Sung, N.; Kim, M. Aged Black Garlic Exerts Anti-Inflammatory Effects by Decreasing NO and Proinflammatory Cytokine Production with Less Cytoxicity in LPS-Stimulated RAW 264.7 Macrophages and LPS-Induced Septicemia Mice. *J. Med. Food* **2014**, *17*, 1057–1063. [CrossRef] [PubMed]
11. Kim, D.; Kang, M.; Hong, S.; Choi, Y.; Shin, J. Anti-inflammatory Effects of Functionally Active Compounds Isolated from Aged Black Garlic. *Phytother. Res.* **2016**, *31*, 53–61. [CrossRef] [PubMed]
12. Choi, I.; Cha, H.; Lee, Y. Physicochemical and Antioxidant Properties of Black Garlic. *Molecules* **2014**, *19*, 16811–16823. [CrossRef] [PubMed]
13. Heitzman, M.E.; Neto, C.C.; Winiarz, E.; Vaisberg, A.J.; Hammond, G.B. Ethnobotany, phytochemistry and pharmacology of (Rubiaceae). *Phytochemistry* **2005**, *66*, 5–29. [CrossRef] [PubMed]
14. Navarro Hoyos, M.; Sánchez-Patán, F.; Murillo Masis, R.; Martín-Álvarez, P.; Zamora Ramirez, W.; Monagas, M.; Bartolomé, B. Phenolic Assesment of *Uncaria tomentosa* L. (Cat's Claw): Leaves, Stem, Bark and Wood Extracts. *Molecules* **2015**, *20*, 22703–22717. [CrossRef] [PubMed]
15. Rojas-Duran, R.; González-Aspajo, G.; Ruiz-Martel, C.; Bourdy, G.; Doroteo-Ortega, V.; Alban-Castillo, J.; Robert, G.; Auberger, P.; Deharo, E. Anti-inflammatory activity of Mitraphylline isolated from *Uncaria tomentosa* bark. *J. Ethnopharmacol.* **2012**, *143*, 801–804. [CrossRef] [PubMed]
16. Pilarski, R.; Filip, B.; Wietrzyk, J.; Kuraś, M.; Gulewicz, K. Anticancer activity of the *Uncaria tomentosa* (Willd.) DC. preparations with different oxindole alkaloid composition. *Phytomedicine* **2010**, *17*, 1133–1139. [CrossRef] [PubMed]
17. Bors, M.; Michałowicz, J.; Pilarski, R.; Sicińska, P.; Gulewicz, K.; Bukowska, B. Studies of biological properties of *Uncaria tomentosa* extracts on human blood mononuclear cells. *J. Ethnopharmacol.* **2012**, *142*, 669–678. [CrossRef] [PubMed]
18. Goncalves, C.; Dinis, T.; Batista, M. Antioxidant properties of proanthocyanidins of bark decoction: A mechanism for anti-inflammatory activity. *Phytochemistry* **2005**, *66*, 89–98. [CrossRef] [PubMed]
19. Allen-Hall, L.; Cano, P.; Arnason, J.; Rojas, R.; Lock, O.; Lafrenie, R. Treatment of THP-1 cells with *Uncaria tomentosa* extracts differentially regulates the expression if IL-1β and TNF-α. *J. Ethnopharmacol.* **2007**, *109*, 312–317. [CrossRef] [PubMed]
20. Domingues, A.; Sartori, A.; Valente, L.; Golim, M.; Siani, A.; Viero, R. *Uncaria tomentosa* Aqueous-ethanol Extract Triggers an Immunomodulation toward a Th2 Cytokine Profile. *Phytother. Res.* **2011**, *25*, 1229–1235. [CrossRef] [PubMed]
21. Gurrola-Díaz, C.; García-López, P.; Gulewicz, K.; Pilarski, R.; Dihlmann, S. Inhibitory mechanisms of two *Uncaria tomentosa* extracts affecting the Wnt-signaling pathway. *Phytomedicine* **2011**, *18*, 683–690. [CrossRef] [PubMed]
22. Mncwangi, N.; Chen, W.; Vermaak, I.; Viljoen, A.; Gericke, N. Devil's Claw—A review of the ethnobotany, phytochemistry and biological activity of *Harpagophytum procumbens*. *J. Ethnopharmacol.* **2012**, *143*, 755–771. [CrossRef] [PubMed]
23. Manon, L.; Béatrice, B.; Thierry, O.; Jocelyne, P.; Fathi, M.; Evelyne, O.; Alain, B. Antimutagenic potential of harpagoside and *Harpagophytum procumbens* against 1-nitropyrene. *Pharmacogn. Mag.* **2015**, *11*, 29. [CrossRef] [PubMed]
24. Fiebich, B.; Muñoz, E.; Rose, T.; Weiss, G.; McGregor, G. Molecular Targets of the Anti-inflammatory *Harpagophytum procumbens* (Devil's claw): Inhibition of TNFα and COX-2 Gene Expression by Preventing Activation of AP-1. *Phytother. Res.* **2011**, *26*, 806–811. [CrossRef] [PubMed]
25. Hostanska, K.; Melzer, J.; Rostock, M.; Suter, A.; Saller, R. Alteration of anti-inflammatory activity of *Harpagophytum procumbens*(devil's claw) extract after external metabolic activation with S9 mix. *J. Pharm. Pharmacol.* **2014**, *66*, 1606–1614. [CrossRef] [PubMed]
26. Schaffer, L.; Peroza, L.; Boligon, A.; Athayde, M.; Alves, S.; Fachinetto, R.; Wagner, C. *Harpagophytum procumbens* Prevents Oxidative Stress and Loss of Cell Viability In Vitro. *Neurochem. Res.* **2013**, *38*, 2256–2267. [CrossRef] [PubMed]

27. Georgiev, M.; Alipieva, K.; Orhan, I. Cholinesterases Inhibitory and Antioxidant Activities of *Harpagophytum procumbens* from In Vitro Systems. *Phytother. Res.* **2011**, *26*, 313–316. [CrossRef] [PubMed]
28. Akter, M.; Oh, S.; Eun, J.; Ahmed, M. Nutritional compositions and health promoting phytochemicals of camu-camu (*Myrciaria dubia*) fruit: A review. *Food Res. Int.* **2011**, *44*, 1728–1732. [CrossRef]
29. Inoue, T.; Komoda, H.; Uchida, T.; Node, K. Tropical fruit camu-camu (*Myrciaria dubia*) has anti-oxidative and anti-inflammatory properties. *J. Cardiol.* **2008**, *52*, 127–132. [CrossRef] [PubMed]
30. Fracassetti, D.; Costa, C.; Moulay, L.; Tomás-Barberán, F. Ellagic acid derivatives, ellagitannins, proanthocyanidins and other phenolics, vitamin C and antioxidant capacity of two powder products from camu-camu fruit (*Myrciaria dubia*). *Food Chem.* **2013**, *139*, 578–588. [CrossRef] [PubMed]
31. Kaneshima, T.; Myoda, T.; Nakata, M.; Fujimori, T.; Toeda, K.; Nishizawa, M. Antioxidant activity of C-Glycosidic ellagitannins from the seeds and peel of camu-camu (*Myrciaria dubia*). *LWT Food Sci. Technol.* **2016**, *69*, 76–81. [CrossRef]
32. Da Silva, F.; Arruda, A.; Ledel, A.; Dauth, C.; Romão, N.; Viana, R.; de Barros Falcão Ferraz, A.; Picada, J.; Pereira, P. Antigenotoxic effect of acute, subacute and chronic treatments with Amazonian camu–camu (*Myrciaria dubia*) juice on mice blood cells. *Food Chem. Toxicol.* **2012**, *50*, 2275–2281. [CrossRef] [PubMed]
33. Garg, A.; Garg, S.; Zaneveld, L.; Singla, A. Chemistry and pharmacology of the citrus bioflavonoid hesperidin. *Phytother. Res.* **2001**, *15*, 655–669. [CrossRef] [PubMed]
34. Devi, K.; Rajavel, T.; Nabavi, S.; Setzer, W.; Ahmadi, A.; Mansouri, K.; Nabavi, S. Hesperidin: A promising anticancer agent from nature. *Ind. Crops Prod.* **2015**, *76*, 582–589. [CrossRef]
35. Saiprasad, G.; Chitra, P.; Manikandan, R.; Sudhandiran, G. Hesperidin alleviates oxidative stress and downregulates the expressions of proliferative and inflammatory markers in azoxymethane-induced experimental colon carcinogenesis in mice. *Inflamm. Res.* **2013**, *62*, 425–440. [CrossRef] [PubMed]
36. Jain, M.; Parmar, H. Evaluation of antioxidative and anti-inflammatory potential of hesperidin and naringin on the rat air pouch model of inflammation. *Inflamm. Res.* **2010**, *60*, 483–491. [CrossRef] [PubMed]
37. Javed, H.; Vaibhav, K.; Ahmed, M.; Khan, A.; Tabassum, R.; Islam, F.; Safhi, M.; Islam, F. Effect of hesperidin on neurobehavioral, neuroinflammation, oxidative stress and lipid alteration in intracerebroventricular streptozotocin induced cognitive impairment in mice. *J. Neurol. Sci.* **2015**, *348*, 51–59. [CrossRef] [PubMed]
38. Rotimi, S.; Bankole, G.; Adelani, I.; Rotimi, O. Hesperidin prevents lipopolysaccharide-induced endotoxicity in rats. *Immunopharmacol. Immunotoxicol.* **2016**, *38*, 364–371. [CrossRef] [PubMed]
39. Xiong, Y.; Chu, H.; Lin, Y.; Han, F.; Li, Y.; Wang, A.; Wang, F.; Chen, D.; Wang, J. Hesperidin alleviates rat postoperative ileus through anti-inflammation and stimulation of Ca^{2+}-dependent myosin phosphorylation. *Acta Pharmacol. Sin.* **2016**, *37*, 1091–1100. [CrossRef] [PubMed]
40. Umar, S.; Kumar, A.; Sajad, M.; Zargan, J.; Ansari, M.; Ahmad, S.; Katiyar, C.; Khan, H. Hesperidin inhibits collagen-induced arthritis possibly through suppression of free radical load and reduction in neutrophil activation and infiltration. *Rheumatol. Int.* **2013**, *33*, 657–663. [CrossRef] [PubMed]
41. Haidari, F.; Heybar, H.; Jalali, M.; Ahmadi Engali, K.; Helli, B.; Shirbeigi, E. Hesperidin Supplementation Modulates Inflammatory Responses Following Myocardial Infarction. *J. Am. Coll. Nutr.* **2015**, *34*, 205–211. [CrossRef] [PubMed]
42. Tits, M. Prodelphinidins from *Ribes nigrum*. *Phytochemistry* **1992**, *31*, 971–973. [CrossRef]
43. Lu, Y.; Yeap Foo, L. Polyphenolic constituents of blackcurrant seed residue. *Food Chem.* **2003**, *80*, 71–76. [CrossRef]
44. Olejnik, A.; Kowalska, K.; Olkowicz, M.; Juzwa, W.; Dembczyński, R.; Schmidt, M. A Gastrointestinally Digested *Ribes nigrum* L. Fruit Extract Inhibits Inflammatory Response in a Co-culture Model of Intestinal Caco-2 Cells and RAW264.7 Macrophages. *J. Agric. Food Chem.* **2016**, *64*, 7710–7721. [CrossRef] [PubMed]
45. Huebbe, P.; Giller, K.; de Pascual-Teresa, S.; Arkenau, A.; Adolphi, B.; Portius, S.; Arkenau, C.; Rimbach, G. Effects of blackcurrant-based juice on atherosclerosis-related biomarkers in cultured macrophages and in human subjects after consumption of a high-energy meal. *Br. J. Nutr.* **2011**, *108*, 234–244. [CrossRef] [PubMed]
46. Lee, S.; Kim, B.; Yang, Y.; Pham, T.; Park, Y.; Manatou, J.; Koo, S.; Chun, O.; Lee, J. Berry anthocyanins suppress the expression and secretion of proinflammatory mediators in macrophages by inhibiting nuclear translocation of NF-κB independent of NRF2-mediated mechanism. *J. Nutr. Biochem.* **2014**, *25*, 404–411. [CrossRef] [PubMed]

47. Hurst, S.; McGhie, T.; Cooney, J.; Jensen, D.; Gould, E.; Lyall, K.; Hurst, R. Blackcurrant proanthocyanidins augment IFN-γ-induced suppression of IL-4 stimulated CCL26 secretion in alveolar epithelial cells. *Mol. Nutr. Food Res.* **2010**, *54*, S159–S170. [CrossRef] [PubMed]
48. Desjardins, J.; Tanabe, S.; Bergeron, C.; Gafner, S.; Grenier, D. Anthocyanin-Rich Black Currant Extract and Cyanidin-3-O-Glucoside Have Cytoprotective and Anti-Inflammatory Properties. *J. Med. Food* **2012**, *15*, 1045–1050. [CrossRef] [PubMed]
49. Garbacki, N.; Tits, M.; Angenot, L.; Damas, J. Inhibitory effects of proanthocyanidins from *Ribes nigrum* leaves on carrageenin acute inflammatory reactions induced in rats. *BMC Pharmacol.* **2004**, *4*, 25. [CrossRef] [PubMed]
50. Bishayee, A.; Mbimba, T.; Thoppil, R.; Háznagy-Radnai, E.; Sipos, P.; Darvesh, A.; Folkesson, H.; Hohmann, J. Anthocyanin-rich black currant (*Ribes nigrum* L.) extract affords chemoprevention against diethylnitrosamine-induced hepatocellular carcinogenesis in rats. *J. Nutr. Biochem.* **2011**, *22*, 1035–1046. [CrossRef] [PubMed]
51. Ullah, N.; Ahmad, M.; Aslam, H.; Tahir, M.; Aftab, M.; Bibi, N.; Ahmad, S. Green tea phytocompounds as anticancer: A review. *Asian Pac. J. Trop. Dis.* **2016**, *6*, 330–336. [CrossRef]
52. Chen, L.; Mo, H.; Zhao, L.; Gao, W.; Wang, S.; Cromie, M.; Lu, C.; Wang, J.; Shen, C. Therapeutic properties of green tea against environmental insults. *J. Nutr. Biochem.* **2017**, *40*, 1–13. [CrossRef] [PubMed]
53. Baeza, G.; Amigo-Benavent, M.; Sarriá, B.; Goya, L.; Mateos, R.; Bravo, L. Green coffee hydroxycinnamic acids but not caffeine protect human HepG2 cells against oxidative stress. *Food Res. Int.* **2014**, *62*, 1038–1046. [CrossRef]
54. Shin, H.; Satsu, H.; Bae, M.; Zhao, Z.; Ogiwara, H.; Totsuka, M.; Shimizu, M. Anti-inflammatory effect of chlorogenic acid on the IL-8 production in Caco-2 cells and the dextran sulphate sodium-induced colitis symptoms in C57BL/6 mice. *Food Chem.* **2015**, *168*, 167–175. [CrossRef] [PubMed]
55. Shi, H.; Dong, L.; Jiang, J.; Zhao, J.; Zhao, G.; Dang, X.; Lu, X.; Jia, M. Chlorogenic acid reduces liver inflammation and fibrosis through inhibition of toll-like receptor 4 signaling pathway. *Toxicology* **2013**, *303*, 107–114. [CrossRef] [PubMed]
56. Strat, K.; Rowley, T.; Smithson, A.; Tessem, J.; Hulver, M.; Liu, D.; Davy, B.; Davy, K.; Neilson, A. Mechanisms by which cocoa flavanols improve metabolic syndrome and related disorders. *J. Nutr. Biochem.* **2016**, *35*, 1–21. [CrossRef] [PubMed]
57. Giribabu, N.; Karim, K.; Kilari, E.; Kassim, N.; Salleh, N. Anti-Inflammatory, Antiapoptotic and Proproliferative Effects of Vitis vinifera Seed Ethanolic Extract in the Liver of Streptozotocin-Nicotinamide-Induced Type 2 Diabetes in Male Rats. *Can. J. Diabetes* **2018**, *42*, 138–149. [CrossRef] [PubMed]
58. Handoussa, H.; Hanafi, R.; Eddiasty, I.; El-Gendy, M.; El Khatib, A.; Linscheid, M.; Mahran, L.; Ayoub, N. Anti-inflammatory and cytotoxic activities of dietary phenolics isolated from *Corchorus olitorius* and *Vitis vinifera*. *J. Funct. Foods* **2013**, *5*, 1204–1216. [CrossRef]
59. Pawlus, A.; Cantos-Villar, E.; Richard, T.; Bisson, J.; Poupard, P.; Papastamoulis, Y.; Monti, J.; Teissedre, P.; Waffo-Téguo, P.; Mérillon, J. Chemical dereplication of wine stilbenoids using high performance liquid chromatography–nuclear magnetic resonance spectroscopy. *J. Chromatogr. A* **2013**, *1289*, 19–26. [CrossRef] [PubMed]

medicines MDPI

Review

Hydroxytyrosol: Health Benefits and Use as Functional Ingredient in Meat

Lorena Martínez, Gaspar Ros and Gema Nieto *

Department of Food Technology, Nutrition and Food Science, Veterinary Faculty University of Murcia, Regional Campus of International Excellence "Campus Mare Nostrum" (Economy based on agri-food), Campus de Espinardo, 30100 Espinardo, Murcia, Spain; lorena.martinez23@um.es (L.M.); gros@um.es (G.R.)
* Correspondence: gnieto@um.es; Tel.: +34-868-889624; Fax: +34-868-884147

Received: 27 December 2017; Accepted: 20 January 2018; Published: 23 January 2018

Abstract: Hydroxytyrosol (HXT) is a phenolic compound drawn from the olive tree and its leaves as a by-product obtained from the manufacturing of olive oil. It is considered the most powerful antioxidant compound after gallic acid and one of the most powerful antioxidant compounds between phenolic compounds from olive tree followed by oleuropein, caffeic and tyrosol. Due to its molecular structure, its regular consumption has several beneficial effects such as antioxidant, anti-inflammatory, anticancer, and as a protector of skin and eyes, etc. For these reasons, the use of HXT extract is a good strategy for use in meat products to replace synthetics additives. However, this extract has a strong odour and flavour, so it is necessary to previously treat this compound in order to not alter the organoleptic quality of the meat product when is added as ingredient. The present review exposes the health benefits provided by HXT consumption and the latest research about its use on meat. In addition, new trends about the application of HXT in the list of ingredients of healthier meat products will be discussed.

Keywords: hydroxytyrosol; antioxidant; antimicrobial; meat; preservative; health

1. Introduction

Meat and meat product consumption provides high-quality proteins (20–25%), minerals (Fe-heme, Mg, K, Zn and Se) and vitamins (A, thiamine, riboflavin, niacin, retinol, B6, folic acid, B12, D and K) necessary for a balanced diet. However, these products usually are rich in saturated fatty acids, and recently, the International Agency for Research on Cancer (IARC) under the World Health Organization (WHO) has classified processed meat as a carcinogen (Group I) and red meat as possible carcinogen (Group 2A) (October 2015) [1]. In fact, carcinogenic compounds in meat could be added during their processing (synthetic additives), but they also can be formed during their storage through lipid and protein oxidation, or during cooking through the Maillard reaction [2,3]. In this way, synthetic additives such as sulphites, BHT (butylated hydroxytoluene) and BHA (butylated hydroxyanisole) are added in meat product formulation to preserve them. The use of these synthetic additives has given rise to social concern by consumers, due to studies that correlates their consumption with disease development (asthma, hyperactivity, cancer, etc.) [4–6]. On the other hand, lipid peroxidation in meat and meat products happens through the radical chain reaction mechanism, although oxygen presence accelerates this process. This oxidation is due to several factors such as polyunsaturated fatty acids concentration (PUFA), the deficit of antioxidants in animal feed (tocopherol, rosmarinic acid) and a high concentration of prooxidants, free radicals or added salt (NaCl). At the same time, these reactions produce reactive oxygen species (ROS) like hydroxyl radical, superoxide anion, ferryl and perferryl species, lipid peroxyl radical and secondary products like reactive carbonyl species (MDA (malondialdehyde) and 4-HNE (4-hydroxynonenal)) responsible for the rancid flavour in aged meat.

Although protein oxidation has received less attention, it has a huge influence on quality of meat [7]. Protein oxidation has been defined as a covalent modification of protein induced either directly by reactive species or secondary products of oxidative stress. The same oxidants that induce the lipid peroxidation produce this alteration, and carbonyl formation is a common reaction in protein oxidation. Furthermore, proteins can react with secondary products of lipid peroxidation like aldehydes and ketones to produce complexes between proteins, proteins and carbonyls or proteins and lipids. In muscle fibres, hydroxyl radical (OH) in presence of Fe or Cu or ROS causes modifications of amino acids, like methionine, lysine, arginine, histidine, tryptophan, valine, serine and proline. This reaction increases proteolytic enzymes and protein polymerization, which produces soluble aggregates, that promotes gelation and emulsification that modifies the texture and toughens the meat [8–10]. But this not only is critical for organoleptic quality, but it might have an impact on human health and safety. For example, during cooking it increases free radical generation while it decreases the antioxidant compounds in meat, which contribute to protein oxidation.

Therefore, natural antioxidants can prevent lipid peroxidation on different ways: preventing chain inhibition by scavenging initiating radicals, breaking chain reaction, decomposing peroxides, decreasing localized oxygen concentrations and binding chain initiating catalyst such as metal ions. Therefore, the use of natural preservatives to keep the shelf life of meat has exhibited similar antioxidant properties compared to some synthetic additives. For this reason, it is a promising tool due to many fruits (grapes, grape seed, pomegranate, date, kinnow mandarin), vegetables (broccoli, potato, drumstick, pumpkin), herbs (olive leaf, acerola, grape seed, cocoa, green coffee, *Ginkgo biloba*, etc.) and spices (rosemary, green tea, black pepper, garlic, oregano, cinnamon, sage, thyme, mint, ginger, clove) reported antioxidant properties in meat products [11–14].

One of most potent natural antioxidant extracts is hydroxytyrosol (or 4-(2-dihydroxyphenyl) ethanol) (HXT)), just below gallic acid (Figure 1). This compound is ten times more antioxidant than green tea and two times more than coenzyme Q10 [15], additionally HXT scavenging ability is comparable to oleorupein and catechol. HXT is a phenylethanoid with demonstrated antioxidant properties in vitro, it is found in olive leaf and oil from this fruit, responsible for intense flavour and aroma, being oleuropein precursor [16,17]. In addition, it has demonstrated this capacity in vivo in several studies in rats, such as Merra et al. or Lemonakis et al. [18,19], that showed the power of HXT to reduce the risk to suffer metabolic syndrome. In its chemical structure, this compound has an additional OH group in its benzene ring, compared to the tyrosol (TYR) (Figure 2). Therefore, it obtains a greater function as a free radical scavenging, increasing its antioxidant power, as well as its efficacy under stress conditions.

In this way, this extract has previously demonstrated its antioxidant capacity in meat products rich in unsaturated fatty acids like sausages and frankfurters with added HXT, nuts and extra virgin olive oil [20,21]. Moreover, HXT is an antioxidant compound linked to certain minerals, such as gluconate Fe (II) in black olives, which catalyzes the oxidation of this compound, so it is possible that HXT influence on biological bioavailability of some minerals and trace elements [17].

The objective of this paper is to review the latest literature about HXT consumption benefits, its extraction from olive leave and other sources and its used as natural antioxidant in meat and meat products as substitute of synthetics additives, with emphasis on new trends and future perspectives in investigation and meat industry.

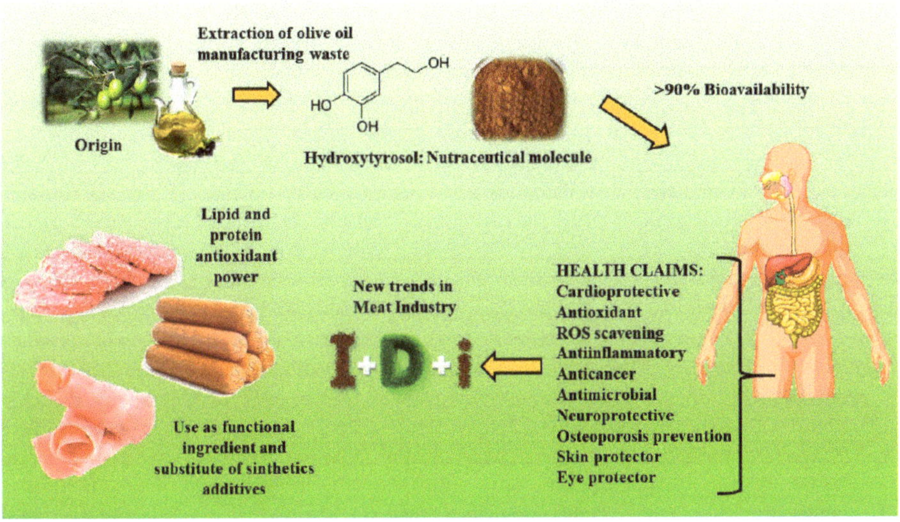

Figure 1. Graphical abstract of the use and health benefits of Hydroxytyrosol to prevent lipid and protein oxidation and substitution of synthetic additives in meat products.

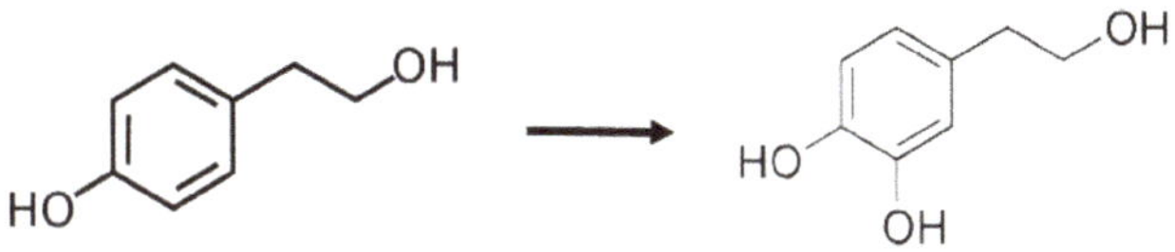

Figure 2. Chemical structures of TYR and HXT: phenolic compound from olive leave and olive oil. TYR: tyrosol (left); HXT: hydroxytyrosol (right).

2. The Role of HXT in Diet

Since many years ago it is known that several aspects about the Mediterranean diet have been associated with a minor risk of cardiovascular diseases and cancer (colorectal, breast, prostate or pancreas, between others) [22] (Figure 1). In particular, olive oil as principal component of this dietary model plays a key role in these benefits, due to its composition of fat, richness in monounsaturated fatty acids (oleic acid) and another micronutrient from non-saponifiable fraction such as squalene, phytosterols, tocopherols and secoiridoids.

HXT is a secoiridoid and a potent antioxidant that acts as main component from phenolic fraction of extra virgin olive oil (EVOO). This compound is derivate from hydrolysis of oleuropein and its concentration in EVOO and table olives can change according to several factors: altitude and latitude of olive tree harvest, the variety of olive, the collection time and the processing conditions [23,24]. For example, the HXT concentration in EVOO is 14.32 $\pm$ 3.01 mg kg^{-1}, while in refined virgin oil is 1.74 $\pm$ 0.84 mg kg^{-1} [25]. In the same way, the concentration in Greek black olives is 100–340 mg kg^{-1}, in Spanish green olives is 170–510 mg kg^{-1} and 250–760 mg kg^{-1} in Greek kalamata olives [26]. Taking into account that the average consumption of EVOO and olives in Spain are 15 g/day^{-1} and 7 g/day, respectively [27], it can be estimated that the HXT consumption per day is 5.6 mg (0.3 mg from EVOO and 5.3 mg from olives), approximately.

In addition, HXT has a bioavailability of 99%, so this compound is easily integrated by human body [28]. In the same way, it was corroborated by Khymenets et al. [29] in their study about human HXT absorption and excretion from a nutraceutical, that HXT is a phenolic compound resistant to gastric juices and to passing through the digestive system, consequently it is bioavailable and is recovered in the urine chiefly as 3′-sulphate. Therefore, it can be confirmed that the consumption of 5.6 mg day^{-1} of HXT can bring great benefits on an organism's functioning.

3. The Role of HXT in Health

HXT has a great bioactive power due to its great antioxidant capacity due to its protective function in cells, its structural affinity to some compounds (for example, with dopamine, it replaces its amine group (NH_2) by hydroxyl group (OH)), it has a simple molecular structure and it is present in organism (e.g., iris of the eye) so it is easy to assimilate by the human body, reaching blood plasma in 15 or 20 min until its elimination 6–8 h later by the renal or digestive system, so it does not present accumulation or toxicity problems. In addition, HXT is an amphipathic, water-soluble and fat-soluble molecule, because of it has a lipophilic end and another hydrophilic end, which makes it a good transporter of substances through the human body, therefore, it can penetrate the cellular membrane easier. These structural and molecular features of HXT make its consumption provide many beneficial effects in the organism [30].

Firstly, in 2012, EFSA (European Food & Safety Authority) accepted that HXT acts as protector of the cardiovascular system, avoiding oxidation of LDL cholesterol by free radicals, maintaining normal blood HDL cholesterol concentrations and preventing atherosclerosis [31]. In addition, HXT consumption can regulate glutathione concentration and provides antioxidant enzymes to adipose tissue [32]. Moreover, in other in vivo study with experimentally induced diabetes mellitus in rats, it was shown that the HXT consumption influenced the major biochemical processes leading to diabetic vasculopathy and reduced cell proliferation in the vascular wall [33]. It is confirmed the prevention against damage by oxidative stress induced by this compound, which acted as regulator of cell protection and damage induction, controls the intracellular redox state. This could influence the prevention of diseases such as cancer, diabetes, inflammation or cardiovascular and neurodegenerative diseases, which aetiology and progression has been linked to the production of ROS on damaged tissues. So, the regular consumption of HXT can help to avoid cardiovascular diseases and diabetes mellitus [34].

Secondly, HXT has the capacity to inhibit COX (cyclooxygenase) and LOX (lipoxygenase) enzymes of arachidonic acid (AA), reducing the oxidative deterioration characteristic of inflammations [35]. At the same time, HXT stimulates the production of chondrocytes by regeneration and repairing the articular cartilage. During physical exercise, HXT helps to increase the production of glutathione and to reduce the production of lactic acid and the consequent muscular atrophy [36].

Because of the connection between cellular oxidation, inflammation and the formation and development of a tumour, it can have a clear idea of the anticancer ability of this extract. Moreover, HXT alters a tumour's eicosanoid biosynthesis and shows an inhibition of tumour cell proliferation [37]. At the same way, the daily consumption of 50 μM–100 μM of HXT, through the intake of EVOO and table olives, has showed antiproliferative activity, apoptotic activity and inhibition of metastasis of leukemia cells (HL60), adenocarcinoma cells (HT29), human colon cancer cells (Caco-2 and HT115) [38,39] and in breast cancer cells (MCF10A, MDA-MB-231 and MCF7) [40].

On the other hand, HXT is protective against neurodegenerative damage and cognitive decline associated with age or diseases like Alzheimer or Parkinson. It is due to the fact that HXT protects brain cells from lipid peroxidation because it is able to cross the blood–brain barrier [41].

Another notable property of HXT is its antimicrobial capacity and acts by inhibiting the growth rate of bacteria in humans, as demonstrated in the research of Medina et al. [42], (against *Clostridium perfringens*, *Escherichia coli*, *Staphylococcus aureus*, *Salmonella enterica*, *Yersinia sp.* and *Shigella sonnei*) and Brenes et al. [43] (against *Helicobacter pylori*). There are also studies with its antifungal properties against *Mycoplasma hominis* and *Pneumoniae fermentans* [44], and against *Fusarium sambucinum*, *Vericillium dahliae* and *Alternaria solani* [45]. Therefore, HXT consumption has an antimicrobial effect that can avoid infections in the respiratory, intestinal and genital systems and it strengthens the immune system.

In addition, HXT can act against virus like HIV. Lee-Huang et al. [46] demonstrated that HXT and oleuropein inhibit the entry and integration of virus, as inside as outside cells.

Finally, HXT also helps to prevent osteoporosis because its consumption has positive effects on the formation and growth of bones [47]. In addition, the retina is also protected by HXT and it is beneficial for ocular health specifically in the regeneration of the retinal pigment epithelium, macular degeneration and glaucoma, caused by oxidative stress [48]. Furthermore, HXT has dermoprotective effects: it protects against UV rays, it reduces the pigmentation of the skin, it protects against oedema and erythema caused by excessive sun exposure, it may even be effective in treating psoriasis, it has anti-aging effect and it stimulates the production of cell-survival promoting proteins [49] (Figure 1).

4. Preparation of HXT Extract

The highest concentration of HXT is found in olive leaves. However, it is lost during oil manufacturing after the waste of the pomace and vegetable water as residues of EVOO, or refined olive oil production. In order to take advantage of this waste and minimize losses to the oil industry, these residues are used by ingredient companies to obtain natural extracts used by the cosmetic, pharmaceutical and food industries (Figure 1).

HXT can be obtained from vegetation water or from olive leave using different ways. It is based in three phases: first, a phenol-rich liquid is obtained as the raw material for the extraction and purification of phenolic compounds; a second phase enables a HXT enriched extract and a HXT with 3,4-dihydroxyphenylglycol (DOPEG) mixture to be obtained, and HXT acetate is produced. In the third phase, highly pure HXT-DOPEG and HXT acetate are obtained. These phases comprise extraction, reaction, concentration, adsorption and desorption, using mixtures of ion exchange resins, adsorption in nonionic resins and a polymer phenolic fraction, membranes of reverse osmosis and evaporators. This methodology is an example of extraction method for HXT from vegetation waters and *Olea europaea* L. subproducts that it is under intellectual property of the Spanish Research Council (Consejo Superior de Investigaciones Científicas, CSIC) [50].

From the industrial point of view, the extraction method depends on the source used for HXT [21]. The first one obtains HXT from olive waters during fruit processing (separating the oil from wet centrifugation). It is used a solvent extraction and purification process, including, crystallization and clarification steps. For that, the original plant material (vegetation water) is dried and suspended in ethanol. The filtered hydroalcoholic solution is concentrated under vacuum until obtain a syrup with a HXT percentage around 20–25%. Among the characteristic polyphenolic compounds from olive oil that this extract contains are large quantities of fulvic acids. HXT can be also obtained from olive leaves (dehydrated) by hydroalcoholic extraction and subsequent hydrolysis. The hydroalcoholic solution obtained contains as main active compound the oleuropein that is present in the leaves.

Another form to obtain HXT extract can also be through olive waters (fruit processing) by liquid–liquid extraction with ethanol. For that purpose, the original plant material (vegetation water) is concentrated in vacuum at temperature of 50–60 °C until a syrup of 65–70% °Bx (w/w) is obtained. This syrup is suspended in ethanol and the supernatant is removed, which is concentrated in vacuum and finally a hygroscopic solid.

5. Use of HXT Extract as Functional Ingredient in Meat

Firstly, AECOSAN (Spanish Agency for Consumer Affairs, Food Safety and Nutrition) accepted using of HXT extract as functional ingredient in 2015 [51], while in 2017, EFSA (European Food & Safety Authority) has confirmed that its use does not provided negative effects on health of consumers [52].

Among all of the literature on this topic, it has been selected as the most innovative and current (Table 1). For example, Rounds et al. [53] researched the antimicrobial activity of HXT (10,000 and 30,000 ppm) in ground beef patties inoculated with *E. coli*. They showed that the cell count was reduced 3% more than the control at the same conditions and the amine formation was 50.6% lower than control.

Table 1. Results on the applicability of HXT on meat and its effect on product quality.

Extract Form	Concentration (ppm)	Meat Product	Test Setup	Tested Parameters	Results	Reference
Commercial	10,000 30,000	Ground beef patties	Ground beef was mixed with extract and inoculated with *E. coli* (10^7 cfu/g). Uniform patties were formed, cooked and shock-cooled.	Total viable count Amine quantification	It was enhanced cell count reduction (3% survivors detectable) Reduction of amine formation (50.6%)	[53]
Commercial	100	Pork meat with $W_1/O/W_2$ emulsions	Ground pork meat and fat were mixed with $W_1/O/W_2$ emulsions and chia oil. Emulsions were vacuum packaged and keep in chilled storage (4 °C) until analyses on the 1st, 7th, 19th, 28th and 39th days.	Light microscopy Antioxidant activity: DPPH Lipid oxidation (TBARs)	Particle size in samples with HXT was higher ($p < 0.05$) Chia oil presence in meat samples increased oxidation, however, HXT acted as antioxidant (8%). HXT presence in meat samples reduced lipid oxidation by more than 50%.	[54]
Concentrate	100.23	Fermented sausages	During the drying process fermented sausages were dipped in extract solutions (2.5–5%) for 1 min at 20 °C and were continued drying.	Total viable count Lactic acid bacteria Micrococci Yeast Moulds pH Water activity Lipid oxidation (TBARs) Volatile compounds Sensory attributes (colour)	No differences No differences Growth reduction affected volatile compound profile No significant differences Reduction of species No significant differences No significant differences Reduced values (12–38%) Reduces volatile compounds from microbial esterification and lipid oxidation Redness increased	[55]
Commercial	100, 200, 400	Lamb meat patties	Minced lamb meat enriched in omega-3 fatty acids (with fish oil) was mixed with natural extracts and stored in high-oxygen modified atmosphere packs for up to 9 days at 4 °C.	In vitro antioxidant activity (ORAC and FRAP) Colour (CIELab) Lipid oxidation (TBARs) Protein oxidation (thiol and carbonyl groups) Sensory analysis	ORAC: No significant differences FRAP: antioxidant activity increases with extract presence Lightness (L*) increased in samples without extract by changes in muscle proteins. Significant differences between samples at day 3, 6 and 9 of storage. No significant differences Natural extracts improvement texture but it alteration odour and flavour.	[56]
Concentrated, undefined	75, 150	Pork sausages	Ground pork (50/50 − meat/fat) was minced and mixed with salt and phenols. Mix was stuffed into 40-mm diameter bovine casings, were left to drip at 15 °C for 6 h and stored without packaging alternating fluorescent light (12 h dark and 12 h light) at 2 °C for 14 days. After, sausages were cooked, stored 72 h at 4 °C and frozen until analysis (80 °C)	Nutritional composition pH Cooking loss Diacylglycerols Lipid oxidation (TBARs) Peroxide value (POV) Cholesterol oxidation products (COPs) Sensory analysis	No differences No differences No differences Phenols had an inhibitory effect on microorganisms and a reduction in lipolytic activity. Oxidation was reduced (>40%) as TBARs as POV. But there are no differences in COPs. Phenols presence was valorated worst by panellists.	[57]

Table 1. *Cont.*

Extract Form	Concentration (ppm)	Meat Product	Test Setup	Tested Parameters	Results	Reference
Commercial 1. HXT 23% from olive waters 2. HXT 7% from olive leaves 3. HXT 7% from olive waters	50	Chicken sausages	Pork fat and chicken meat were minced and mixed with walnuts, EVOO and three HXT extracts. Samples were cooked for 3 h at 72 °C, packaged in MAP (10% O_2/20% CO_2/10% N_2) and stored at 4 °C for 21 days.	Nutritional composition Colour (CIELab) Cooking loss Lipid oxidation (TBARs) Protein oxidation (thiol groups) Scanning electron microscopy Sensory analysis	No differences L* and b* were lower in samples with HXT and EVOO, while a* was higher Cooking loss values were higher in samples with HXT In samples with HXT TBARs value was lower and in samples with HXT and EVOO, lipid oxidation was 71% lower than control. HXT reduced protein oxidation between 13–25%. Sausages incorporated HXT showed different structures. Samples with HXT 7% from olive water was accepted, while other samples with HXT presented lowest acceptability.	[21]
Commercial, 7% from olive waters	50	Chicken Frankfurters	Back fat and chicken meat were minced and mixed with walnuts, EVOO and HXT. Samples were cooked for 3 h at 72 °C, packaged in MAP (10% O_2/20% CO_2/10% N_2) and stored at 4 °C for 21 days.	Nutritional composition Mineral content Fatty acid profile. Sensory analysis	No differences Ca, K, Fe, Mg, P, Mn and Zn concentrations were higher in samples with HXT. No differences Extracted flavour and odour parameters were increased in samples with HXT but it was accepted by panellists.	[20]
Olive cake applied in chicken feed	4.6 9.5	Chicken meat	297 chickens were feeding until 21 days of age with three treatments: basal diet, diet supplemented with 82.5 g/kg olive phenols and diet supplemented with 165 g/kg olive phenols. Chickens were weighed at 28, 35 and 42 days of age and slaughtered at 42th. Carcasses were maintained at −20 °C for three months until consumption and at −80 °C for other analyses.	Chicken weight Colour (CIELab) Cooking loss Nutritional composition pH Lipid oxidation (TBARs) Antioxidant capacity (DPPH) Sensory analysis	The chicken weight was higher L* and b* was higher while a* was lower No differences No differences No differences Lipid oxidation was lower Samples with HXT showed a high antioxidant capacity No differences, so HXT did not alter the sensory quality.	[58]

However, the antimicrobial capacity of HXT has already been demonstrated in several matrices, so after this researcher focused on studying the shelf life of meat products in which synthetic additives have been replaced by compounds derived from olive: HXT, tyrosol, oleorupein, verbascoside and pinoresinol. Such as, in the work of Chaves-López et al. [55], they elaborated fermented sausages with HXT (100.23 ppm) and proved that lipid oxidation was lower (12–38%), while volatile compounds were reduced and colour redness was increased. On the other hand, Muíño et al. [56] analysed lamb meat patties enriched with omega 3 (fish oil) and HXT (100, 200 and 400 ppm). They found that antioxidant activity of patties increased with HXT presence and lipid oxidation was lower at day 3, 6 and 9 of storage compared with control samples. In addition, patties with HXT kept the colour and texture stable while the odour and flavour were modified by the extract. Similar results were obtained in pork sausages enriched with HXT (75 and 150 ppm) and stored for 14 days, even though Balzan et al. [57] also showed how this extract had an inhibitory effect on lipolytic activity and microorganism growth. Finally, on chicken frankfurters, Nieto et al. [20,21] proved that a small quantity of HXT (50 ppm) is enough to maintain the colour and reduced the lipid and protein oxidation until 21 days if it is combined with other ingredients like EVOO (extra virgin olive oil) and/or walnuts. At the same way, they compared three extracts: HXT 23% from olive waters, HXT 7% from olive leaves and HXT 7% from olive waters; and they reported that HXT 7% from olive waters was more sensory acceptable than the others.

In addition, meat can be enriched exogenously through the use of natural extracts to replace synthetics additives or endogenously through the animal diet. It is the case of Branciari et al. [58] whose research was based on feeding 297 chickens during 21 days with three treatments: basal diet, diet supplemented with 82.5 g/kg of "paté cake" rich on olive phenols (4.6 ppm HXT), and diet supplemented with 165 g/kg of the same product (9.5 ppm HXT). They showed that chicken feeding with olive phenols had a higher weight; they had a higher antioxidant capacity while lipid oxidation was lower. It is important to remark that the sensory quality of meat was not modified by olive feed.

Taking into account previous studies, HXT can be used as exogenously as endogenously to report benefits to the meat and meat products.

6. New Trends

New trends in the use of HXT in meat focus on the maintenance of its antioxidant power and eliminating its intense flavour and smell, as shown in the studies of Cofrades et al. [54] or Freire et al. [59]. At first, it was proved that HXT added to the ground pork meat in $W_1/O/W_2$ emulsions reduced lipid oxidation by more than 50%. In the same way, Freire et al. showed that using cold-set gelled double emulsions enriched with perilla oil (*Perilla frutescens* as a source of n-3 fatty acids) and HXT as animal fat replacer during 30 days of storage, it was found HXT maintained the stability of emulsions and increased its antioxidant capacity while it was reduced lipid oxidation and bacterial growth. That kind of emulsion has the characteristic of encapsulating the extract to avoid the strong flavour and odour of HXT on meat. However, there are no studies about sensorial changes after the application of the HXT extracts.

On the other hand, Moudache et al. [60] have studied another application of HXT: an antioxidant food packaging material applied to fresh minced pork and whose plastic film contained olive leave extract. This researcher showed that active films with olive leave extract, rich in HXT, had a positive effect on the oxidation stability of meat fat. In addition, this active packaging does not need being in contact with meat, so it does not alter the sensorial quality of the product.

7. Conclusions and Perspectives

As reviewed, the beneficial effects of HXT has been extensively investigated during the last twenty years, so many researchers of pharmaceutical industry have been focused on use of this compound due to its nutraceutical power. In parallel, researchers in the food and meat industries have been focused on the elimination of preservatives and dyes in order to achieve the 'clean label'. However,

HXT has a strong flavour so cannot be added directly to the meat. For this reason, researchers have currently been focused on the encapsulation of this extract and the production of emulsion gels to prevent the sensorial alteration of meat products. However, nothing has been concluded in this field about the organoleptic quality of the product. Therefore, it can be concluded that the best way to obtain its benefits on meat is endogenously, through the animal diet, or through its application in new packaging systems.

Author Contributions: Lorena Martínez collected the information and drafted the article. Gema Nieto and Gaspar Ros interpreted and reviewed the article.

Conflicts of Interest: The authors declare no conflicts of interest.

References

1. The International Agency for Research on Cancer (IARC). *Q&A on the Carcinogenicity of the Consumption of Red Meat and Processed Meat*; Press Release N°240; Monographs-Q&A; IARC: Geneva, Switzerland, 2015; Volume 114.
2. Lund, M.N.; Ray, C.A. Control of Maillard reactions in foods: Strategies and chemical mechanisms. *J. Agric. Food Chem.* **2017**, *65*, 4537–4552. [CrossRef] [PubMed]
3. Capuano, E.; Fogliano, V. Acrylamide and 5-hydroxymethylfurfural (HMF): A review on metabolism, toxicity, occurrence in food and mitigation strategies. *LWT Food Sci. Technol.* **2011**, *44*, 793–810. [CrossRef]
4. Soubra, L.; Sarkis, D.; Hilan, C.; Verger, P.H. Dietary exposure of children and teenagers to benzoates, sulphites, butylhydroxyanisol (BHA) and butylhiddroxytoluen (BHT) in Beirut (Lebanon). *Regul. Toxicol. Pharmacol.* **2007**, *47*, 68–77. [CrossRef] [PubMed]
5. Chang, T.W.; Pan, A.Y. Chapter 2: Cumulative Environmental Changes, Skewed Antigen Exposure and the Increase of Allergy. *Adv. Inmunol.* **2008**, *98*, 39–83.
6. Clough, S.R. Sodium Sulfite. In *Encyclopedia of Toxicology*, 3rd ed.; Elsevier: Amsterdam, The Netherlands, 2014; pp. 341–343.
7. Nieto, G.; Jongberg, S.; Andersen, M.L.; Skibsted, L.H. Thiol oxidation and protein cross-link formation during chill storage of pork patties added essential oil of oregano, rosemary, or garlic. *Meat Sci.* **2013**, *95*, 177–184. [CrossRef] [PubMed]
8. Xiong, Y.L. Chapter 4: Protein oxidation and implications for muscle food quality. In *Antioxidants in Muscle Foods: Nutritional Strategies to Improve Quality*; Decker, E.A., Faustman, C., Lopez-Bote, C.J., Eds.; John Wiley & Sons, Inc.: Hoboken, NJ, USA, 2010; pp. 85–112, ISBN 0-471-31454-4.
9. Xiong, Y.L.; Blanchard, S.P.; Ooizumi, T.; Ma, Y. Hydroxyl radical and ferryl-generating systems promote gel network formation of myofibrillar protein. *J. Food Sci.* **2010**, *75*, C215–C221. [CrossRef] [PubMed]
10. Estévez, M. Protein carbonyls in meat systems: A review. *Meat Sci.* **2011**, *89*, 259–279. [CrossRef] [PubMed]
11. Jian, J.; Xiong, Y.L. Natural antioxidants as food and feed additives to promote health benefits and quality of meat products: A review. *Meat Sci.* **2016**, *120*, 107–117. [CrossRef] [PubMed]
12. Ahmad Shah, M.; Don Bosco, S.J.; Ahmad Mir, S. Plant extracts as natural antioxidants in meat and meat products. *Meat Sci.* **2014**, *98*, 21–33. [CrossRef] [PubMed]
13. Nieto, G.; Díaz, P.; Bañón, S.; Garrido, M.D. Dietary administration of ewe diets with a distillate from rosemary leaves (Rosmarinus officinalis L.): Influence on lamb meat quality. *Meat Sci.* **2010**, *84*, 23–29. [CrossRef] [PubMed]
14. Nieto, G.; Estrada, M.; Jordán, M.J.; Garrido, M.D.; Bañón, S. Effects in ewe diet of rosemary by-product on lipid oxidation and the eating quality of cooked lamb under retail display conditions. *Food Chem.* **2011**, *124*, 1423–1429. [CrossRef]
15. Lee Richards, K. The Most Powerful Natural Antioxidant Discovered to Date—Hydroxytyrosol. Pro-Health, 2014. Available online: http://www.prohealth.com/library/print.cfm?libid=17054 (accessed on 12 January 2018).
16. Yadav, A.S.; Singh, R.P. Natural preservatives in poultry meat products. *Nat. Prod. Radiance* **2004**, *3*, 300–303.
17. Wang, D.; Williams, B.A.; Ferruzzi, M.G.; D'Arcy, B.R. Microbial metabolites, but not other phenolics derived from grape seed phenolic extract, are transported through differentiated Caco-2 cell monolayers. *Food Chem.* **2013**, *138*, 1564–1573. [CrossRef] [PubMed]

18. Merra, E.; Calzaretti, G.; Bobba, A.; Storelli, M.M.; Casalino, E. Antioxidant role of hydroxytyrosol on oxidative stress in cadmium-intoxicated rats: Different effect in spleen and testes. *Drug Chem. Toicol.* **2014**, 1–7. [CrossRef] [PubMed]
19. Lemonakis, N.; Poudyal, H.; Halabalaki, M.; Brown, L.; Tsarbopoulos, A.; Skaltsounis, A.L.; Gikas, E. The LC-MS-based metabolomics of hydroxytyrosol administration in rats reveals amelioration of the metabolic syndrome. *J. Chromatogr. B* **2017**, *1041*, 45–59. [CrossRef] [PubMed]
20. Nieto, G.; Martínez, L.; Castillo, J.; Ros, G. Effect of hydroxytyrosol, walnut and olive oil on nutritional profile of Low-Fat Chicken Frankfurters. *Eur. J. Lipid Sci. Technol.* **2017**, *119*, 1600518. [CrossRef]
21. Nieto, G.; Martínez, L.; Ros, G. Hydroxytyrosol extracts, olive oil and walnuts as functional components in chicken sausages. *J. Sci. Food Agric.* **2017**. [CrossRef] [PubMed]
22. Trichopoulou, A.; Lagiou, P.; Kuper, H.; Trichopoulos, D. Cancer and Mediterranean dietary traditions. *Cancer Epidemiol. Biomark. Prev.* **2000**, *9*, 869–873.
23. Ragusa, A.; Centonze, C.; Grasso, M.E.; Latronico, M.F.; Mastrangelo, P.F.; Fanizzi, F.P.; Maffia, M. Composition and statistical analysis of biophenols in Apulian Italian EVOOs. *Foods* **2017**, *6*, 90. [CrossRef] [PubMed]
24. Fuentes, E.; Paucar, F.; Tapia, F.; Ortiz, J.; Jimenez, P.; Romero, N. Effect of the composition of extra virgin olive oils on the differentiation and antioxidant capacities of twelve monovarietals. *Food Chem.* **2018**, *243*, 285–294. [CrossRef] [PubMed]
25. Owen, R.W.; Giacosa, A.; Hull, W.E.; Haubner, R.; Würtele, G.; Spiegelhalder, B.; Bartsch, H. Olive-oil consumption and health: The possible role of antioxidants. *Lancet Oncol.* **2000**, *1*, 107–112. [CrossRef]
26. Blekas, G.; Vassilakis, C.; Harizanis, C.; Tsimidou, M.; Boskou, D.G. Biophenols in table olives. *J. Agric. Food Chem.* **2002**, *50*, 3688–3692. [CrossRef] [PubMed]
27. MAPAMA (Ministerio de Agricultura y Pesca, Alimentación y Medio Ambiente). Informe del consume de alimentación en España. In *Taller del Centro de Publicaciones del MAPAMA*; MAPAMA: Madrid, Spain, 2016; NIPO 013-17-143-0.
28. Schaffer, S.; Müller, W.E.; Eckert, G.P. Cytoprotective effects of olive mill wastewater extract and its main constituent hydroxytyrosol in PC12 cells. *Pharm. Res.* **2010**, *62*, 322–327. [CrossRef] [PubMed]
29. Khymenets, O.; Crespo, M.C.; Dangles, O.; Rakotomanomana, N.; Andres-Lacueva, C.; Visioli, F. Human hydroxytyrosol's absorption and excretion from a nutraceutical. *J. Funct. Foods* **2016**, *23*, 278–282. [CrossRef]
30. Fernández-Bolaños, J.G.; López, O.; López-García, M.A.; Marset, A. Chapter 20, Biological properties of Hydroxytyrosol and its derivates. In *Olive Oil—Constituents, Quality, Health Properties and Bioconversions*; InTech: London, UK, 2012; pp. 375–398. [CrossRef]
31. EFSA Panel on Dietetic Products; Nutrition and Allergies (NDA). Scientific Opinion on the substantiation of a health claim related to polyphenols in olive and maintenance of normal blood HDL-cholesterol concentrations (ID 1639, further assessment) pursuant to Article 13 of Regulation (EC) No 1924/2006. *EFSA J.* **2012**, *10*, 2848.
32. Schaffer, S.; Podstawa, M.; Visioli, F.; Bogani, P.; Müller, W.E.; Eckert, G.P. Hydroxytyrosol-Rich Olive Mill Waste water Extract Protects Brain Cells in Vitro and ex Vivo. *J. Agric. Food Chem.* **2007**, *55*, 5043–5049. [CrossRef] [PubMed]
33. López-Villodres, J.A.; Abdel-Karim, M.; De La Cruz, J.P.; Rodríguez-Pérez, M.D.; Reyes, J.J.; Guzmán-Moscoso, R.; Rodríguez-Gutiérrez, G.; Fernández-Bolaños, J.; González-Correa, J.A. Effects of hydroxytyrosol on cardiovascular biomarkers in experimental diabetes mellitus. *J. Nutr. Biochem.* **2016**, *37*, 94–100. [CrossRef] [PubMed]
34. Merola, N.; Castillo, J.; Benavente-García, O.; Ros, G.; Nieto, G. The effect of consumption of citrus fruit and olive leaf extract on lipid metabolism. *Nutrients* **2017**, *9*, 1062. [CrossRef] [PubMed]
35. Silva, S.; Sepodes, B.; Rocha, J.; Direito, R.; Fernandes, A.; Brites, D.; Freitas, M.; Fernandes, E.; Bronze, M.R.; Figueira, M.E. Protective effects of hydroxytyrosol-supplemented refined olive oil in animal models of acute inflammation and rheumatoid arthritis. *J. Nutr. Biochem.* **2015**, *26*, 360–368. [CrossRef] [PubMed]
36. Siriani, R.; Chimento, A.; De Luca, A.; Casaburi, I.; Rizza, P.; Onofrio, A.; Iacopetta, D.; Puoci, F.; Andò, S.; Maggiolini, M.; et al. Oleuropein and hydroxytyrosol inhibit MCF-7 breast cancer cell proliferation interfering with ERK1/2 activation. *Mol. Nutr. Food Res.* **2010**, *54*, 833–840. [CrossRef] [PubMed]

37. Ragione, F.D.; Cucciolla, V.; Borriello, A.; Pietra, V.D.; Pontoni, G.; Racioppi, L.; Manna, C.; Galletti, P.; Zappia, V. Hydroxytyrosol, a natural molecule occurring in olive oil, induces cytochrome c-dependent apoptosis. *Biochem. Biophys. Res. Commun.* **2000**, *278*, 733–739. [CrossRef] [PubMed]
38. Fabiani, R.; De Bartolomeo, A.; Rosignoli, P.; Servili, M.; Montedoro, G.F.; Morozzi, G. Cancer chemoprevention by hydroxytyrosol isolated from virgin olive oil through G1 cell cycle arrest and apoptosis. *Eur. J. Cancer Prev.* **2002**, *11*, 351–358. [CrossRef] [PubMed]
39. Hashim, Y.Z.; Rowland, I.R.; McGlynn, H.; Servili, M.; Selvaggini, R.; Taticchi, A.; Esposto, S.; Montedoro, G.; Kaisalo, L.; Wähälä, K.; et al. Inhibitory effects of olive oil phenolics on invasion in human colon adenocarcinoma cells in vitro. *Int. J. Cancer* **2008**, *122*, 495–500. [CrossRef] [PubMed]
40. Warleta, F.; Sánchez-Quesada, C.; Campos, C.; Allouche, Y.; Beltrán, G.; Gaforio, J.J. Hydroxytyrosol protects against oxidative DNA damage in human breast cells. *Nutrients* **2011**, *3*, 839–857. [CrossRef] [PubMed]
41. Cabrerizo, S.; De La Cruz, J.P.; López-Villodres, J.A.; Muñoz-Martín, J.; Guerrero, A.; Reyes, J.J.; Labajos, M.T.; González-Correa, J.A. Role of the inhibition of oxidative stress and inflammatory mediators in the neuroprotective effects of hydroxytyrosol in rat brain slices subjected to hypoxia reoxygenation. *J. Nutr. Biochem.* **2013**, *24*, 2152–2157. [CrossRef] [PubMed]
42. Medina, E.; De Castro, A.; Romero, C.; Brenes, M. Comparison of the concentrations of phenolic compounds in olive oils and other plant oils: Correlation with antimicrobial activity. *J. Agric. Food Chem.* **2006**, *54*, 4954–4961. [CrossRef] [PubMed]
43. Brenes, M.; Medina, E.; Romero, C.; De Castro, A. Antimicrobial activity of olive oil. *Agro Food Ind. Hi-Tech* **2007**, *18*, 6–8.
44. Furneri, P.M.; Piperno, A.; Sajia, A.; Bisignano, G. Antimycoplasmal activity of hydroxytyrosol. *Antimicrob. Agents Chemother.* **2004**, *48*, 4892–4894. [CrossRef] [PubMed]
45. Yangui, T.; Dhouib, A.; Rhouma, A.; Sayadi, S. Potential of hydroxytyrosol rich composition from olive mill wastewater as a natural disinfectant and its effect on seeds vigour response. *Food Chem.* **2009**, *117*, 1–8. [CrossRef]
46. Lee-Huang, S.; Huang, P.L.; Zhang, D.; Lee, J.W.; Bao, J.; Sun, Y.; Chang, Y.T.; Zhang, J.; Huang, P.L. Discovery of small-mollecule HIV-1 fusion and integrase inhibitors oleuropein and hydroxytyrosol. *Biochem. Biophys. Res. Commun.* **2007**, *354*, 872–878. [CrossRef] [PubMed]
47. Hagiwara, K.; Goto, T.; Araki, M.; Miyazaki, H.; Hagiwara, H. Olive polyphenol hydroxytyrosol prevents bone loss. *Eur. J. Pharmacol.* **2011**, *662*, 78–84. [CrossRef] [PubMed]
48. Zhu, L.; Liu, Z.; Feng, Z.; Hao, J.; Shen, W.; Li, X.; Sun, L.; Sharman, E.; Wang, Y.; Wertz, K.; et al. Hydroxytyrosol protects against oxidative damage by simultaneous activation of mitochondrial biogenesis and phase II detoxifying enzyme systems in retinal pigment epithelial cells. *J. Nutr. Biochem.* **2010**, *21*, 1089–1098. [CrossRef] [PubMed]
49. Viola, P.; Viola, M. Virgin olive oil as a fundamental nutritional component and skin protector. *Clin. Dermatol.* **2009**, *27*, 159–165. [CrossRef] [PubMed]
50. Consejo Superior De Investigaciones Científicas (Csic). *Method for Obtaining Hydroxytyrosol Extract, Mixture of Hydroxytyrosol and 3,4-dihydroxyphenylglycol Extract, and Hydroxytyrosyl Acetate Extract, from By-Products of the Olive Tree, and the Purification Thereof; WO2013007850 A1*; Universidad De Sevilla: Seville, Spain, 2013.
51. AECOSAN (Agencia Española de Consumo, Seguridad Alimentaria y Nutrición) (Food Safety and Nutrition Section of the Scientific Committee). Report of the Scientific Committee of the Spanish Agency for Consumer Affairs, Food Safety and Nutrition (AECOSAN) on a request for initial assessment for marketing of synthetic hydroxytyrosol under Regulation (EC) No 258/97 concerning novel foods and novel food ingredients. *Rev. Com. Cient. AECOSAN* **2015**, *21*, 11–25.
52. EFSA Panel on Dietetic Products, Nutrition and Allergies (NDA). Safety of hydroxytyrosol as a novel food pursuant to Regulation (EC) No 258/97. *EFSA J.* **2017**, *15*, 4728.
53. Rounds, L.; Havens, C.M.; Feinstein, Y.; Friedman, M.; Ravishankar, S. Concentration dependent inhibition of *Escherichia coli* O157:H7 and heterocyclic amines in heated ground beef patties by apple and olive extracts, onion powder and clove bud oil. *Meat Sci.* **2013**, *94*, 461–467. [CrossRef] [PubMed]
54. Cofrades, S.; Santos-López, J.A.; Freire, M.; Benedí, J.; Sánchez-Muniz, F.J.; Jiménez-Colmenero, F. Oxidative stability of meat systems made with $W_1/O/W_2$ emulsions prepared with hydroxytyrosol and chia oil as lipid phase. *LWT Food Sci. Technol.* **2014**, *59*, 941–947. [CrossRef]

55. Chaves-Lopez, C.; Serio, A.; Mazzarrino, G.; Martuscelli, M.; Scarpone, E.; Paparella, A. Control of household mycoflora in fermented sausages using phenolic fractions from olive mill wastewaters. *Int. J. Food Microbiol.* **2015**, *207*, 49–56. [CrossRef] [PubMed]
56. Muíño, I.; Díaz, M.T.; Apeleo, E.; Pérez-Santaescolástica, C.; Rivas-Cañedo, A.; Pérez, C.; Cañeque, V.; Lauzurica, S.; De la Fuente, J. Valorisation of an extract from olive oil waste as a natural antioxidant for reducing meat waste resulting from oxidative processed. *J. Clean. Product.* **2016**, *140*, 924–932. [CrossRef]
57. Balzan, S.; Taticchi, A.; Cardazzo, B.; Urbani, S.; Servili, M.; Di Lecce, G.; Berasategi-Zabalza, I.; Rodríguez-Estrada, M.T.; Novelli, E.; Fasolato, L. Effect of phenols extracted from a by-product of the oil mill on the shelf-life of raw and cooked fresh pork sausages in the absence of chemical additives. *LWT Food Sci. Technol.* **2017**, *85*, 89–95. [CrossRef]
58. Branciari, R.; Galarini, R.; Giusepponi, D.; Trabalaza-Marinucci, M.; Forte, C.; Roila, R.; Miraglia, D.; Servili, M.; Acuti, G.; Valiani, A. Oxidative status and presence of bioactive compounds in meat from chickens fed polyphenols extracted from olive oil industry waste. *Sustainability* **2017**, *9*. [CrossRef]
59. Freire, M.; Bou, R.; Cofrades, S.; Jiménez-Colmenero, F. Technological characteristics of cold-set gelled double emulsion enriched with n-3 fatty acids: Effect of hydroxytyrosol addition and chilling storage. *Food Res. Int.* **2017**, *100*, 298–305. [CrossRef] [PubMed]
60. Moudache, M.; Nerín, C.; Colon, M.; Zaidi, F. Antioxidant effect of an innovative active plastic film containing olive leaves extract on fresh pork meat and its evaluation by Raman spectroscopy. *Food Chem.* **2017**, *2291*, 98–103. [CrossRef] [PubMed]

MDPI
St. Alban-Anlage 66
4052 Basel
Switzerland
Tel. +41 61 683 77 34
Fax +41 61 302 89 18
www.mdpi.com

Medicines Editorial Office
E-mail: medicines@mdpi.com
www.mdpi.com/journal/medicines

www.ingramcontent.com/pod-product-compliance
Lightning Source LLC
LaVergne TN
LVHW070626100526
838202LV00012B/739